PREVENTION
IS PRIMARY

PREVENTION IS PRIMARY

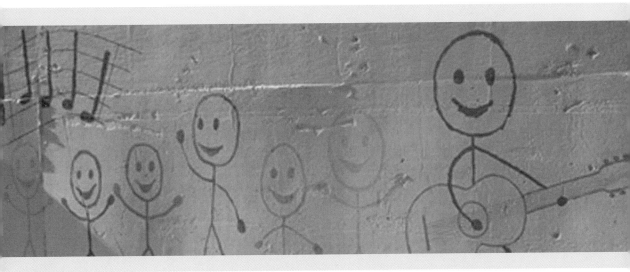

STRATEGIES FOR COMMUNITY WELL-BEING

Second Edition

Larry Cohen • Vivian Chávez • Sana Chehimi

Editors

Foreword by Georges C. Benjamin

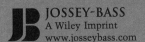

JOSSEY-BASS
A Wiley Imprint
www.josseybass.com

Prevention Institute
Prevention and equity at the center of community well-being

Library of Congress Cataloging-in-Publication Data

   Prevention is primary : strategies for community well-being / Larry Cohen, Vivian Chávez, Sana Chehimi,
editors ; foreword by Georges C. Benjamin. — 2nd ed.
      p.   cm.
   Includes bibliographical references and indexes.
   ISBN 978-0-470-55095-3 (pbk.); ISBN 9780470873342 (ebk); ISBN 9780470873359 (ebk);
   ISBN 9780470873366 (ebk)
      1. Medicine, Preventive—United States.   2. Community health services—United States.   3. Medical
policy—United States.   4. Social medicine—United States.   I. Cohen, Larry, 1947 May 21- II. Chávez,
Vivian.   III. Chehimi, Sana.
   [DNLM: 1. Primary Prevention—organization & administration—United States.   2. Community Health
Services—organization & administration—United States.   3. Health Policy—United States.   4. Social
Justice—United States. WA 108 P942235 2010]
   RA445.P6585 2010
   362.1—dc22
                                                                              2010023126

Printed in the United States of America
SECOND EDITION
PB Printing   10 9 8 7 6 5 4 3 2 1

CONTENTS

v

TABLES, FIGURES, AND EXHIBITS

TABLES

FIGURES

EXHIBITS

We dedicate this book to Dr. Beverly Coleman-Miller, a physician and nurse who understood prevention with every bone in her body. She made magic and inspired us with her vision and commitment. She emphasized that every heartbeat matters, and in our limited heartbeats every one of us can have a profound impact in improving the world. In Beverly's memory, we hope that this book will move hearts and make magic.

ACKNOWLEDGMENTS

We gratefully acknowledge the following individuals and institutions for their contributions to this edition of *Prevention Is Primary*.

To the entire Prevention Institute team of staff, interns, and fellows for their continuing and unwavering support and assistance. In particular, a great big thank-you to:

Alice Ricks, for her role as a graduate student editor, researcher, and writer.

Andy Riesenberg, for providing significant editorial assistance and writing on several chapters.

Ann Whidden, for extensive writing and editorial assistance, particularly on the preventing violence chapter.

Linda Shak and Nicole Schneider for editorial assistance and writing on the mental health chapter.

Melissa Murrin and Katherine Rea, for their role as student researchers on several chapters.

Omar Sahak, for providing content, editing, writing, and organizational assistance.

Shakirah Simley, for pitching in wherever needed and providing support on several chapters.

To San Francisco State University and the Department of Health Education, gratitude for a vision grounded in social justice and a mission enriched with multicultural perspectives.

To past, present, and future students, thank you for trusting Vivian Chávez with the creative freedom to teach prevention.

To Dan Perales and the San Jose State University MPH Distance Education Program, our appreciation for your using the first edition of *Prevention Is Primary* as an underlying framework. To Barbara Krimgold and Kalahn Taylor-Clark, our thanks for your facilitating the collaboration with past and current Kellogg Health Scholars, whose contributions to chapters and sidebars are evidenced throughout the second edition.

And last, but certainly not least, our heartfelt gratitude to all of the readers of the first edition whose enthusiasm and support made the text such a hit and this edition a reality.

Larry Cohen
Vivian Chávez
Sana Chehimi
Editors

FOREWORD

Georges C. Benjamin

The United States spends $2.4 trillion annually on health care delivery and millions more on alternative treatments. The sum of these expenditures means we spend more per capita than any other industrialized nation; yet we rank fiftieth in the world in terms of life expectancy.

The current U.S. health care delivery system does little to promote health. It has great difficulty delivering consistent quality and struggles to eliminate disparities in health outcomes. Almost 50 million Americans do not have health insurance. These people often receive medical care late in the course of their disease, often without having had the opportunity for preventive care. Hundreds of thousands of underinsured individuals also frequently suffer the same fate.

In 2010, the nation passed historic legislation to expand quality, affordable health insurance coverage to more than 30 million Americans. The supporters of this legislation recognized that having an insurance card is not enough and added $15 billion in provisions to promote wellness and to fund prevention. Basic elements of healthy communities, such as healthy food, opportunities for physical activity, and clean air and water, are too often missing in low-income communities and communities of color. These disparities demonstrate the schism between the extraordinary potential of primary prevention and the reality of health policy and practice at the population level. As the nation becomes older, more ethnically diverse, and more deeply plagued by chronic illness, these disparities will become more apparent and will widen.

Public health improvement is part of a continuum that includes health promotion and disease prevention as well as timely and appropriate clinical care. It is delivered in a social and economic context that affects health and quality of life. Understanding this context improves our ability to efficiently address our most pressing health concerns.

Good public health practice creates a community benefit. It is science-based and prevention-oriented. A good public health system should reduce morbidity and mortality and improve quality of life. It might even right a wrong. It can save money, but, like most things, it usually requires an investment in time, money, and effort.

A 2009 survey by Lake Research Partners and Public Opinion Strategies showed bipartisan support for prevention, with 71 percent of Americans favoring an increased investment in disease prevention. Despite this support, getting people to practice prevention continues to be a problem. Whether this is due to a lack of knowledge, lack of belief in preventive measures, or inability to connect the dots from preventive measures to outcomes, this text strives to fill that void. It does so by addressing prevention in its purest form: primary prevention.

The authors of the chapters assembled here are foremost authorities in the field of population health. They represent an important collection of experts in a range of public health and prevention disciplines. Examples include Deborah Prothrow-Stith, who was a trailblazer in defining violence as a public health problem and in proposing prevention strategies for its reduction; and Howard Frumkin and Andrew Dannenberg, who have been effective advocates for changing the way we design, build, and rebuild communities. Their work offers clear guidance about the intersection between the built environment and health. The authors from Prevention Institute, led by Larry Cohen, along with his coeditors Vivian Chávez and Sana Chehimi, are an exceptional group who have made it their life's work not only to think about prevention in the academic sense but to go one step further and put their ideas into practice by working directly with communities.

This book tackles emerging issues such as community resilience and revisits old strategies such as social justice and community organizing. The latter are viewed as primary prevention tools. The need to invest in strategies to empower communities more effectively was brought into our communal consciousness during Hurricanes Katrina and Rita, which hit the Gulf Coast of the United States in 2005, and which were followed by a number of social failures.

Using prevention as a tool to improve health and reduce costs is being increasingly touted as a component of the solution to controlling health care costs and improving national health. Primary prevention is about cost avoidance as well. The challenge is to understand its use, practice it, and evaluate its success. This book is designed to help readers understand the complex concepts of primary prevention in their purest form and incorporate them into practice. The old adage that "an ounce of prevention is worth a pound of cure" is the substance of this book; this book is also about proving the adage to be true.

REFERENCES

Holmes, M., Ricketts, T. C., & King, J. (2009, March). Updating uninsured estimates for current economic conditions: State specific estimates. Cecil G. Sheps Center for Health Services Research and North Carolina Institute of Medicine.

Lake Research Partners and Public Opinion Strategies. (July 13, 2009). New national polling data on health care system reform. http://old.preventioninstitute.org/documents/AmericasAgenda-PACMemo.pdf

World Health Organization. (2004). *The world health report 2004: Changing history.* Retrieved November 14, 2006, from http://www.who.int/whr/2004/en/index.html

THE CONTRIBUTORS

Dolores Acevedo-Garcia, PhD, is associate professor in the Bouvé College of Health Sciences and associate director of the Institute on Urban Health Research at Northeastern University. Prior to joining Northeastern in September 2009, she was associate professor in the Department of Society, Human Development and Health at the Harvard School of Public Health (HSPH). She is project director for DiversityData, a multiyear project studying racial and ethnic equity in U.S. metropolitan areas, supported by the W.K. Kellogg Foundation. Her research focuses on the effect of social determinants (such as residential segregation and immigrant adaptation) on racial and ethnic health disparities; the role of nonhealth policies (such as housing and immigrant policies) in reducing those disparities; and the health and well-being of children with special needs.

Deborah Balfanz, PhD, is on staff at the Stanford Health Improvement Program (HIP) division within the Stanford Prevention Research Center at the Stanford University School of Medicine. Her role includes coordinating several behavior-change programs that guide participants through gradual lifestyle change. In addition to her work with individuals, Balfanz and her colleagues have worked with the YMCA of the USA (Y-USA) on projects to bring about more global change. She coauthored *Building Generation Play: Addressing the Crisis of Inactivity Among America's Children*, a paper that outlined the relationship between inactivity among children and the rising childhood obesity epidemic. With Y-USA, Balfanz and her colleagues have developed the Community Healthy Living Index (CHLI), a tool that allows communities to assess their own opportunities for healthy eating and active living and then guides them through a change process.

Bonnie Benard, MSW, is a senior program associate in WestEd's Health and Human Development Program in Oakland, California. She writes widely, leads professional development, and makes presentations in the field of prevention and resilience and youth development theory, policy, and practice. Her book *Fostering Resiliency in Kids: Protective Factors in the Family, School, and Community* is credited with introducing resilience theory and application to the fields of prevention and education. Her most recent book, *Resiliency: What We Have Learned*, synthesizes the latest developments in resilience research and describes how it has been applied most successfully to support young people. Benard's work in resilience led to the development of the Resilience and Youth Development Module of the California Department of Education's *Healthy Kids Survey*, which polls students on their perceptions of supports and opportunities in their schools, homes, communities, and peer groups.

Georges C. Benjamin, MD, is executive director of the American Public Health Association (APHA). At APHA, Benjamin publishes the nonprofit's monthly publication, *The Nation's Health*, the association's official newspaper and *The American Journal of Public Health*, the profession's premier scientific publication. He is the author of more than one hundred scientific articles and book chapters. Formerly, he was secretary of the Maryland Department of Health and Mental Hygiene, where he oversaw the expansion and improvement in the state's Medicaid program. Benjamin was chief of the acute illness clinic at Madigan Army Medical Center, where he managed a 72,000-patient visit ambulatory care service and later was chief of emergency medicine at the Walter Reed Army Medical Center. Benjamin chaired the department of community health and ambulatory care at the District of Columbia General Hospital, became acting commissioner for public health for the District, and later directed the emergency ambulatory bureau of the District's fire department, one of the busiest ambulance services in the nation. Benjamin serves on the boards of Research! America, Partnership for Prevention, and the Reagan-Udall Foundation, and is a member of the Institute of Medicine of the National Academies. In 2008 he was named one of the top twenty-five minority executives in health care by *Modern Healthcare Magazine* in addition to being voted amongst the one hundred most powerful people in health care in 2007 through 2009 and one of the nation's Most Powerful Physician Executives in 2009.

Vivian Chávez, DrPH, is an associate professor in the Department of Health Education at San Francisco State University. Her current research examines the role of expressive arts, somatic movement and cultural humility in the classroom as well as in public health practice. She is a registered yoga teacher whose scholarship includes innovative pedagogy to integrate the mind/body split characteristic of higher education. Chávez is a media advocacy trainer and coauthor of *Drop That Knowledge: Youth Radio Stories* with Elizabeth Soep.

Sana Chehimi, MPH, is a program manager at Prevention Institute, where she oversees projects related to healthy eating and active living by developing tools and strategies to promote healthier, more equitable food environments. Chehimi oversees national media advocacy efforts supporting prevention and health reform and also leads a statewide Rapid Response Media Network, providing tools and resources for effective media advocacy to promote healthy eating and active living. She leads the development of the Environmental Nutrition and Activity Community Tool (ENACT), a Web-based resource designed to improve local nutrition and physical activity environments and oversees the institute's media advocacy efforts through the Rapid Response Media Network. She has authored numerous reports and publications for the organization.

Molly Chidsey, BA, is the sustainability coordinator for Metro, the regional government in Portland, Oregon. With Multnomah County's Sustainability Program, Chidsey led efforts to prevent waste, increase recycling, reduce toxics, and make purchases more sustainable. She led development of several projects, including a waste prevention and recycling plan for county facilities, a toxics reduction strategy in partnership with the City of Portland, and a city-county sustainable procurement strategy. She also coordinated a voluntary mercury-free medicine campaign with health care facilities and the international Health Care Without Harm coalition.

Larry Cohen, MSW, is founder and executive director of Prevention Institute, a national nonprofit center dedicated to improving community health and well-being by building momentum for effective primary prevention. He was founding director of the Contra Costa County Prevention Program, where he engaged the American Cancer Society and the American Heart and Lung Associations in forming the first coalition in the United States to change tobacco policy by passing the nation's first multi-city smoking ban. The coalition ignited other statewide and national efforts, including smoking bans on airplanes and restrictions in public places, restaurants, and workplaces. Cohen also created the Food and Nutrition Policy Consortium, whose work led to a county food policy that sparked momentum for the U.S. food labeling law. He helped shape strategy to secure passage of bicycle and motorcycle helmet laws, strengthen child and adult passenger restraint regulations, and set fluoridation requirements in California. Among his previous publications are *A Time of Opportunity: Local Solutions to Reduce Inequities in Health and Safety* for the Institute of Medicine Roundtable on Health Disparities and *Good Health Counts: A 21st Century Approach to Health and Community for California*. Cohen currently heads Urban Networks to Increase Thriving Youth through Violence Prevention (UNITY), a national initiative designed to strengthen and support the forty-five largest cities in the United States to more effectively prevent violence. Cohen developed one of the first courses in the country on preventing violence for UC Berkeley's School of Public Health. He has authored several seminal texts, including *A Public Health Approach to the Violence Epidemic in the United States*, and *Poised for Prevention: Advancing Promising Approaches to Primary Prevention of Intimate Partner Violence*. Among his numerous awards are the Injury Control and Emergency Health Services Section Public Service Award from the APHA, the Secretary's Award for Health Promotion from the U.S. Department of Health and Human Services, and recognition from the American Cancer Society and the Society for Public Health Education.

Dionne Smith Coker-Appiah, PhD, is an assistant professor in the Department of Psychiatry at Georgetown University School of Medicine. Coker-Appiah, a licensed psychologist, has expertise in adolescent health and using community-based participatory research (CBPR) approaches. Her research focuses on adolescent dating violence prevention, adolescent mental health, and adolescent sexual health. She has collaborated on research projects in the United States that focus on mental health utilization among African American women (In Their Own Voices), adolescent HIV/AIDS prevention (Project GRACE), and adolescent dating violence prevention (Project LOVE). She has conducted quantitative and qualitative research among African Americans in rural and urban settings. Coker-Appiah publishes in peer-reviewed journals, consults, and presents her research at local, national, and international conferences. She has won numerous awards for her scholarship, maintains memberships in professional development organizations, and volunteers with community-based organizations.

Andrew L. Dannenberg, MD, is associate director for science in the Division of Emergency and Environmental Health Services at the National Center for Environmental Health (NCEH) of the Centers for Disease Control and Prevention. He oversees NCEH activities on the health aspects of community design (the built environment), such as land use, transportation, and urban planning. He is exploring the use of a health impact assessment as a tool to inform community planners and the use of model zoning codes to promote health. Dannenberg is an adjunct professor of epidemiology and of environmental and occupational health at the Rollins School of Public Health at Emory University. He has served as director of CDC's Division of Applied Public Health Training with oversight responsibility for the Epidemic Intelligence Service and other training programs, as preventive medicine residency director and injury prevention epidemiologist at the Johns Hopkins School of Public Health, and as a cardiovascular epidemiologist at the National Institutes of Health.

Rachel Davis, MSW, is managing director at Prevention Institute, overseeing management of projects related to prevention of violence, community health and reducing inequity, health care reform, and mental health. She creates tools and materials to support local and state initiatives and educates government agencies, foundations, and community groups throughout the country. Davis is project director for UNITY, Prevention Institute's CDC-funded national initiative to strengthen and support the forty-five largest U.S. cities in more effectively preventing violence. Davis codeveloped THRIVE (Toolkit for Health and Resilience in Vulnerable Environments), an interactive web-based tool to help identify and foster factors in the community environment that improve health outcomes and reduce inequity. Her publications include *First Steps: Taking Action Early to Prevent Violence.* She coauthored *A Time of Opportunity: Local Solutions to Reduce Inequities in Health and Safety, Health for All: California's Strategic Approach to Eliminating Racial and Ethnic Disparities in Health,* and *Good Health Counts: A 21st Century Approach to Health and Community for California.* Prior to joining Prevention Institute in 1997, Davis was a social worker for the San Francisco Unified School District.

Lori Dorfman, DrPH, directs the Berkeley Media Studies Group, a project of the Public Health Institute, where she oversees BMSG's research on the news, media advocacy training for advocates, and professional education for journalists. Her recent research examines how local television news and newspapers portray a variety of public health issues, including racial discrimination, children's health, nutrition and agriculture, paid family leave, youth and violence, intimate-partner violence, and alcohol, tobacco, and other drugs. Dorfman cowrote major texts on media advocacy, *Public Health and Media Advocacy: Power for Prevention* and *News for a Change: An Advocates' Guide to Working with the Media,* and teaches a course for master's students on mass communication and public health at UC-Berkeley's School of Public Health. She conducts media advocacy training for grassroots organizations and public health leaders, consults for government agencies and community programs across the United States and internationally, and publishes articles on public health and mass communication.

Jonathan M. Ellen, MD, is professor and vice chair of the Department of Pediatrics at the Johns Hopkins University's School of Medicine and director of the Johns Hopkins Center for Child and Community Health Research. His research has focused on prevention of sexually transmitted diseases (STIs), including HIV, among adolescents on the effectiveness of innovative community-based strategies for controlling STIs. He has cochaired the Community Prevention Leadership Group for Adolescent HIV Prevention Trials Network, leads multisite research HIV prevention protocols, has consulted with STI investigators internationally, has been invited to lecture at international meetings, and advises the CDC and the Jamaican Ministry of Health in Jamaica on STI prevention and control.

Catherine S. Erickson, MPH, has participated in research related to fresh-food access in low-income neighborhoods and links between the sustainable agriculture and health care communities.

Stephanie Ann Farquhar, PhD, is associate professor of Community Health at Portland State University. She is a researcher on a NIH grant that seeks to reduce pesticides exposure and occupational stressors among indigenous farmworkers in Oregon. Farquhar is on the board of directors of Upstream Public Health, and served as a commissioner on the city and county Sustainable Development Commission. In partnership with Multnomah County Health Department and community organizations, Farquhar examined the role of Community Health Workers and popular education in Latino and African American communities in Portland through a three-year CDC grant. Farquhar has been the recipient of a W.K. Kellogg Foundation Community Health Scholars postdoctoral fellowship.

Nicholas Freudenberg, DrPH, is Distinguished Professor of Public Health at Hunter College, City University of New York and director of the CUNY Doctoral Program in Public Health. He is founder and director of Corporations and Health Watch. Freudenberg has published four books and more than one hundred articles and chapters on urban health, incarceration and health, public health policy, and health and social justice. For the last thirty years, he has worked with and for a variety of community organizations, advocacy groups, government agencies, and others to plan, implement and evaluate community health interventions in urban settings.

Howard Frumkin, MD, DrPH, is director of the National Center for Environmental Health and Agency for Toxic Substances and Disease Registry (NCEH/ATSDR) at the CDC. Frumkin is an internist, environmental and occupational medicine specialist, and epidemiologist. His research interests include public health aspects of urban sprawl and the built environment; air pollution; metal and PCB toxicity; climate change; health benefits of contact with nature; and environmental and occupational health policy, especially regarding minority workers and communities, and those in developing nations. Before joining the CDC in 2005, he was professor and chair of the Department of Environmental and Occupational Health at the Rollins School of Public Health of Emory University and professor of medicine at Emory. He is the author or coauthor of more than one hundred scientific journal articles and chapters. His books include *Environmental Health: From Global to Local, Urban Sprawl and Public Health, Emerging Illness and Society*, and *Safe and Healthy School Environments*.

Sandro Galea, DrPH, is professor of epidemiology at the University of Michigan School of Public Health and director of its Center for Global Health. Galea is primarily interested in the social and economic production of health, particularly mental health and behavior in urban settings. Galea has authored or coauthored more than two hundred scientific journal articles, more than twenty-five chapters and commentaries and four books. His work has been published in medical and public health journals including the *New England Journal of Medicine, American Journal of Epidemiology, American Journal of Public Health*, and *Epidemiology*. Galea's work has been featured by several media outlets including the *New York Times* and NBC Dateline among others. He was named one of *Time* magazine's epidemiology "innovators" in 2006. He has received research grants from the NIH, the Robert Wood Johnson Foundation, and the CDC.

Wayne H. Giles, MD, is the director of the Division of Adult and Community Health, National Center for Chronic Disease Prevention and Health Promotion. Giles directs programmatic and research activities in community health promotion, arthritis, aging, health care utilization, and racial and ethnic disparities in health. His experience includes examinations of the prevalence of hypertension in Africa, clinical trials evaluating the effectiveness of cholesterol-lowering agents, and studies examining racial differences in the incidence of stroke. He has more than one hundred publications in peer reviewed journals and has authored several book chapters. He has been awarded the Centers for Disease Control and Prevention's Charles C. Shepard Award in Assessment and Epidemiology and the Jeffrey P. Koplan Award.

Nancy M. Goff, MPH, coordinates outreach for the Oregon Environmental Public Health Tracking Program as well as Oregon's new Health Impact Assessment Initiative, making environmental and health data and information available for more informed decision making at the individual, community, organizational, and policy levels. To build capacity to conduct health impact assessments around the state of Oregon, she trains community leaders and public health practitioners. Previously, Goff worked on a community-based participatory research project involving farmworker health at Portland Columbia River Crossing project with the Multnomah County Health Department.

Joseph P. Gone, PhD, is assistant professor in the Department of Psychology (clinical area) and the Program in American Culture (Native American Studies) at the University of Michigan, Ann Arbor. As a cultural psychologist, Gone studies how to provide culturally appropriate helping services to Native Americans that avoid the neo-colonial subversion of indigenous thought and practice. His published articles and chapters concern the ethnopsychological investigation of self, identity, personhood, and social relations in American Indian cultural contexts vis-à-vis the mental health professions, especially as these pertain to therapeutic processes and practices such as psychotherapy and traditional healing.

Soowon Kim, PhD, is a program manager at Stanford University School of Medicine's Health Improvement Program, where she designs and evaluates health promotion efforts inside and outside of Stanford. She focuses on providing practical guidance to those developing health promotion programs and public policy by addressing the multiple pathways through which biological, behavioral, and contextual contributors affect individual and population health. She also participates in evaluating Y-USA's broader community effort, the Healthier Communities Initiatives, which facilitate community health improvements through collaboration.

Barbara Krimgold serves as national program director of the W.K. Kellogg Foundation's Kellogg Health Scholars Program and Kellogg Fellows in Health Policy Research Program at the Center for Advancing Health in Washington. She was codirector of the Diversity Data project, which launched the website DiversityData.org and produced the report "Children Left Behind: How U.S. Metropolitan Areas Are Failing America's Children." Her particular focus is on understanding the economic determinants of health inequities and developing policy menus designed to achieve greater health equity and life opportunity and on changing the direction of U.S. health and social policy.

Bonnie Lefkowitz is a health policy writer and consultant with twenty-four years of experience as a federal researcher, administrator and policy analyst. She is the author of the recent book *Community Health Centers: A Movement and the People Who Made it Happen.*

Leandris Liburd, PhD, is chief of the Community Health and Program Services Branch at the CDC where she directs a broad range of public health programs addressing community health promotion and the elimination of health disparities. Her principal research is the intersection of race, class, and gender in chronic disease risks, management, and prevention, and the social determinants of health. Liburd spent twelve years in the Division of Diabetes Translation at CDC as a community interventionist and later as chief of the Community Interventions Section. During her tenure in the Division of Diabetes Translation, her work was focused on developing community models for diabetes prevention and control programs in racial and ethnic communities. Liburd has written extensively. Her edited volume, *Diabetes and Health Disparities: Community-based Approaches for Racial and Ethnic Populations*, was published in September 2009.

Nancy McArdle, MPP, is a researcher and author with more than twenty years experience analyzing housing policy and demographics, migration and settlement patterns, racial segregation, and the intersection between civil rights and opportunity. McArdle was a research analyst at Harvard's Joint Center for Housing Studies and research director of the Harvard Civil Rights Project's Metro Boston Equity Initiative. She has served as an expert witness, providing analysis and testimony at trial in several major legal cases involving housing and school segregation. McArdle is currently codeveloper and principal data analyst of DiversityData.org. She is a recent contributor to *Twenty-First Century Color Lines: Multiracial Change in Contemporary Society* and *The Integration Debate: Competing Futures for American Cities.* She serves on the board of directors of the Fair Housing Center of Greater Boston.

GiShawn A. Mance, PhD, is a Visiting Assistant Professor at American University in Washington. Her primary research interest examines contextual and cultural influences on symptom presentation for youth exposed to chronic stressors. Mance specializes in empirically-supported treatments for youth who have witnessed or experienced multiple traumas that create vulnerability to depression, and in adapting evidence-based interventions to meet the cultural and contextual needs of communities.

Leslie Mikkelsen, MPH, as managing director at Prevention Institute advances the conceptual work of the organization and supervises the Supporting Healthy Eating and Active Living projects and team. She develops tools and materials to support local and state initiatives, and guides government bureaus, foundations and community organizations throughout the country on effective environmental approaches, coalition building, and interdisciplinary partnerships. Mikkelsen is the cofounder and project director for the Strategic Alliance for Healthy Food and Activity Environments, a statewide advocacy network for creating healthy food and physical activity opportunities. Her research and publications aided in the development of ENACT and the ENACT Local Policy Database. She is a policy consultant to the national Healthy Eating Active Living Convergence Partnership, where she directs research and helps shape national strategy related to policy priorities that support healthy food and activity environments. Leslie has written many articles, including *Setting the Record Straight: Nutritionists and Health Professionals Define Healthful Food* and *Where's the Fruit? Fruit Content of the Most Highly Advertised Children's Food and Beverages*. Mikkelsen worked for the Alameda County, California and New York City food banks. She received the APHA Food and Nutrition Section 2008 Catherine Cowell Award for Excellence in Public Health Nutrition.

Meredith Minkler, DrPH, is professor of health and social behavior and director of the DrPH program at the School of Public Health at UC Berkeley. She has three decades of experience in community building and organizing and community-based participatory research (CBPR) activities in underserved communities. Her current research includes documenting the impacts of CBPR on public policy, empowerment intervention studies with youth and the elderly, and national studies of health disparities in older Americans. Minkler has written more than one hundred articles and book chapters and has written, cowritten, or edited seven books, including *Community Organizing and Community Building for Health, Community-Based Participatory Research for Health* (with Nina Wallerstein), *Grandmothers as Caregivers* (with Kathleen Roe), and *Critical Perspectives on Aging* (with Carroll L. Estes).

Peter Murchie, MPH, has worked for the World Health Organization, the International Joint Commission, and the U.S. Environmental Protection Agency using collaborative approaches to solve environmental health issues. At the U.S. EPA, Murchie helped start and led the West Coast Collaborative, a partnership among leaders from federal, state, and local government, the private sector, and environmental groups working to reduce heavy duty engine emissions along the West Coast. Murchie was a member of the U.S. EPA Regional Climate and Clean Energy Team and the Mobile Source Workgroup of the Green House Gas Reporting Rulemaking. Presently, Murchie leads an effort at the Policy Consensus Initiative and the National Policy Consensus Center at PSU that supports state and local leaders in using public-private collaboration to implement climate and clean energy strategies and projects.

Marion Nestle, PhD, is Paulette Goddard Professor in the Department of Nutrition, Food Studies, and Public Health (the department she chaired from 1988–2003) and professor of sociology at New York University. Nestle was senior nutrition policy advisor in the Department of Health and Human Services and managing editor of the 1988 *Surgeon*

General's Report on Nutrition and Health. She has been a member of the FDA Food Advisory Committee and Science Board, the USDA/DHHS Dietary Guidelines Advisory Committee, and American Cancer Society committees that issue dietary guidelines for cancer prevention. Her research focuses on how science and society influence dietary advice and practice. She is the author of *Pet Food Politics: The Chihuahua in the Coal Mine, What to Eat, Food Politics: How the Food Industry Influences Nutrition and Health,* and *Safe Food: Bacteria, Biotechnology, and Bioterrorism.* Her forthcoming book, coauthored with Malden Nesheim, is *Feed Your Pet Right.*

Theresa L. Osypuk, SD, is a social epidemiologist researching racial, socioeconomic, and nativity disparities in health, their geographic patterns, and causes. She is particularly interested in why place affects health and health disparities, including the role of racial residential segregation, neighborhood context, and social policies. Osypuk's research has appeared in leading epidemiology, social epidemiology, public health, and urban studies journals. Osypuk is an assistant professor in the Bouvé College of Health Sciences at Northeastern University.

Donald Parker, BA, works for Project Momentum, Inc. a community-based organization founded in 2005 to address the many social, environmental, and health issues that face the mostly rural community of Edgecombe County, North Carolina. Donald has served as a community advisory board member for Project LOVE and Project EAST (another HIV/AIDS research project that helps reduce the stigma of HIV/AIDS) and is a steering committee member and data collection supervisor for Project GRACE. Donald's work spans HIV/AIDS education, adolescent dating violence, and research on health disparities in rural counties in North Carolina.

Neha Patel, MS, is a work group process manager for Zero Waste Alliance's Outdoor Industry Association Eco Index project. Neha worked for eight years as the program director for the Oregon Center for Environmental Health's Health Care Without Harm campaign with measured reductions in mercury, PVC use, and waste, and increased integration of green building techniques, environmentally preferable purchasing and sustainable food procurement within the hospital sector.

Daniel Perales, DrPH, is full professor of public health in the Department of Health Science at San Jose State University. He teaches health promotion planning and evaluation in the university's MPH program and social marketing and epidemiology in the undergraduate program. His twenty years of research include observational studies of bicycle safety helmet use and a needle exchange HIV/AIDS harm reduction program. He has evaluated programs in tobacco control, adolescent pregnancy prevention, nutrition education and food security, child immunization, and coalition development and maintenance. In 1995 and 1996, he served on the APHA's Strategic Planning Committee. Perales is former treasurer and upcoming president of the Society for Public Health Education in 2010–2011. He sat on the editorial board of *Health Education and Behavior*, the editorial advisory board of the journal *Health Promotion Practice*, and the editorial board of the *Californian Journal of Health Promotion*. He has served on the Prevention Institute's board of directors since 2003.

Deborah Prothrow-Stith, MD, works at Spencer Stuart, an executive search firm, and serves as adjunct faculty in the Health Policy and Management Department at Harvard School of Public Health. She has been associate dean for diversity and Henry Pickering Walcott Professor of Practice of Public Health at Harvard School of Public Health. As commissioner of public health for the Commonwealth of Massachusetts, she established the first Office of Violence. She continues to develop programs and nurture partnerships with community-based programs locally, nationally, and internationally that include the Community Violence Prevention Project, the Girls and Violence Project, and Partnerships for Preventing Violence, a six-part satellite broadcast training providing education, justice, and health professionals with a thorough understanding of comprehensive, effective, school-centered violence prevention approaches. Prothrow-Stith developed and wrote *The Violence Prevention Curriculum for Adolescents*. She has written or cowritten more than eighty articles and books on medical and public health issues. Prothrow-Stith has received numerous professional awards.

Juliet Sims, MPH, is a program coordinator at Prevention Institute. Sims' research and advocacy efforts focus on developing tools, resources, and strategies to advance environmental and policy change in the realm of healthy eating and active living. She supports the Institute's media advocacy efforts, including its Rapid Response Media Network, and she facilitates development of ENACT. Sims developed "Setting the Record Straight: Nutrition and Health Professionals Define Healthful Food," a definition of healthful food that looks beyond nutrients to acknowledge that truly healthful food comes from a system where food is produced, processed, transported, and marketed in environmentally sound, sustainable, and just ways. Prior to joining Prevention Institute, she worked in clinical nutrition.

Michael S. Spencer, PhD, is associate dean for Educational Programs and associate professor at the University of Michigan School of Social Work. His research examines the causes and consequences of disparities in the health, mental health, and service use of people of color. Spencer is the principal investigator of the NIH-funded REACH Detroit Family Intervention, a community-based participatory research project whose goal is to reduce health disparities, particularly diabetes, among African American and Latino Eastside and Southwest Detroit residents through the promotion of a healthy lifestyle and self-management of health. Spencer teaches courses in contemporary cultures in the United States, multicultural and multilingual organizing, facilitation training for dialogues in diversity and social justice, social work practice in communities and social systems, and community development.

Makani Themba-Nixon is executive director of the Praxis Project, a nonprofit organization dedicated to helping communities use media and policy advocacy to advance health equity and justice. She was previously director of the Grass Roots Innovative Policy Program (GRIPP), a national project to build capacity among local organizing groups to engage policy advocacy to address institutional racism in welfare and public education. She served as staff for the California state legislature, was media director for the Southern Christian Leadership Conference in Los Angeles, and worked five years for the Marin Institute for the Prevention of Alcohol and Other Drug Problems, including three years as director of its Center for Media and Policy Analysis. Themba-Nixon has published numerous articles and case studies on race, media, policy advocacy, and public health. Her latest book, cowritten with Hunter Cutting, is *Talking the Walk: Communications Guide for Racial Justice*. She is the author of *Making Policy, Making Change*, which examines media and policy advocacy for public health through case studies and practical information. She is coauthor of *Media Advocacy and Public Health: Power for Prevention*, a contributor to the volumes *We the Media and State of the Race: Creating Our 21st Century*, among other edited book projects.

M. Taqi Tirmazi is a W.K. Kellogg Postdoctoral Fellow at Morgan State University School of Community Health and Policy. He is conducting a community-based participatory research project that examines the contextual factors associated with the preconception and interconception health of African American youth in Baltimore. Tirmazi has studied the impact of demographic, social, educational, and environmental factors on the acculturation and psychosocial adaptation of immigrant Muslim youth in the United States, the impact of social and physical determinants on the mental health of urban black youth, maternal depression among African American mothers, hip hop and youth development, elderly Muslims and mental health, socialization of adolescent Muslim girls, and acculturation of immigrant Muslim youth. At Utrecht University, he conducted a comparative study on the ethnic and religious identity of Muslim youth in the Netherlands and United States.

Nina Wallerstein, DrPH, is Professor, Masters in Public Health Program, Department of Family and Community Medicine; and director of the Center for Participatory Research, Office of Community Health, Health Sciences Center, University of New Mexico. She has worked in empowerment and popular education and CBPR since the mid-1970s. Recent books include *Community-Based Participatory Research in Health: From Process to Outcomes, 2nd edition* (edited with Meredith Minkler) and *Problem-Posing at Work: A Popular Educator's Guide* (with Elsa Auerbach).

Anita M. Wells, PhD, is an assistant professor and the graduate program coordinator in the Department of Psychology at Morgan State University in Baltimore. Wells' work is grounded in the theory that social, psychological, and biological factors all interact, often in complex ways, to produce health outcomes. Her areas of research are cancer health disparities, health promotion, and mental health and well-being. She investigates health decision-making among African Americans, the impact of trauma and violence on mental health, and the relationship between health policy and health outcomes. Wells has conducted community based research with African American populations since 1995.

Dan Wohlfeiler, MPH, is chief of the Office of Policy and Communications of the Sexually Transmitted Disease Control branch of the California Department of Health Services. From 1990 to 1998, he served as education director of San Francisco's STOP AIDS Project, a leading HIV-prevention organization run by and for gay and bisexual men in San Francisco. He is a nationally recognized expert on structural interventions for HIV prevention and offers training through the California STD/HIV Prevention Training Center. His current interests focus on structural and network-level interventions for STD/HIV prevention.

Ashby Wolfe, MD, joined Prevention Institute in 2005 as a contributing editor for the first edition of *Prevention Is Primary*. She is a family physician in the Department of Family and Community Medicine at the UC Davis Medical Center in Sacramento, California. She has worked in family practice as a researcher and clinician and holds a particular interest in the development of policies and programs to improve the quality of care for underserved and low-income populations. She has experience with health policy at the local, state, and federal levels. Wolfe served as acting medical officer for the Centers for Medicare and Medicaid Services Region IX office in San Francisco during 2006–2007, and has worked with a number of health care organizations, provider groups and patient organizations in an effort to reduce disparities in care for vulnerable populations. She has worked on several outreach campaigns for the Department of Health and Human Services and has experience developing and evaluating quality improvement initiatives.

Ellen Wu, MPH, is the executive director of the California Pan-Ethnic Health Network (CPEHN), a statewide network of multicultural health organizations working to ensure that all Californians have access to quality health care and can live healthy lives. CPEHN played a critical role in mobilizing the health community to defeat Proposition 54, which would have prohibited the collection of race and ethnicity data by government agencies, and in the chartering of SB 853, a bill that ensured language services to all limited-English proficient health plan members. During Wu's tenure, CPEHN has doubled in size, expanding its advocacy capacity and increasing its impact. Wu helped establish Having Our Say, a coalition of community organizations working to ensure communities of color have a voice in health care reform, and the Healthy Places Coalition, which advances public health involvement in land use planning. Prior to joining CPEHN, Wu consulted with the community health center network, was a program officer at the Tides Foundation, and served as director of health education and cultural linguistic services for the Alameda Alliance for Health. Wu is an adjunct faculty member at San Francisco State University and serves on numerous boards and advisory committees that include the Department of Public Health, the California Budget Project, and Healthy Families. Wu has coauthored studies on cultural competency and health care reform and is a frequent presenter on health disparities.

Mysha Wynn, MAEd, is founder and executive director of Project Momentum, Inc., a community-based organization that collaborates with UNC researchers in efforts to address health disparities in Edgecombe County, North Carolina. Wynn's work spans mental health, teaching, HIV/AIDS education, and research on health disparities in rural counties in North Carolina. Wynn was community mentor for Coker-Appiah at the University of North Carolina through the Kellogg Health Scholars Program, sits on the community advisory board of Project LOVE, and is a subcontractor for Project GRACE.

INTRODUCTION

Larry Cohen, Vivian Chávez, Sana Chehimi

It is simply undeniable that prevention works. From mandatory seat belt use to regulation of chemicals in children's toys, from fluoridated water to childhood immunizations, our daily lives are filled with reminders that prevention saves lives and reduces unnecessary suffering. Although only three years have passed since publication of the first edition of this text, the role of prevention, in policy and in practice, has undergone a significant transformation, with unprecedented visibility and unheralded support.

A new and vigorous commitment to reforming the U.S. healthcare system provided unprecedented opportunities to promote prevention and community wellness strategies that could simultaneously improve health and conserve resources. Public health and equity advocates, many of whom were readers or contributors to this text, were instrumental in ensuring that the health, equity and well-being of our communities were seen as key elements in discussions about the health of our economy. Thanks in no small part to these efforts, the American Recovery and Reinvestment Act (ARRA) of February 2009 included a landmark investment in prevention and wellness, totaling more than $1 billion. Nearly $400 million of this funding was earmarked for the "Communities Putting Prevention to Work" initiative, which aims to create healthier communities across the nation through exactly the kinds of innovative and proven prevention approaches described throughout this text.

Equity and community prevention were also built into the health reform legislation. Although overall the debate on health reform was contentious, the provisions on prevention were barely debated, perhaps because there was bipartisan recognition that we must refocus our health system to keep people healthy *in the first place* and cannot continue to simply treat problems after the fact. The funding commitment to prevention in ARRA and health reform is nothing less than a down payment on the nation's future; it represents the critical understanding that prevention requires a government commitment to community wellness, safety, and equity in *all* policies. This greater focus on prevention will save both lives and money; recent studies forecast a savings of $5 for each $1 invested in prevention (Trust for America's Health, Prevention Institute, The Urban Institute, New York Academy of Medicine, 2008).

By making a strong case for primary prevention, our hope is that this edition of *Prevention Is Primary: Strategies for Community Well-Being* changes the ways in which a new generation of community and public health leaders approach health. Shaping and maintaining quality prevention initiatives is not easy. It requires an understanding of the underlying determinants of health and inequities and knowledge of how to apply primary prevention strategies. During the past few years, the notion of social determinants of health and the need to address the underlying causes of health and health inequities has received more attention. At the same time, we are increasingly aware that the health sector cannot work alone. Instead, it is imperative that we work hand-in-hand with other practitioners and sectors, including transportation, agriculture, and economic development, to name a few.

Prevention Is Primary deliberately builds on cross-disciplinary wisdom and experiences of a variety of sectors and defines a coherent set of principles and approaches that guide the practice of prevention across a wide range of contemporary health and social issues. The social and health concerns of our time were not created in isolation, and they cannot be ameliorated in isolation, either. We all share responsibility for addressing monumental concerns, which include global warming, violence, and inequitable distribution of resources. These concerns cannot be simply siloed into issue areas or disciplines. The task for emerging public health practitioners is to recognize the connection between issues and to develop practices that are synchronous, collaborative, and concerted. This kind of prevention approach holds the promise of addressing multiple concerns simultaneously. Even more important, this holistic view sees communities, practitioners, families, and legislators as partners who are interconnected, interdependent, and equally invested in building healthy, thriving communities.

The text is organized in three sections: "Defining the Issues," "Key Elements of Effective Prevention Efforts," and "Prevention in Context." The sections are arranged in sequence, and we suggest readers move through them sequentially. Each section includes its own introduction, which provides the context and analysis for each of the included chapters. A number of chapters are complemented by sidebars that further contextualize primary prevention from a variety of disciplines and perspectives. These sidebars represent the perspectives of the editors or sidebar contributors, not necessarily the chapter authors.

Part One, "Defining the Issues," begins with a thorough definition of what primary prevention is and, equally important, what it is not. It continues by describing the overarching framework and principles guiding quality prevention efforts, including a focus on social justice, health equity, and community resilience.

Part Two, "Key Elements of Effective Prevention Efforts," describes the transition from prevention theory to implementation and practice, that is, from interdisciplinary collaboration to the evaluation of primary prevention efforts.

Part Three, "Prevention in Context," explores the application of prevention efforts to a wide range of contemporary health and social issues and demonstrates both current successes and the potential inherent in prevention practice.

Although we recognize we are members of a global community with transnational connections and implications, we focus predominantly in this book on the United States. We also recognize primary prevention efforts will not resolve every health and social problem, and yet these efforts are nonetheless a much-needed complement to care and treatment.

As much as this book is about health, it is equally about social justice and equity. We draw our inspiration in putting this text together from the many other social movements in which ordinary people united to fight for what they believed in (for example, the Suffragette movement, the ongoing Civil Rights movement, and the Peace Movement). As the civil rights leader Fannie Lou Hamer of the Student Nonviolent Coordinating Committee stated, "I'm sick and tired of being sick and tired" (DeMuth, 1964, p. 549). She then transformed her despair at U.S. injustice into voter registration leadership. For the new generation of leaders, the readers this book is intended for, health and justice must be inseparable. As César Chávez explained, "We can choose to use our lives for others to bring about a better and more just world for our children" (National Farm Worker Ministry, 2005, p. 1). "Our movement," Chávez stated, referring to the United Farm Workers, "is spreading like flames across a dry plain" (1966, p. 14). Our hope is that this book becomes a small spark in the movement for good health for all.

REFERENCES

Albee, G. W. (1983). Psychopathology, prevention, and the just society. *Journal of Primary Prevention, 4*, 5–40.

Chávez, C. E. (1966, March 17). The plan of Delano. *El Malcriado*, pp. 11–14.

DeMuth, J. (1964, June 1). Tired of being sick and tired. *The Nation*, pp. 548–551.

McGinnis, J. M., & Foege, W. H. (1993). Actual causes of death in the United States. *Journal of the American Medical Association, 270*, 2207–2212.

Mokdad, A. H., Marks, J. S., Stroup, D. F., & Gerberding, J. L. (2004). Actual causes of death in the United States, 2000. *Journal of the American Medical Association, 291*, 1238–1245.

National Farm Worker Ministry. (2005, November 22). *Litany of Christian hope*. Retrieved October 7, 2006, from http://www.nfwm.org/worshipresources/litanies.shtml

Trust for America's Health, Prevention Institute, The Urban Institute, New York Academy of Medicine. (2008). *Prevention for a healthier America. Investments in disease prevention yield significant savings, stronger communities*. Retrieved October 7, 2006, from http://preventioninstitute.org/component/jlibrary/article/id-75/127.html

PREVENTION IS PRIMARY

PART ONE

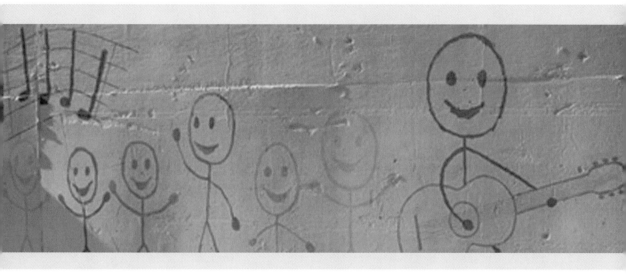

DEFINING THE ISSUES

Typically, medical approaches treat people after they get sick and look at one individual at a time. But a better option for societal health and well-being would be to create quality prevention techniques to keep people from getting sick in the first place. What is quality prevention? It is far more than a message in a brochure or information received during a medical visit. The three chapters in Part One explain the fundamental concepts needed to complement medical treatment with quality prevention efforts and to improve and maintain societal health.

Chapter One, "The Imperative for Primary Prevention," by Larry Cohen and Sana Chehimi, establishes the need to address factors that cause unnecessary illness, injury, and death. The authors show that primary prevention provides an important solution to an overburdened health care system where, as health care services weaken, everyone is increasingly at risk and marginalized populations are most vulnerable. A prevention-oriented approach to health and well-being is needed to help eliminate the injustice of the greatest impact of illness and injury falling on disfranchised populations. The authors note that primary prevention is far from a new idea and highlight its long and proven record of success. The chapter emphasizes the importance of a comprehensive approach and presents the *Spectrum of Prevention*, a framework for putting primary prevention into practice.

Health inequities, which are gaps between health outcomes by race, ethnicity, and other factors, are often stark for people of color. In Chapter Two, "Achieving Health Equity and Social Justice," Wayne Giles and Leandris Liburd reveal that health inequities are primarily the result of social structures and processes rather than individual genetic factors. A new sidebar by Dolores Acevedo-Garcia, Nancy McArdle, Theresa L. Osypuk, Bonnie Lefkowitz, and Barbara Krimgold provides an excerpted analysis from the diversitydata.org Web site's report "Children Left Behind: How Metropolitan Areas Are Failing America's Children."

While access to quality medical services for people of color (and associated inequities) are well-documented and contribute to disparities, addressing medical care inequities is just one part of a larger solution. Modifying key elements of the community environment can reduce the number of people who become ill or injured to begin with. Therefore, adoption of a primary prevention-oriented framework that includes comprehensive efforts directed at the broader social and policy environments, which promote health and prevent disease, offers the opportunity for improving health and equity.

In Chapter Three, "Individual, Family, and Community Resilience," Bonnie Benard describes *resilience* (the ability of individuals, families, and communities to face and overcome challenges and obstacles) as a key building block of prevention. The more *traditional approach* to community health focuses primarily on risk factors. The traditional approach can have the effect of stigmatizing and demoralizing individuals and communities. *Protective factors*, such as strong social networks and partnerships, caring relationships between community members, and education and literacy, help people grow stronger. These factors also give communities the ability to build their own capacity to effect change and prevent illness and injury.

1

The Imperative for Primary Prevention

Larry Cohen
Sana Chehimi

LEARNING OBJECTIVES

- Understand the importance of an up-front, primary prevention approach and be able to distinguish it from secondary prevention, tertiary prevention, and patient-provider education that occurs after the onset of illness and disease
- Conceptualize that primary prevention extends beyond the individual by improving health outcomes of entire communities
- Understand prevention as an upstream, or proactive, comprehensive solution
- Describe the six synergistic levels of the *Spectrum of Prevention* as a multifaceted and sustainable framework for achieving community change

Some years ago, a prominent individual suffered a major heart attack across the street from the local county hospital. Although the initial prognosis was poor, the care provided by the hospital resulted in a quick and near-complete recovery. The county board of supervisors proudly emphasized the hospital's success during its next meeting. In the presence of the media, the supervisors congratulated key health officials on the outstanding care and treatment provided, noting in particular the high quality of the hospital staff, medical equipment, and training. As the proceedings were winding down, one supervisor asked, "But what about prevention? Do we have quality prevention?" Without missing a beat, the health director answered, "Yes." Pointing to a pile of brochures titled *Staying Heart Healthy*, he proclaimed, "We have these!"

This isn't an isolated case. Many aspects of health in the United States, from how resources are allocated to who has access to care, suffer from a lack of focus on prevention. Far too often, prevention is an afterthought (Cowen, 1987). The predominant approach to health and well-being in this country focuses on medical treatment and services—after the fact—for the many Americans who are sick and injured each year. Unfortunately, there is a lack of corresponding emphasis on quality community prevention efforts, those that prevent people from getting sick and injured *in the first place*. Furthermore, prevention is often relegated to a message in a brochure or to a few moments during a medical visit. Such approaches are not quality prevention efforts. Human behavior is complicated, and awareness of a health risk does not automatically lead to taking protective action (Ghez, 2000).

Effectively addressing the range of health and social problems of the twenty-first century requires a fundamental paradigm shift that generates equity for the most vulnerable members of society and maximizes limited resources. This paradigm shift results in moving from medical treatment after the fact to prevention in the first place—and from targeting individuals to moving toward a comprehensive community focus. The imperative for this shift in thinking is best described by the psychologist and noted prevention advocate George Albee (1983), who noted that "no mass disorder afflicting mankind is ever brought under control or eliminated by attempts at treating the affected individual" (p. 24).

This chapter moves prevention beyond brochures by presenting an alternative to the dominant individual-based prevention and treatment model. We begin by defining *primary prevention* and offering recent and historical examples of prevention successes, demonstrating that prevention is the basis of public health and that prevention works. We then make the case for primary prevention, emphasizing that prevention supports the health care infrastructure, is an effective use of health care resources, and assists those most in need by decreasing disparities in health. Finally, we describe the six complementary levels of the *Spectrum of Prevention*, which provide a multifaceted and sustainable framework for achieving community change.

MOVING UPSTREAM WITH PRIMARY PREVENTION

In a 2002 speech to the Commonwealth Club in San Francisco, Gloria Steinem observed, "We are still standing on the bank of the river, rescuing people who are drowning. We have not gone to the head of the river to keep them from falling in. That is the twenty-first-century task." Steinem's remark refers to a popular analogy, "moving upstream," which is used to highlight the importance and relevance of primary prevention (Ardell, 1977/1986).

MOVING UPSTREAM

While walking along the banks of a river, a passerby notices that someone in the water is drowning. After pulling the person ashore, the rescuer notices another person in the river in need of help. Before long, the river is filled with drowning people, and more rescuers are required to assist the initial rescuer. Unfortunately, some people are not saved, and some victims fall back into the river after they have been pulled ashore. At this time, one of the rescuers starts walking upstream. "Where are you going?" the other rescuers ask, disconcerted. The upstream rescuer replies, "I'm going upstream to see why so many people keep falling into the river." As it turns out, the bridge leading across the river upstream has a hole through which people are falling. The upstream rescuer realizes that fixing the hole in the bridge will prevent many people from ever falling into the river in the first place.

The act of "moving upstream" and taking action before a problem arises in order to avoid it entirely, rather than treating or alleviating its consequences, is called primary prevention. The term *primary prevention* was coined in the late 1940s by Hugh Leavell and E. Guerney Clark from the Harvard and Columbia University Schools of Public Health, respectively. Leavell and Clark described primary prevention as "measures applicable to a particular disease or group of diseases in order to intercept the causes of disease before they involve man . . . [in the form of] specific immunizations, attention to personal hygiene, use of environmental sanitation, protection against occupational hazards, protection from accidents, use of specific nutrients, protection from carcinogens, and avoidance of allergens" (Goldston, 1987, p. 3). Although Leavell and Clark's definition is mostly disease-oriented, the applications of primary prevention extend beyond medical problems. These include the prevention of other societal concerns that affect health and well-being and that range from violence to environmental degradation. Primary prevention efforts are proactive by definition and should generally be aimed at populations, not just at individuals. Returning to the upstream analogy, fixing the hole in the bridge will benefit not only those at greatest risk of falling in but everyone who crosses the river—as well as the rescuers on the riverbank and those who help pay for rescue costs.

Leavell and Clark further identified two other degrees of prevention termed *secondary* and *tertiary prevention*. Secondary prevention consists of a set of measures used for early detection and prompt intervention to control a problem or disease and minimize the poor health consequences, while tertiary prevention focuses on the reduction of further complications of an existing disease or problem, through treatment and rehabilitation (Spasoff, Harris, & Thuriaux, 2001).

Leavell and Clark's "overarching concept of prevention," described in Exhibit 1.1 through the example of childhood lead poisoning, actually refers to three distinctive activities that might be better termed "prevention, treatment, and rehabilitation" (Goldston, 1987, p. 3). As noted by Albee (1987, p. 12), "all three forms of preventive intervention are useful and defensible." However, whereas primary prevention alone is not enough to address pervasive health and social problems, it remains the foremost method we can employ in order to eliminate future health and social problems. Albee goes on to note that "any reduction in incidence [of disease] must rely heavily on proactive efforts with large groups, and such actions involve primary prevention approaches" (p. 12).

EXHIBIT 1.1　THREE LEVELS OF PREVENTION FOR CHILDHOOD LEAD POISONING

Lead poisoning occurs when the body absorbs too much lead by breathing it in or swallowing it. Children are exposed to lead primarily through the lead-based paint that is frequently found in older homes and through soil that has been previously contaminated by lead-based paint. Lead affects nearly every system in the body and in high enough quantities can cause irreversible neurocognitive damage in developing children under six.

Primary Prevention

Data from the National Health and Nutrition Examination Survey (NHANES) showed that blood lead levels in children younger than thirteen years of age declined nearly 90 percent from 1976 to 2002 (Jacobs, Wilson, Dixon, Smith & Evens, 2009). This dramatic decrease is attributed to population-based environmental policies that banned the use of lead in gasoline, paint, drinking-water pipes, and food and beverage containers. The decrease in blood lead level from 1990 to 2000 is associated with trends in housing demolition and substantial housing rehabilitation (Jacobs, Wilson, Dixon, Smith & Evens, 2009). Primary prevention is the only way to reduce the neurocognitive effects of lead poisoning (Lee & Hurwitz, 2002).

Secondary Prevention

Lead-level screening programs for at-risk children are followed by the treatment of children with high levels and removal of lead paint from households. Screening can prevent recurrent exposures and the exposure of other children to lead by triggering the identification and remediation of sources of lead in children's environments (New York State Department of Health, 2004).

Tertiary Prevention

Tertiary prevention refers to the treatment, support, and rehabilitation of children with lead poisoning who manifest complications of the disease. Lead chelation of the blood and soft tissues of exposed individuals can reduce morbidity associated with lead poisoning. Chelation can reduce the immediate toxicity associated with acute ingestion of lead but has limited ability to reverse the neurocognitive effects of chronic exposure (Lee & Hurwitz, 2002).

THE HISTORY OF EFFECTIVE PREVENTION EFFORTS

In practice, primary prevention involves policies and actions that fix the metaphorical holes in the bridge that lead to sickness and injury. Primary prevention works to reduce the ailments that would otherwise require treatment.

One well-known and very successful modern example of primary prevention is the National Minimum Age Drinking Act of 1984, which required all states to raise the minimum age to purchase alcohol to twenty-one or risk losing major transportation funding. The National Highway Traffic Safety Administration (NHTSA) estimates that as a result of minimum-drinking-age laws, 18,220 lives were saved between 1975 and 1999 (U.S. Department of Transportation, 1999), and 4,242 people between eighteen and twenty years old were saved between 2004 and 2008 (NHTSA, 2009).

This law is far from the first example of primary prevention. In fact, public health has always been founded on prevention. The first public health measures were vast environmental improvements aimed at keeping entire populations healthy. *The Sanitary Conditions of the Labouring Population of Great Britain*, a seminal report published in 1842 by the English civil servant Edwin Chadwick, noted that widespread preventive measures were necessary to preserve the health of England's workforce (Duffy, 1990). Initial public health efforts focused primarily on improving water supplies, refuse and sewage disposal, housing, ventilation, disinfection, and general cleanliness in a community (Vetter & Matthews, 1999). Labor, housing standards, and other health regulations were also developed during this period in an effort to curtail disease and premature death (Duffy, 1990).

What many experts recognize as the seminal event of the prevention movement was a simple but exceptionally effective action taken by John Snow, a physician, during

England's 1854 cholera outbreak. Cholera spreads rapidly, causing diarrhea, vomiting, and, if untreated, eventual death from dehydration. During the 1854 outbreak, five hundred people from an impoverished section of South London died within a ten-day period as a result of the disease. Many people needed treatment. However, instead of just treating his patients individually, Snow, who is credited with some of the initial investigative work in epidemiology for his work during an earlier cholera outbreak, also decided to "move upstream" and locate the source of the problem (Summers, 1989).

By studying the trends of the particular outbreak, Snow mapped the origin to a specific water pump on Broad Street. He used the information he had collected about the source of cholera to prevent its spread. Instead of warning locals not to drink water from the contaminated pump or attempting to treat the water for drinking, Snow took his initial efforts a step further and had the pump's handle removed to prevent new cases of cholera from the pump (Summers, 1989).

Snow's story illustrates the importance of taking environmental factors into account when diseases or other problems occur in a community and the importance of also displaying the common sense associated with prevention.

EXAMPLES AND CHALLENGES OF PRIMARY PREVENTION

Actions like Snow's are behind many public health successes. Many injuries have been averted and lives saved by such primary prevention measures. In addition to the minimum-drinking-age law, recent examples of primary prevention include the following:

- **Antismoking legislation**. California's aggressive antitobacco effort under Proposition 99 has resulted in 33,000 fewer deaths from cardiovascular disease in the first three years (Kuiper, Nelson, & Schooley, 2005).
- **Routine immunizations**. As childhood immunizations against diphtheria, tetanus, pertussis (whooping cough), polio, measles and tuberculosis have become increasingly routine, an estimated 2.5 million young lives are being saved every year. (UNICEF, 2009).
- **Water fluoridation**. Water fluoridation has been effective in reducing tooth decay by 50 to 60 percent (Centers for Disease Control and Prevention, 2009).
- **Motorcycle helmet laws**. Motorcycle helmet laws, enacted in six states (California, Maryland, Nebraska, Oregon, Texas, and Washington) since 1989, have successfully reduced motorcycle fatalities by an average of 27 percent in the first year (NHTSA, 2008b). On the other hand, states that have weakened their motorcycle helmet laws since 1997 to cover only those under a specific age showed an average increase in fatalities of more than 50 percent in the first year (NHTSA, 2008b).

These examples provide compelling evidence that primary prevention is effective. But despite this evidence, there is resistance to primary prevention. Unfortunately, primary prevention is often treated as if it were a distraction from the real and urgent pressure to meet the needs of those who are presently ill.

Why is this the case? One reason is that until prevention efforts succeed, it is generally difficult to conceptualize what prevention looks like. Meanwhile, the need to provide treatment services to affected individuals is clear. Thus it is easy to understand that someone who experiences domestic violence may need counseling and other supportive services, but harder to understand how to change whole populations to prevent occurrences of domestic violence before they begin.

We can learn how to overcome obstacles and to create effective prevention initiatives by studying previous successes. Most prevention efforts, including those mentioned in this chapter, were at their initiation viewed as "impossible." The first antismoking advocates routinely heard "You're crazy!" and "That will never work!" as they attempted to pass no-smoking laws for restaurants and public places. Indeed, in light of the powerful tobacco industry and the skepticism of the general public, the passage of no-smoking laws seemed ambitious at best. Today, however, we often take for granted what once seemed impossible. Many (but certainly not all) public spaces are smoke-free, from airplanes to hospitals and increasingly bars and restaurants (Loftus, 2002).

Another common but unfounded criticism is that the impact of primary prevention is invisible: How can we know if an illness or injury has been prevented or simply did not occur? Although prevention is often difficult to quantify on an individual level, when viewed in aggregate at the population level, the significant impact of prevention becomes immediately quantifiable. Consider the impact that mandatory use of seat belts and infant and child safety seats has had in the primary prevention of death and injury from automobile crashes. Between 1978 and 1985, every state, beginning with Tennessee (see box about Dr. Robert Sanders in Chapter Six for more on these efforts), passed laws requiring safety seats for child passengers (Harvard Injury Control Research Center, 2003–2006). Between 1975 and 2008, mandatory car seat use resulted in the prevention of close to eight thousand deaths and injuries in the United States (NHTSA, 2009).[1] Early prevention at the community level has a substantial impact.

THE CASE FOR PRIMARY PREVENTION

Primary prevention offers the hope of eliminating unnecessary illness, injury, and even death. Nearly 50 percent of annual deaths in the United States—and the impaired quality of life that frequently precedes them—are preventable in part because they are attributable to external environmental or behavioral factors (McGinnis & Foege, 1993; McGinnis, Williams-Russo & Knickman, 2002; Mokdad, Marks, Stroup, & Gerberding, 2004; Thorpe, Florence, & Joski, 2004). A focus on primary prevention can reverse this current trend by converting some of the resources used to treat injuries and illnesses into efforts that effectively prevent them in the first place.

According to the noted public health expert Henrik Blum (1981), medical care and interventions "play key restorative or ameliorating roles. But they are predominantly applied only after disease occurs and therefore are often too late and at a great price" (p. 43). Despite the widely held belief in the United States that the state of being healthy is derived primarily from health care, Blum notes that, in reality, there are four major determinants of health: environment, heredity, lifestyle, and health care services. Of these four, Blum found that "by far the most potent and omnipresent set of forces is the one labeled 'environmental,' while behavior and lifestyle are the second most powerful force" (p. 43).

HEALTH CARE NEEDS PREVENTION

"Simply put, in the absence of a radical shift towards prevention and public health, we will not be successful in containing medical costs or improving the health of the American people," noted then-Senator and Presidential Candidate Barack Obama (2008). Although they are often viewed as an after-the-fact add-on to treatment, primary prevention strategies are a natural complement to medical care and treatment. As the capacity of the U.S. health care system approaches a breaking point (Cooper, Getzen, McKee, & Prakash, 2002), prevention becomes even more critical. This is demonstrated in Exhibit 1.2. A systematic investment in prevention decreases the burden on the health care system, translating into higher-quality care and treatment services for those truly in need.

EXHIBIT 1.2   TRANFORMING THE U.S. HEALTH CARE SYSTEM INTO A HEALTH SYSTEM

A U.S. health system that addresses health along a continuum beginning with prevention is vital to improving population health. Most major diseases and conditions are largely preventable. Thus, primary prevention could support healthy development and minimize the risk of a lifetime of treatment for injury and chronic disease. A system that values and promotes disease prevention would help to contain mounting health care costs. Medical treatment is critical, but it is not enough to keep people healthy in the first place.

Why a Comprehensive Approach to Health Through Prevention Is Needed

- Health and wellness are determined by far more than what occurs in the hospital and doctor's office. Despite high levels of spending, access to health care—although vital to the U.S. population and economy—does not affect health status as much as one might expect. In fact, access to care is estimated to contribute only to 10 percent of individuals' health outcomes (McGinnis, Williams-Russo & Knickman, 2002). Meanwhile, behavioral factors account for 40 percent; genetic predispositions, 30 percent; social circumstances, 15 percent; and toxins and infectious agents, 5 percent (McGinnis, Williams-Russo & Knickman, 2002).

- Current health care spending is rising alarmingly. In 2007, the U.S. spent $2.2 trillion on health care, approximately $7,421 per person. This amount was more than twice as much as most other industrialized countries (Centers for Medicare and Medicaid Services, 2008). The percentage of gross domestic product (GDP) devoted to health care expenditures in the United States has risen from 7.2 percent in 1970 to 16.3 percent in 2007. Projected spending may reach 20.3 percent of GDP by 2018 (Centers for Medicare and Medicaid Services, 2008).

- The health care system is prone to making avoidable mistakes. Medical errors and hospital-acquired infections cause more deaths than AIDS, breast cancer, firearms, diabetes, and auto accidents combined; recent estimates place the number of annual deaths attributable to medical error at 195,000 and the number attributable to hospital infections at 103,000 (American College of Emergency Physicians, 2004).

- Treatment costs will continue to rise unless incidences of disease and injury are reduced. Since the 1960s, major advances in heart attack treatment have occurred and death rates from coronary heart disease have declined (Brown, 2009; Lloyd-Jones et al., 2010). During the same period, the costs for treating heart attacks increased from $5,700 in 1977 to $54,400 in 2007 (without adjusting for inflation) (Brown, 2009). Providing greater access to medical care will do little to reduce these costs but instead will increase associated medical payments for treatments (Brown, 2009). Although advances in medical treatment may extend someone's life by years, his or her quality of life and levels of productivity are not guaranteed. Health promotion and disease prevention could reduce outright the burden of illness, acute events, injury, and their sequelae.

PRIMARY PREVENTION HELPS THOSE MOST AT RISK

> All members of a community are affected by the health status of its least healthy members.
>
> —*Institute of Medicine, 2002, p. 37*

The burden of illness and lack of access to care in the United States is not borne equally across the population. Both frequency of illness and quality of care are often a reflection of socioeconomic status, ethnicity, and race (Agency for Healthcare Research and Quality, 2000). According to the Centers for Disease Control and Prevention (CDC), "The demographic changes that are anticipated over the next decade magnify the importance of addressing disparities in health status" (2006). A greater proportion of the total U.S. population will experience poorer health status; therefore, since we are all cared for by the same system—and so share limited resources—the future health of America will be influenced substantially by our success in improving the health of members of these relatively less healthy groups. A national focus on disparities in health status is particularly important as major changes unfold in the way in which health care is delivered and financed.

African Americans, Hispanics, American Indians, Alaska Natives, and Pacific Islanders consistently face higher rates of morbidity and mortality, and compelling evidence indicates that race and ethnicity correlate with persistent and often increasing health disparities compared to the U.S. population as a whole. Research has now shown that after adjusting for individual risk factors, differences remain in health outcomes among various communities (PolicyLink, 2002). Primary prevention can serve to eliminate underlying health disparities through its upstream population focus; as Albee (1996) notes, "Logically, prevention programs should include efforts at achieving social equality for all" (p. 1131). For example, improving access to healthy foods in order to prevent the onset of diabetes due to poor nutrition for at-risk individuals in a community would result in positive health benefits for other community members as well.

Furthermore, inequalities affect entire societies, not just those who disproportionately share the burden of disease. Wilkinson and Pickett (2009) present a compelling argument for the ways in which income inequality is correlated with worse health outcomes in unequal societies. The fact that some people earn higher incomes than others does not protect them from the corrosive effects of income inequality; in other words, everyone suffers from inequality. Wilkinson and Pickett report that psychosocial factors, including stress, anxiety, shame, self-deprivation, among others, prevail in societies where a social gradient exists. Moreover, countries with greater income inequality have greater rates of homicide, conflict in childhood (for example, bullying), substance abuse, imprisonment, teenage pregnancies, and obesity. Quality of life also suffers for all, as countries with greater differences between "haves" and "have nots" are more likely to have citizens who are less likely to trust one another. Unfortunately, the United States is among the worst of unequal societies. The richest 20 percent in the United States earn more than 8 times what the poorest 20 percent earn. Moreover, the U.S. states with greater income inequality have residents with worse health status. States with more difference in the incomes of the very wealthy and the very poor have a larger population of people who are sicker. If there were even a 1 percent redistribution of income from the richest to the poorest, this move toward equity could improve death rates for all (Berkman & Kawachi, 2000).

PRIMARY PREVENTION IS A GOOD INVESTMENT

Currently, health care spending is growing at an unsustainable rate driven up by rising costs and a growing burden of disease. The costs are bankrupting families and small businesses, putting corporations and industry at a competitive disadvantage, and straining public resources. The long-term solution must involve both cost containment and reduced demand for services. However, of the more than $2.2 trillion in health care spent nationally every year, fewer than four cents of every dollar are spent on prevention and public health (Lambrew, 2007). Table 1.1 lays out specific cost savings associated with different forms of primary prevention.

Table 1.1   A lesson in responsible spending

	Every $1 invested in:	Produces savings of:
Government	Water fluoridation	$37.24 in communities with more than 20,000 people (Griffin, Jones, & Tomar, 2001).
	High-quality preschool programs	$16.41 from averted crime, remedial services, and child welfare services (High/Scope Educational Research Foundation, 2005).
	Breastfeeding support by employers	$3 in reduced absenteeism and health care costs for mothers and babies, and improved productivity (United States Breastfeeding Committee, 2002).
	Women, Infants, and Children (WIC) services	$2.91 in Medicaid for newborn medical care (Buescher, Larson, Nelson, Lenihan, 1993).
Community	Child safety seats	$41.52 in direct medical and other costs to society (Children's Safety Network, 2005).
	Bicycle helmets	$30 in direct medical and other costs to society (National Highway Traffic Safety Administration, 2008a).
	California Tobacco Control Program	$50 in total personal health care spending (Lightwood, Dinno, & Glantz, 2008).
	Walking and biking trails	$2.60 in direct medical costs of physical inactivity (Wang et al, 2004).
	Physical activity programs for older adults	$4.50 on hip fractures (National Governors Association, 2009).
	Worksite wellness programs	$15.60 in reduced absenteeism (Aldana, Merrill, Price, Hardy, Hager, 2005).
	Family- and school-based addiction prevention programs	$10 in employer and community benefit (Iowa State University News Service, 2009).

(Continued)

Table 1.1 ***(Continued)***

	Every $1 invested in:	Produces savings of:
Clinical	The seven-vaccine routine childhood immunization schedule	$16.50 in direct medical and other costs to society (Zhou et al., 2005).
	The chickenpox vaccine	$4.37 in direct medical costs and other costs to society (Zhou, Ortega-Sanchez, Guris, Shefer, Lieu, & Seward, 2008).
	Screening and brief counseling interventions for alcohol misuse among pregnant women	$4.30 in healthcare costs (Fleming et al., 2002).
	Hospital needlestick prevention program	$6.20 in medical and associated costs (Hatcher, 2002).
	Vaccinations for older adults	$2.44 in hospitalization costs due to influenza (Maciosek, Solberg, Coffield, Adwards & Goodman, 2006).
	Hospital program (handwashing promotion, education of staff) to prevent the spread of infection	$6.00 in hospital medical costs (Macartney, Gorelick & Manning, 2000).

Primary prevention has a track record of improving health and reducing costs and has the potential to save more lives if applied comprehensively and strategically. A landmark 2008 study, *Prevention for a Healthier America: Investments in Disease Prevention Yield Significant Savings, Stronger Communities*—produced through a partnership between Trust for America's Health, the New York Academy of Medicine, the Urban Institute, The California Endowment, the Robert Wood Johnson Foundation, and Prevention Institute (2008)—validates that prevention saves money. The study demonstrates that investments of $10 per person per year in programs to increase physical activity, improve nutrition, and prevent tobacco use could save the country more than $16 billion in annual health care costs within five years. Out of the potential $16 billion in savings, Medicare could save more than $5 billion, Medicaid could save more than $1.9 billion, and private payers could save more than $9 billion. Furthermore, the return on investment for prevention is substantial; for every $1 invested in community-based prevention, the return amounts to $5.60 in the fifth year. Prevention investments result in savings for both public and private health care payers.

Prevention can also help improve productivity and competitiveness. Good health is fundamental to broad-based economic sustainability. In order to remain competitive with other countries, the United States needs a healthy workforce and, because employers are the main purchasers of health insurance for workers, health care costs must remain within the range of other industrialized nations. The United States has the highest per capita health care spending in the world, nearly double the spending in Switzerland, which has the next highest. In recent years, many companies have moved their operations overseas, laying-off thousands of workers in the process, in part, to be spared the burden of skyrocketing health care costs. Comprehensive year-round health programs have the potential to yield cost savings of $3 for every $1 spent (University of Michigan Health Management Research Center, 2000). By adopting worksite wellness programs—with elements such as fitness classes, stress management, ergonomic equipment policies, and on-site farmers' markets (at over 20 Kaiser Permanente sites in California)—companies have improved employee health and productivity, while reducing employee absenteeism and the business costs associated with poor health conditions. As Safeway's Chief Executive Steve Burd notes, "If we can create a health care plan that contains costs or drives them down, that improves the health of the employee and extends their life, and avoids catastrophic illness and doesn't cost them any more money, why would anybody quarrel with that plan?" (Colliver, 2007).

MAKING HEALTH MANLY

"Health matters are women's matters." "Only women pamper their bodies." There is substantial evidence, at least in the United States, that asking for help and caring for one's health are widely considered to be the province of women (Courtenay, 2000c). Collective beliefs and assumptions such as these are what social scientists refer to as *social norms* (Berkowitz, 2003) or *subjective norms* (Ajzen, 2001).

Given the existence of these norms, it is not surprising that in most Western industrialized countries, women are the greatest consumers of health-related products and services. Women are often first to take responsibility, not only for the health and well-being of themselves and their offspring, but also for the health of men. This helps explain why single men have the greatest health risks—and why the benefits of marriage are consistently found to be greater for men than for women (who can suffer substantial stress in caring for their spouses) (Courtenay, 2000a).

Ultimately, men need to take greater responsibility for their own health. But here is the problem: men receive strong social prohibitions against doing *anything* that women do (Courtenay, 2000c).

Men and boys who engage in behaviors representing feminine gender norms risk being perceived as "wimps" or "sissies." Consequently, men often seek to prove their manhood by *actively rejecting* doing anything that women do—and this includes caring for their health (Courtenay, 2000b). Not surprisingly, there is solid

birth (Wolf, 2003). Rates have declined dramatically over the past century for a number of reasons, including lack of accommodations for working mothers who are breastfeeding, social mores about the acceptability of breastfeeding in public, and the development and marketing of baby formulas as a primary source of infant nutrition (Wolf, 2003). As more evidence becomes available to clinicians, breastfeeding is again being promoted in order to improve the public's health.

The cultural context surrounding breastfeeding, however, is still a significant barrier in the United States. As sociologist Joan Retsinas noted, "While it is known that breastfeeding is better, our society is not structured to facilitate that choice" (quoted in Wright, 2001, p. 1). Groups like the Women, Infants and Children's (WIC) Program funded by the U.S. Department of Agriculture to improve birth outcomes and early childhood health have prioritized breastfeeding for low-income women and children through nutritional support programs (Ahluwalia & Tessaro, 2000).

Making progress requires more than simply helping mothers with the skills to successfully breastfeed. Creating and maintaining widespread social norms for breastfeeding is critical. This requires activities along each level of the Spectrum of Prevention.

The first level of the Spectrum, *strengthening individual knowledge and skills*, emphasizes enhancing individual skills that are essential in healthy behaviors. Clinical services are one common opportunity for delivering these skills, although there are many avenues of importance. Individual skill building is essential to the success of breastfeeding for new mothers. Women need support before and after their child is born in order to successfully initiate and maintain breastfeeding. Often an ob-gyn, presenting expectant parents with information on the benefits of breastfeeding for themselves and their infants, can have an early influence on the decision to breastfeed. In-hospital support, round-the-clock hotlines, and lactation counselors help troubleshoot the challenges a mother encounters and motivate her to continue in her breastfeeding commitment.

The second level of the Spectrum, *promoting community education*, entails reaching people with information and resources in order to promote their health and safety. Typically, many health education initiatives focus on developing brochures, holding health fairs, and conducting community forums and events. Such onetime exposures can be a valuable element of a broader campaign but often don't have a big impact. We need to understand that today the mass media are the primary sources of education for almost everyone. Although there have been creative efforts to use the media to improve health, the massive expenditures of corporations far overshadow public health efforts in the mass media. As Ivan Juzang (2002) of MEE Productions points out, word of mouth can be a powerful and effective tool. It's the best advertising money can't buy. Creating positive word of mouth allows your prevention message to live on, even after a formal campaign is over, as community members take ownership of the message and begin to initiate their own activities that support it.

Educating a larger community about the benefits of breastfeeding helps create community environments that encourage breastfeeding and view it as normal. Posters have been used in health care settings to signal the value of breastfeeding. One example of a large-scale community media campaign is the one coordinated by the U.S. Department of Health and Human Services and the Ad Council (U.S. Department of Health and Human Services, Office of Women's Health, 2001).

Locally, the news media can provide rich—and free—opportunities to emphasize public health. A great example of this was the Berkeley, California, Public Health Department's event to enter the *Guinness Book of World Records* by bringing together the largest number of breastfeeding mothers in history (BBC News, 2002).

Advocates also cite corporate advertising as one of the roadblocks in encouraging social change toward increased breastfeeding. Manufacturers often idealize the use of formula for infant nutrition by touting convenience; Derrick Jellife coined the term *commerciogenic malnutrition* to describe the impact of industry marketing practices on infant health ("Baby Milk Action," n.d.). A resulting boycott, and the media attention it engendered, created large-scale awareness that the decline in breastfeeding was not simply a matter of unfettered individual choice.

The third level of the Spectrum is *educating providers*. Because health care providers are a trusted source of health-related information, they are a key group to reach with strategies for prevention. Similarly, teachers and public safety officials are often identified as key groups to reach with new information and methods. The notion of who is a provider should be approached more broadly, however, and extends beyond the "usual suspects" to include faith leaders; postal workers and other public servants; business, union, and community leaders; and cashiers—and anyone who is in a position to share information or influence others.

Because of their contact with expectant mothers, a first place to start is with the ob-gyn and pediatric staff. Maternity staff have been trained that a good practice is to encourage breastfeeding within a half hour of birth. In California, Riverside County's Nutrition Services Department has created a marketing team modeled on pharmaceutical company representatives that visit prenatal and pediatric care providers to supply them with educational materials, displays, takeaway cards, and training to ensure they have the resources necessary to help their patients choose to breastfeed their babies and continue to do so. An additional approach is the involvement of business leaders who can assist mothers in transitioning back into the workplace. Training includes helping business leaders understand their role when mothers return to work and how to set up facilities that allow breastfeeding in the workplace. Another innovative model of provider education, developed in some African American communities, involves sharing information about the benefits of breastfeeding with beauty shop employees and their clients, who in turn share it with their neighbors (Best Start Social Marketing, 2003).

Level four of the Spectrum, *fostering coalitions and networks*, focuses on collaboration and community organizing. Fostering collaborative approaches brings together the participants necessary to ensure an initiative's success and increase the "critical mass" behind a community effort. Coalitions and expanded partnerships are vital in successful public health movements, including breastfeeding promotion. The metaphor of a jigsaw puzzle is appropriate, with each piece having value but taking on a greater significance when all the pieces are put together in the right way. Collaboration is not an intrinsic outcome like the other levels of the Spectrum, but rather a tool used to achieve an objective. Often the best way to ensure a comprehensive strategy is to build a diverse coalition.

Collaborations may take place at several levels: at the community level grassroots partners may work together in community organizing; at the organizational level nonprofits may work together to coordinate the efforts of business, faith, or other interest groups; and at the governmental level different sectors of government may link with one another. Typical partnerships include elements of all three. In health fields, interdisciplinary and intergovernmental partnerships are probably less common than collaborations between community-based organizations and grassroots efforts, which hold enormous promise for advancing the work of primary prevention (Cohen, Baer, & Satterwhite, 2002). Often the best way to ensure a comprehensive strategy is to build a diverse coalition. *Eight Steps to Effective Coalition Building* (Cohen et al., 2002) is a framework that guides advocates and practitioners through the process of coalition building, from deciding whether or not a coalition is appropriate to selecting the best membership and conducting ongoing evaluation.

An important objective of coalition building is to identify and work toward goals that can have greater impact on the community overall than any coalition participant might achieve alone. A key part of leadership, then, is finding an interest common to most or all groups and facilitating work toward achieving vital shared goals.

Returning to our example, collaboration between organizations and the fostering of coalitions are vital in the promotion of breastfeeding. To effect not only individual behavioral changes but social norm changes as well, leadership is needed from health experts, grassroots advocates, social service workers, politicians, business groups, and the media. On the international level, a broad collaboration of community members around the world led to the effective challenge of corporations promoting infant formula ("Challenging Corporate Abuses," 1993). At the local level, building on public knowledge of the importance of breastfeeding and engaging the business and medical community led to changes in the organizational practices of businesses and hospitals.

The fifth level of the Spectrum, *changing organizational practices*, deals with organizational change from a systems perspective. Reshaping the general practices of key organizations can affect both health and norms. Such change reaches the members, clients, and employees of the company as well as the surrounding community and serves as a model for all. Changing organizational practices is easier than changing policy in many cases, so can serve as the testing ground for policy change. Government and health institutions are key places to make change because of their role as standard setters. Other critical arenas include media, business, sports, faith organizations, and schools. Nearly everyone belongs to or works in an organization, so this approach gives collaborators an immediate place to initiate change surrounding a particular issue.

Two key areas for changing organizational practices that support breastfeeding are the Baby-Friendly Hospital Initiative and workplace policies around maternity leave and lactation support. As part of the Baby-Friendly Hospital Initiative, participating hospitals provide an optimal environment for the mother to learn the skills of breastfeeding, including allowing mothers to keep their newborns in the same room rather than in the hospital nursery, and encouraging initiation of breastfeeding within a half hour after birth. These hospitals stop the standard practice of sending mothers home with discharge packs that include artificial baby formula. This initiative has resulted in significant increases in breastfeeding initiation rates (Phillip et al., 2001).

For mothers who work, breastfeeding can be difficult unless their employers adopt policies that facilitate breastfeeding. Such organizational policies include allowing enough maternity leave to solidly establish breastfeeding practices and designing environments that make it easier for mothers to pump and store breast milk while at work. Media portrayals of breastfeeding as normal, as opposed to portraying breasts as almost entirely sexualized, could also facilitate breastfeeding.

The sixth level of the Spectrum, *influencing policy and legislation*, has the potential for achieving the broadest impact across a community. Policy is the set of rules that guide the activities of governmental or quasi-governmental organizations. Policy thus sets the foundation or framework for action. By mandating what is expected and required, sound policies can lead to widespread behavioral changes on a communitywide scale that may ultimately become the social norm. Over the course of the past several years, major health improvements have occurred as a result of policy changes, including a reduction in diseases associated with cigarette smoking, a decrease in workplace and roadway accidents due to dramatically greater use of safety equipment, and reductions in lead poisoning.

Although policy is frequently thought of as either state or federal, evidence indicates that highly effective prevention policy can be developed on the community level and that local policy development is integral to the success of prevention programs (Holder et al., 1997). As a result, sound policies can lead to widespread behavior change on a communitywide scale. As noted by the Municipal Research and Services Center of Washington (2000), "Policy making is often undervalued and misunderstood, yet it is the central role of the city, town, and county legislative bodies."

Using our breastfeeding example, policies that support breastfeeding mothers include laws mandating maternity leave and requiring workplaces to make accommodations for employees who breastfeed. Additional legislation at the state level can help modify the existing structure of a system in order to promote the healthier choice for a mother and her newborn infant. A California policy proposed in 2004 would have provided comprehensive education about infant feeding options to new mothers and would have banned the marketing of infant formulas in California hospitals. However, despite widespread support, the bill failed to receive adequate votes for passage.

Local, state, and federal policies are still needed to protect a woman's right to breastfeed in public and to encourage and achieve adequate nutrition for our society's children in their earliest years of life. Although many barriers to breastfeeding exist, the sixth level of the Spectrum is an essential piece to achieving such social change.

One reason the Spectrum can be a powerful tool for prevention is that it is helpful in designing efforts that change norms. Norms shape behavior and are key determinants of whether our behaviors will be healthy or not. More than habits, often based in culture and tradition, norms are regularities in behavior to which people generally conform (Ullmann-Margalit, 1990).

Typically, the tipping factor for normative change requires efforts at the broadest levels of the Spectrum to change organizational practices or policies, because such actions change the community environment. (The other elements of the Spectrum are usually important also, contributing to and building on this momentum for change.) As Schlegel (1997) points out, policy change can trigger norm change by altering what is considered acceptable behavior, encouraging people to think actively about their own behavior, and providing relevant information and a supportive environment to promote change. The emergence of new social norms occurs when enough individuals have made the choice to change their current behavior.

Norm change regarding smoking behaviors is probably the most frequently cited example of this tipping factor and makes the importance of interplay between elements of the Spectrum visible. After the Surgeon General's report in 1964 found that smoking harms health—and after numerous reports of research implied that secondhand smoke was risky (*promoting community education*)—local communities formed coalitions to shape policy in restaurants, public places, and workplaces (*influencing policy*). The ensuing policy controversy received media attention that explained the law and that explained why smoking is risky (*promoting community education*), and the newfound attention led to more requests for training for health and civic leaders (*educating providers*). Doctors started to change their practices. More offered stop-smoking clinics and warned patients about the dangers of smoking (*strengthening individual knowledge and skills*). Once passed, the implementation of the policy required changing organizational practices to comply with the policy. This led to training, conducted by coalition partners for government employees, restaurateurs, and business owners. This spurred an increase in people wanting to quit, and quit-smoking clinics became busier. As the number and extent of policies grew, momentum built for further changes. "What's next?" asked policymakers and enterprising reporters. And the process started again. Policies were adopted that banned vending machines, boosted tobacco taxes, and forbade smoking in bars and public recreation areas. Individual choice still exists, and people still behave according to their own personal preferences. What has changed is society's perception about what is acceptable smoking behavior. This shift in the social norms changes the preference and improves the health of millions.

A well-designed strategy, while seizing opportunities that may arise, always considers a variety of levels of the Spectrum. Also, data and evaluation are key. They are not levels of the Spectrum because they are not inherently outcome-related activities, but they are critical in informing and enhancing the Spectrum strategy.

HUMAN RIGHTS FRAMEWORK AND PRIMARY PREVENTION

Vivian Chávez

Human rights are basic standards without which people cannot survive and develop in dignity. They are inherent to the human person, inalienable and universal. A human rights framework is central to health equity. A human rights framework declares that all people deserve to be treated with dignity, compassion, and support, wherever they are on the Spectrum of Prevention.

Learning about human rights can put power in people's hands to achieve social change by knowing their human rights and claiming them. Every woman, man, youth and child has the human right to the highest attainable standard of physical and mental health, without discrimination of any kind. Human rights relating to health are set out in basic human rights treaties and include:

- The human right to the highest attainable standard of physical and mental health, including reproductive and sexual health.
- The human right to equal access to adequate health care and health-related services, regardless of sex, race, or other status.
- The human right to equitable distribution of food.
- The human right to access to safe drinking water and sanitation.
- The human right to an adequate standard of living and adequate housing.
- The human right to a safe and healthy environment.
- The human right to a safe and healthy workplace, and to adequate protection for pregnant women in work proven to be harmful to them.
- The human right to freedom from discrimination and discriminatory social practices, including female genital mutilation, prenatal gender selection, and female infanticide.
- The human right to education and access to information relating to health, including reproductive health and family planning to enable couples and individuals to make their own responsible decisions about all matters of reproduction and sexuality.
- The human right of the child to an environment appropriate for physical and mental development.

Adapted from UNICEF, *Convention on the Rights of the Child* (http://www.unicef.org/crc/index_framework.html), and *The Human Right to Health: The People's Movement for Human Rights Education* (http://www.pdhre.org/rights/health.html)

Berkman, L. F., & Kawachi, I. (Eds.). (2000). *Social Epidemiology*. New York: Oxford University Press.

Berkowitz, A. D. (2003). Applications of social norms theory to other health and social justice issues. In H. W. Perkins (Ed.), The social norms approach to preventing school- and college-age substance abuse (pp. 259–279). San Francisco: Jossey-Bass.

Best Start Social Marketing. (2003, December). *Using loving support to build a breastfeeding-friendly community: Follow-up report to Indiana WIC Program*. Retrieved July 29, 2006, from http://www .indianaperinatal.org/files/education/EMPR1003.pdf

Blum, H. L. (1981). Social perspective on risk reduction. *Family and Community Health, 3*, 41–50.

Borger, C., Smith, S., Truffer, C., Keehan, S., Sisko, A., Poisal, J., & Clemens, M. K. (2006). Health spending projections through 2015: Changes on the horizon. *Health Affairs, 25*, W61–W73.

Brown, D. (2009, July 26). A case of getting what you pay for: With heart attack treatments, as quality rises, so does costs. *The Washington Post*, Retrieved July 27, 2009 from http://www.washington-post.com/

Buescher, P. A., Larson, L. C., Nelson, M. D., Lenihan, A. J. (1993). Prenatal WIC participation can reduce low birth weight and newborn medical costs: A cost-benefit analysis of WIC participation in North Carolina. *Journal of American Dietetic Association, 93*, 163–166.

Centers for Disease Control and Prevention. (2003). *The power of prevention: Reducing the health and economic burden of chronic disease*. Atlanta, GA: Author. Retrieved from http://www.cdc.gov/ nccdphp/publications/PowerOfPrevention/pdfs/power_of_prevention.pdf

Centers for Disease Control and Prevention, Office of Minority Health. (2006). *Eliminating racial and ethnic health disparities*. Atlanta, GA: Author. Retrieved July 11, 2006, from http://www.cdc .gov/omh/AboutUs/disparities.htm

Centers for Disease Control and Prevention. (2009). *Community water fluoridation*. Atlanta, GA: Author. Retrieved December 29, 2009, from http://www.cdc.gov/fluoridation/faqs.htm

Centers for Medicare and Medicaid Services (2008). *National health expenditures by type of service and source of funds*. Washington, DC, Centers for Medicare and Medicaid Services. Retrieved July 7, 2009, from http://www.cms.hhs.gov/NationalHealthExpendData/downloads/dsm-07.pdf

Challenging corporate abuses: An interview with Elaine Lamy. (1993, August). *Multinational Monitor, 15*(7–8). Retrieved July 28, 2006, from http://multinationalmonitor.org/hyper/issues/ 1993/08/mm0893_08.html

Children's Safety Network. (2005). *Child safety seats: How large are the benefits and who should pay?* Newton, MA, Children's Safety Network.

Cohen, L., Baer, N., & Satterwhite, P. (2002). Eight steps to effective coalition building. In M. E. Wurzbach (Ed.), *Community health education and promotion: A guide to program design and evaluation* (2nd ed., pp. 144–161). Gaithersburg, MD: Aspen.

Cohen, R. A., & Martinez, M. E. (2005). *Health insurance coverage: Estimates from the National Health Interview Survey*. Retrieved June 1, 2006, from http://www.cdc.gov/nchs/nhis.htm

Colliver, V. (2007, February 11). Preventive health plan may prevent cost increases: Safeway program includes hot line, lifestyle advice. *San Francisco Chronicle*, p. F1.

Cooper, R. A., Getzen, T. E., McKee, H. J., & Prakash, L. (2002). Economic and demographic trends signal an impending physician shortage. *Health Affairs, 21,* 140–154.

Courtenay, W. H. (2000a). Behavioral factors associated with disease, injury, and death among men: Evidence and implications for prevention. *Journal of Men's Studies, 9,* 81–142.

Courtenay, W. H. (2000b). Constructions of masculinity and their influence on men's well-being: A theory of gender and health. *Social Science and Medicine, 50,* 1385–1401.

Courtenay, W. H (2000c). Engendering health: A social constructionist examination of men's health beliefs and behaviors. *Psychology of Men and Masculinity, 1,* 4–15.

Courtenay, W. H. (2000d). Teaming up for the new men's health movement. *Journal of Men's Studies, 8,* 387–392.

Courtenay, W. H. (2003). Key determinants of the health and well-being of men and boys. *International Journal of Men's Health, 2,* 1–30.

Courtenay, W. H. (2004). Making health manly: Social marketing and men's health. *Journal of Men's Health & Gender, 1*(2–3), 275–276.

Cowen, E. L. (1987). Research on primary prevention interventions: Programs and applications. In S. E. Goldston (Eds.), *Concepts of primary prevention: A framework for program development* (pp. 33–50). Sacramento: California Department of Mental Health.

Davidoff, A. J. & Kenney, G. (2005). *Uninsured Americans with chronic health conditions: Key findings from the national health interview survey.* Retrieved July 27, 2009 from http://www.urban.org/publications/411161.html

Dorfman, L., Wallack, L, Woodruff, K. (2005). More than a message: Framing public health advocacy to change corporate practices. *Health Education & Behavior, 32*(3), 320–336.

Duffy, J. (1990). *The sanitarians: A history of American public health.* Champaign: University of Illinois Press.

Fleming, M. F., Mundt, M. P., French, M. T., Manwell, L. B., Stauffacher, E. A., & Barry, K. L. (2002). Brief physician advice for problem alcohol drinkers: long-term efficacy and benefit-cost analysis. A randomized controlled trial in community-based primary care settings. *Alcohol: Clinical and Experimental Research, 26,* 36–43.

Ghez, M. (2000). Getting the message out: Using media to change social norms on abuse. In C. M. Renzetti, J. L. Edleson, & R. K. Bergen (Eds.), *Sourcebook on violence against women* (pp. 417–438). Thousand Oaks, CA: Sage.

Goldston, S. E. (Ed.). (1987). *Concepts of primary prevention: A framework for program development.* Sacramento: California Department of Mental Health.

Griffin, S. O., Jones, K., Tomar, S. (2001). An economic evaluation of community water fluoridation. *Journal of Public Health Dentistry, 61*(2), 78–86.

Harkin, T. (2005, February 17). Remarks at the annual conference of the American College of Preventive Medicine, Washington, DC.

Harvard Injury Control Research Center. (2003–2006). Child safety seats. In *Success stories in injury prevention.* Boston: Author. Retrieved July 11, 2006, from http://www.hsph.harvard.edu/hicrc/success.html

Hatcher, I. B. (2002). Reducing sharps injuries among health care workers: A sharps container quality improvement project. *Joint Commission journal on quality improvement, 28*(7), 410–414.

High/Scope Educational Research Foundation. (2005). *The High/Scope Perry Preschool Study through Age 40.* Ypsilanti, MI: Schweinhart, L. J.

Hoffman, K. & Tolbert, J. (2008, October). *The Uninsured: A Primer.* The Henry J. Kaiser Family Foundation. Available at: http://www.kff.org/uninsured/upload/7451–04.pdf

Holder et al. (1997). Summing up: Lessons from a comprehensive community prevention trial. *Addiction, 92,* 293–302. http://www.nhtsa.dot.gov/portal/site/nhtsa/menuitem.d7975d55e8abbe089 ca8e410dba046a0/

Institute of Medicine. (2000). *Promoting health: Intervention strategies from social and behavioral research* (B. D. Smedley & L. S. Syme, Eds.). Washington, DC: National Academies Press.

Institute of Medicine. (2002). *Unequal treatment: Confronting racial and ethnic disparities in health care* (B. D. Smedley, A. Y. Stith, & A. R. Nelson, Eds.). Washington, DC: National Academies Press.

Iowa State University News Service. (2009, January 20). *ISU report to United Nations conference says drug prevention programs help the economy,* [Press release]. Ames, Iowa: Iowa State University. Retrieved July 27, 2009 from http://www.public.iastate.edu/~nscentral/news/2009/jan/prevention .shtml.

Jacobs, D. E., Wilson, J., Dixon, S. L., Smith J., Evens, A. (2009). The relationship of housing and population health: A 30-year retrospective analysis. *Environmental Health Perspectives, 117,* 597–604.

Juzang, I. (2002, November 20–22). Presentation at the Preventing Obesity in the Hip-Hop Generation Workshop sponsored by the California Adolescent Nutrition and Fitness Program (CANFit) and Motivational Educational Entertainment (MEE) Productions, San Diego, CA.

Kuiper, N. M., Nelson, D. E., & Schooley, M. (2005). *Evidence of effectiveness: A summary of state tobacco control program evaluation literature.* Atlanta, GA: Centers for Disease Control and Prevention, Office on Smoking and Health. Retrieved July 11, 2006, from http://www.cdc.gov/ tobacco/sustainingstates/pdf/lit_Review.pdf

Lambrew J. M. (2007). A wellness trust to prioritize disease prevention. Washington DC: The Hamilton Project, Brookings Institution. Retrieved July 11, 2006, from http://www3.brookings.edu/ views/papers/200704lambrew.pdf

Leape, L. (2006). System analysis and redesign: The foundation of medical error prevention. In M. Cohen (Ed.), *Medication Errors.* Washington DC: American Pharmacist Association.

Lee, D. A., & Hurwitz, R. L. (2002). Childhood lead poisoning: Exposure and prevention. In B. D. Rose (Ed.), *UpToDate* [CD-ROM]. Wellesley, MA: UpToDate.

Lightwood, J. M., Dinno, A., & Glantz, S. A. (2008). Effect of the California tobacco control program on personal health care expenditures. *PLoS Medicine,* 5(8): e178. doi:10.1371/journal.pmed.0050178. Retrieved January 7, 2010, from http://www.plosmedicine.org/article/info%3Adoi%2F10.1371%2F journal.pmed.0050178

Lindblom, E. (2005, February 24). *Comprehensive statewide tobacco prevention programs save money.* Washington, DC: Campaign for Tobacco-Free Kids.

Lloyd-Jones, D., et al. (2010). Heart disease and stroke statistics—2010 update. A report from the American Heart Association Statistics Committee and Stroke Statistics Subcommittee. *Circulation, 121*:e46-e215.

Loftus, M. J. (2002, Spring). Making smoking history. *Public Health*. Retrieved November 13, 2006, from http://www.whsc.emory.edu/_pubs/ph/spring02/smoking.html

Macartney K. K., Gorelick, M. H., Manning, M. L. (2000). Nosocomial respiratory syncytial virus infections: The cost-effectiveness and cost-benefit of infection control. *Pediatrics, 106*(3), 520–526.

Maciosek, M. V., Solberg, L. I., Coffield, A. B., Adwards, N. M., & Goodman, M. J. (2006). Influenza vaccination health impact and cost effectiveness among adults aged 50 to 64 and 65 and older. *American Journal of Preventive Medicine, 31*(1), 72–29.

McCaig, L. F., & Burt, C. W. (2005, May). *National hospital ambulatory medical care survey: 2003 emergency department summary*. Hyattsville, MD: National Center for Health Statistics.

McGinnis, J. M., & Foege, W. H. (1993). Actual causes of death in the United States. *Journal of the American Medical Association, 270*, 2207–2212.

McGinnis, J. M., Williams-Russo, P., & Knickman, J. R. (2002). The case for more active policy attention to health promotion. *Health Affairs, 2*, 78–93.

McGlynn et al. (2003). The quality of health care delivered to adults in the United States. *New England Journal of Medicine, 348*, 2635–2645.

Messonnier, M. L., Corso, P. S., Teutsch, S. M., Haddix, A. C., & Harris, J. R. (1999, April). An ounce of prevention: What are the returns? A handbook. *American Journal of Preventive Medicine, 16*, 248–263.

Mokdad, A. H., Marks, J. S., Stroup, D. F., & Gerberding, J. L. (2004, March 10). Actual causes of death in the United States, 2000. *Journal of the American Medical Association, 291, 1238*–1245.

Municipal Research and Services Center of Washington. (2000, September). *Policy making introduction*. Retrieved July 27, 2006, from http://www.mrsc.org/Subjects/Governance/legislative/intro.aspx

National Governors Association. Healthy aging and states: Making wellness the rule, not the exception. Retrieved May 3, 2009, from http://www.subnet.nga.org/ci/1-aging.html

National Highway Traffic Safety Administration. (2003). *Traffic safety facts, 2003* (DOT HS 809 775). Washington, DC: Author. Retrieved July 11, 2006, from http://www.nrd.nhtsa.dot.gov/pdf/nrd-30/NCSA/TSFAnn/2003HTMLTSF/TSF2003.htm

National Highway Traffic Safety Administration. (2008b). *Traffic safety fact laws: Motorcycle helmet use laws*. Washington, DC: Author. Retrieved December 28, 2009, from http://www.nhtsa.dot.gov/staticfiles//DOT/NHTSA/Communication%20&%20Consumer%20Information/Articles/Associated%20Files/810887.pdf

National Highway Traffic Safety Administration. (2008a). *Traffic safety facts*. Washington, DC. DOT HS 811 172.

National Highway Traffic Safety Administration. (2009, June). *Traffic safety facts, 2009* (DOT HS 811 153). Washington, DC: Author. Retrieved October 11, 2009, from http://www.nrd.nhtsa.dot.gov/pdf/nrd-30/NCSA/TSFAnn/2003HTMLTSF/TSF2003.htm

2

Achieving Health Equity and Social Justice

Wayne H. Giles
Leandris C. Liburd

Sidebar Contributors
Dolores Acevedo-Garcia, Nancy McArdle, Theresa L. Osypuk,
Bonnie Lefkowitz, Barbara Krimgold

LEARNING OBJECTIVES

- Articulate the difference between health disparities and health equity.
- Understand that health disparities are largely socially constructed on the basis of race and ethnicity, gender, education, employment, income and geography and not the result of heredity.
- Describe the determinants of health disparities and the recommended steps to reduce health disparities.
- Become familiar with a framework for a comprehensive public health strategy to eliminate health disparities.

WHAT IS HEALTH EQUITY?

The terms *health disparities* and *health equity*, although clearly not household expressions, are fairly common to many health practitioners, program managers, policymakers, and researchers (Braveman, 2006). The terms health disparities and health inequities are generally used in the United States, although health equity is more common in Europe. The definitions for these terms have evolved over time, but there is little consensus on usage or meaning. One of the best definitions was developed by Margaret Whitehead in the early 1990s. Whitehead defined health disparities as "differences in health that are not only avoidable and unnecessary but in addition unjust and unfair." Health equity is defined as "providing all people with fair opportunities to attain their full health potential to the extent possible" (Braveman, 2006, p. 167). The central implication for primary prevention in this definition is that disparities in health reflect conditions that are avoidable, unjust, and unfair.

Paula Braveman and her colleagues at the World Health Organization state that health equity exists when individuals' "needs, rather than their social privileges, guide the distribution of opportunities for well-being" (World Health Organization, 1996, p. 15). Braveman and Tarimo add that "in virtually every society in the world, social privilege varies among groups of people categorized not only by economic resources but also by gender, by geographic location, by ethnic or religious differences, and by age" (2002, p. 1623). Pursuing equity means trying to reduce avoidable gaps in health status and services between groups with different levels of social privilege (Braveman, Krieger, & Lynch, 2000). A key aspect of this definition is social privilege. Disparities are not merely differences in health between groups but differences between groups with varying levels of social privilege. *Social privilege* can be defined as one's relative position in a hierarchy determined by prestige, power, or wealth. In the United States, for instance, high socioeconomic position tends to result in better health (Braveman et al., 2000).

As one conceptualizes health equity, it is important to realize that there are at least two types of equity, horizontal and vertical (Krieger, Williams, & Moss, 1997). *Horizontal equity*, which means equal treatment for equal needs, would ensure that all people with an equally severe heart attack, for example, would be treated in the same way. In many instances however, this is not the case. Those without health insurance, the poor, and racial and ethnic minorities may receive less aggressive treatments than their more socially privileged counterparts. One survey found that African American women who suffer a heart attack were 75 percent less likely to receive invasive care than Caucasian men (Giles, Anda, Casper, Escobedo, & Taylor, 1995).

Vertical equity refers to different levels of treatment for different needs. That is, one would expect a greater expenditure of resources to treat the people most in need. Here again, research has shown that this is frequently not the case. We find, for example, that poorer individuals, who have many more chronic conditions (and who are more in need), are less likely to receive preventive health care than wealthier individuals, who often have fewer chronic conditions (National Center for Health Statistics, 2009).

Vertical equity may be related to the health care financing schemes characterized by O'Rourke and Iammarino (2006) as *progressive* and *regressive*. A *progressive* approach takes a rising percentage of payments as income increases, whereas a *regressive* approach takes a falling percentage as income increases. The primary financing system employed in the United States is a regressive approach that, according to O'Rourke and Iammarino "guarantees and perpetuates inequities" (p. 59). In other words, people with the highest income pay a smaller percentage of their total income for health insurance, while low-income families pay a higher percentage, thereby reducing their disposable income, which in turn "exacerbates the effects of poverty" (p. 59). This cycle can contribute to the observed patterning of health disparities.

HOW METROPOLITAN AREAS ARE FAILING AMERICA'S CHILDREN

Dolores Acevedo-Garcia, Nancy McArdle, Theresa L. Osypuk, Bonnie Lefkowitz, and Barbara Krimgold

Across metropolitan America, black and Hispanic children face particularly severe challenges as they strive to achieve their health potential and enjoy the full range of life's opportunities, especially when compared to white and Asian children. Not only do black and Hispanic children live in families that experience many disadvantages, those disadvantages are exacerbated by vast inequalities in neighborhood and school environments. These inequalities cannot be explained solely by income differences, as poor black and Hispanic children tend to encounter environments considerably worse than do poor white and Asian children. More hopefully, however, the conditions that contribute to these inequalities suggest some possible policy solutions.

Children Left Behind: How U.S. Metropolitan Areas Are Failing America's Children is the first in a series of reports from diversitydata.org and focuses on the one hundred metropolitan areas with the largest child populations. It paints a stark picture of disparities across all dimensions of well-being, including housing, neighborhood conditions, residential integration, education, and health.

Specific report findings are as follows:

- Across various indicators—including family income and homeownership, average neighborhood income and homeownership rates, residential and school segregation, and school poverty—black children consistently fared

DETERMINANTS OF HEALTH DISPARITIES

Typically, when policymakers and public health professionals attempt to address health disparities, they focus on the elimination of inequities within the organized health care system. We agree that all persons are entitled to receive high-quality health care regardless of gender, race, socioeconomic status, or other social variables that have historically driven unequal treatment. However, the elimination of health disparities requires attention to the physical, mental, and dental health of all communities—and to the social and political context in which health occurs or is threatened. The prevention of health disparities requires interventions that are holistic and that address the allocation of public health and medical resources, quality of care, and the environments in which people live. In addition, public health interventions intending to eliminate health disparities need to systematically address their underlying determinants. Only by addressing the full continuum of health can one expect to effectively eliminate disparities.

ACCESS TO CARE

Although medical care plays an important role in health, its contribution is weaker than usually assumed. According to Blum (1981), there are four major determinants of health: environment, heredity, lifestyle, and health care services. Of these four, "by far the most potent and omnipresent set of forces is the one labeled 'environmental,' while behavior and lifestyle are the second most powerful force" (p. 43). Clinical care has played a small role in improving population health during the last two hundred years; better nutrition, sanitation, and living conditions have played a much greater role (Blum, 1981). Nevertheless, timely and appropriate preventive medical services and effective therapies to manage acute and chronic illnesses can improve health, enhance quality of life, and reduce disparities (Williams, 2003). Yet access to health care in this country is severely limited, and people fall into three categories: the *insured*, the *underinsured*, and the *uninsured*.

Socially disadvantaged groups have lower levels of health insurance coverage and hence less access to health care (National Center for Health Statistics, 2009). O'Rourke and Iammarino (2006) argue, for example, that *underinsured* is merely a "euphemism meaning that you are insured only as long as nothing serious happens" (p. 59). Furthermore, socially disadvantaged groups differ greatly in their use of health care. Multiple barriers at the institutional and personal level can lead to lower utilization of care, such as language and cultural barriers, prior experiences, and organizational characteristics of the health care system that make it easier for socioeconomically advantaged individuals to receive care (for example, more accessible office hours and the availability of transportation).

Differences in the way health care providers and their institutions respond to social groups may also lead to variations of care. For example, there is compelling evidence that white women and minorities receive less intensive and poorer-quality care than their white male counterparts (Giles et al., 1995; Institute of Medicine, 2002). Some of the strongest evidence exists for differences in the receipt of cardiovascular care based upon race or ethnicity (Institute of Medicine, 2002). Black patients are less likely to receive coronary artery bypass graft (CABG), catheterization, percutaneous transluminal coronary angiography, and thrombolytic therapy (Institute of Medicine, 2002). These differences remain even after controlling for factors such as the severity of disease, access to care, where care is received, and the presence of clinical comorbidities (Institute of Medicine, 2002). Other studies have also documented that African Americans largely receive less-intensive treatment and therapies for cancer, end-stage renal disease, asthma, diabetes and HIV/AIDS compared to whites (Institute of Medicine, 2002).

STRESS

Exposure to chronic stress is a risk factor for a number of health problems, and coping responses can ameliorate at least some of the negative effects associated with stress (Politzer et al., 2001; Myers 2009). Increasingly, research is suggesting that the differential exposure to psychosocial stress is a key component of the expression of health disparities by race, ethnicity, and socioeconomic status (Myers, 2009). Politzer and colleagues have noted that compared to their economically and socially advantaged counterparts, disadvantaged minorities, individuals of low socioeconomic status, and those living in rural areas have higher levels of stress and fewer resources to cope with stress.

For example, several studies have indicated that

> Those from the lower social classes, especially ethnic minorities, often report a greater number of negative life events, greater and more frequent exposure to generic life stressors (i.e., stressors that are a usual part of modern life—financial, occupational, relationships, parental, etc.), perceive these events as more stressful, and report greater psychological distress from these stressful life experiences than their Caucasian American counterparts [Myers, 2009, p. 14].

The types of stressors, the availability of resources to cope with stress, and the patterned nature of responses to environmental challenges are shaped by the larger social and economic environments in which people live. For example, if someone lives in an environment where there is a liquor store on every corner and that individual is under increasing amounts of stress, the method used to cope with stress may include increased consumption of alcohol. In contrast, another individual who lives in an environment with walking and biking paths might deal with the same level of stress by becoming increasingly physically active. Disadvantaged community members are challenged in being able to access and sustain tangible resources that ease stress, such as income, childcare, and transportation; intrapersonal perspectives (for example, optimistic future orientation and personal agency); sociocultural supports (for example, family networks, *familismo*, biculturalism,

The Centers for Disease Control and Prevention's Racial and Ethnic Approaches to Community Health (REACH) program has demonstrated that coupling national vision with local interventions can be an extremely effective strategy in reducing long-standing disparities in health. As partners in this national program, REACH communities across the country have achieved dramatic improvements in health. For example, partners have achieved increased rates of cholesterol and cancer screening, more blood sugar testing and fewer diabetes-related complications, improved immunization coverage, and positive changes in lifestyle behaviors, such as cigarette smoking and exercise (Bachar et al., 2006; Giles & Liburd, 2006; Nguyen et al., 2006; CDC, 2007a; CDC, 2007b). (For detailed information about the REACH 2010 program and communities, see http://www.cdc.gov/reach)

In South Carolina, the REACH 2010 Charleston and Georgetown Diabetes Coalition, coordinated by the Medical University of South Carolina, has improved outcomes for thirteen thousand urban and rural African American residents with Type 2 diabetes (CDC, 2007a; CDC, 2007b). The Coalition works simultaneously to build people's skill at managing their own diabetes, improve diabetes care provided by local clinicians, and foster grassroots support for diabetes prevention and treatment. Some of the Coalition's strategies include: organizing walk-talk groups, grocery store tours, and health fairs; creating educational environments where health professionals and people with diabetes learn together; and providing diabetes medicine and supplies.

The impact of four hundred years of slavery and social inequality has not been erased from African American communities in the South. In recognition of this history, the programs sponsored by REACH 2010 in South Carolina not only build discrete diabetes self-management skills, but also empower residents by engaging them in a learning process that is transferable to other areas of their lives. In other words, the health education programs have become a source of continued learning for adults who have not historically had access to the same level of health information as their white counterparts. Furthermore, having opportunities to interact with health care providers outside of the hierarchical structure of the clinical setting has demystified the position of power held by physicians, while also teaching adults with Type 2 diabetes that they are entitled to a particular quality of health care that has historically been withheld from them (Airhihenbuwa & Liburd, 2006). For example, African Americans served by REACH 2010 are learning that the devastating outcomes of Type 2 diabetes, such as end-stage renal disease and lower-extremity amputations, are not inevitable and that proven strategies exist to prevent these outcomes. Those served by REACH 2010 are also learning that such strategies are available and accessible to them.

In 2004, just five years after the program began, REACH 2010 had already demonstrated significant improvements in diabetes-related outcomes for African Americans in Charleston and Georgetown, South Carolina. A much higher percentage of REACH community residents now received recommended preventive care—including annual blood sugar testing (97 percent, up from 77 percent), cholesterol testing (81 percent, up from 47 percent), kidney testing (53 percent, up from 13 percent), and foot exams (97 percent, up from 64 percent). In fact, the initial 21 percent disparity in hemoglobin A1C testing between African Americans and whites had, within only two years, been virtually eliminated. Furthermore, local clinicians documented a twofold increase in the percentage of patients following the American Diabetes Association's self-management guidelines (up from 41 percent to 94 percent). Finally, emergency room visits by uninsured people with diabetes dropped by 50 percent, and lower extremity amputations among African American men decreased dramatically—from 80 per 1,000 hospitalizations in 1999 to 33 per 1,000 hospitalizations in 2004 (CDC, 2007a).

In New York City, REACH 2010 efforts include the Northern Manhattan Start Right Coalition, which serves African American and Latino residents of Harlem and Washington Heights (CDC, 2007a; CDC, 2007b). By partnering with established community programs, such as early childhood education centers and supplemental food assistance agencies, the Coalition sought to eliminate immunization disparities between children of color and their white peers. As of 2006, the Coalition had achieved this goal: African American and Latino children living in REACH communities were being immunized at rates equaling or exceeding city and national averages.

Several REACH 2010 projects focus their interventions beyond the clinical care setting (CDC, 2007a; CDC, 2007b). In Charlotte, North Carolina, interventions focus on making the local environment a healthier place to live, while also facilitating community education opportunities. Among other accomplishments, Charlotte's program spurred the opening of a farmer's market; this increased the availability of affordable fresh fruits and vegetables in an African American community, while simultaneously creating new markets for local farmers to sell their produce (Liburd, Jack, Williams, & Tucker, 2005). Evidence from other urban communities shows that consumption of healthier foods increases when such foods are made available (Zenk et al., 2005). In Charlotte, 73 percent of REACH community residents now report eating more fruits and vegetables, whereas 67 percent have reduced their fat intake.

A final example of REACH 2010 addressing the social determinants of cardiovascular disease and diabetes comes from South Los Angeles, California (CDC, 2007a; CDC, 2007b). There, the African Americans Building a Legacy of Health Coalition has improved the food and physical activity environment by increasing local engagement, advocating for new policies and programs, and prioritizing community development initiatives. Among other outcomes, the Coalition has been instrumental in getting the City Council to support incentives for store owners who stock healthy foods, in increasing the availability of physical activity opportunities, and in developing workplace wellness initiatives. In 2008, the City Council passed a groundbreaking one-year moratorium on new fast-food restaurants, with the Coalition playing a key leadership role.

CONCEPTUAL FRAMEWORK

Figure 2.4 provides a conceptual framework for a comprehensive public health strategy to eliminate disparities in health. The current reality with regard to disparities is noted in the middle panel. Unfavorable social, political, and environmental conditions exist in many communities, and these may be due to historical injustices, discrimination, racism, and sexism. They result in unhealthy environments for many Americans, experienced through poor housing conditions, lack of transportation, few opportunities for employment, and lack of access to healthy foods and physical activity. These unfavorable environments then lead to adverse behaviors that promote disparities, including unhealthy eating, lack of physical activity, and an increasing likelihood of sexually transmitted diseases. These adverse behaviors then lead to the development of major risk factors, including high blood pressure, high cholesterol, diabetes, and obesity and overweight. The risk factors favor the development of diseases, including HIV/AIDS, tuberculosis, cancer, heart disease, and stroke. These higher rates of disease lead to increased disability and recurrence of disease, which may be reflected in reduced health status and health-related quality of life. The final result is higher mortality and a shorter life span among the affected groups.

The middle pattern depicts the current reality and the top panel depicts a vision of the future where social, political, and environmental conditions are favorable to the promotion of health and the elimination of disparities. Including increased opportunities for employment, education, and wealth, this vision of the future favors the development of behavior patterns that promote health and eliminate disparities, such as lower rates of tobacco use, increased physical activity, and healthy eating. These behaviors lead to low population risks for disease, lower disease outcomes, low risk of recurrent disease, and full functional capacity, all of which contribute to an improved overall quality of life.

To move from the present reality to the vision of the future requires policy and environmental changes that promote social, political, and environmental conditions favorable to disparity elimination. This might entail policies that promote equal access to employment and education and policies and environments that ensure community members have access to safe places to engage in physical activity and access to healthy nutrition. In addition, these policies and practices may increase community awareness related to health and should lead to increased risk factor detection and control, better emergency and acute care as people develop conditions, improved rehabilitation and long-term care, and improved end-of-life care.

The bottom panel illustrates the size of the population targeted by each type of intervention. Policy and environmental strategies will target the entire population, whereas those related to the health care system will each address smaller and smaller subsets of the population. Thus the greater impact occurs with strategies that focus on the primary prevention of diseases at the policy and environmental-change levels. However, when addressing health disparities, it is imperative to engage in the full continuum of intervention activities, which include the prevention of risk factors, treatment of risk factors, detection of disease,

Figure 2.4   Framework for a comprehensive public health strategy to eliminate health disparities

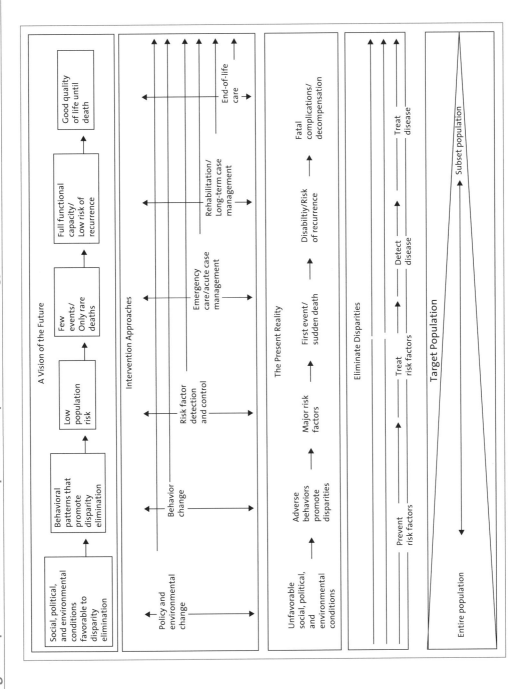

and treatment of disease. It is through policy and environmental-policies changes, behavior changes, risk factor detection and treatment, emergency care, and rehabilitation that this full continuum is addressed.

CONCLUSION

Taking the necessary steps toward eliminating health disparities across vulnerable populations challenges traditional public health sensibilities. Relying solely on public health programs that encourage individuals to adopt healthy behaviors is inadequate; emphasis on setting up social conditions that promote health must occur at the same time. Reducing disparities in health requires national leadership that provides direction and financial resources, government action at the regional and local levels, and active support and commitment from community organizations and individuals. This combination of national vision and resources with local action allows for flexibility in planning and implementation at the local level. To substantially reduce disparities, interventions aimed at improving health must be coupled with interventions seeking to reduce social disadvantages.

A deeper understanding of the context in which health disparities occur is needed as a first step in developing interventions that effectively eliminate avoidable, unjust, and unfair conditions. The public health community must move toward more innovative, broadly focused strategies for prevention. In training the next generation of public health workers, we must include intervention research on the social determinants of health and breakdown along the silos that inhibit transdisciplinary research and practice. Public health workers must also support and work with community institutions dedicated to achieving social equality for disenfranchised communities and challenge unjust policies that perpetuate health inequalities. Historically black colleges and universities, Hispanic colleges and universities, tribal colleges, the business sector, and national and regional minority organizations with state and local chapters are all possible collaborators.

Taken together, a sustained focus on achieving favorable social, political, and environmental conditions that promote good health, coupled with access to affordable and high-quality health care and with communities informed about how to prevent disease and injuries, will set this nation on the path to the elimination of health disparities.

DISCUSSION QUESTIONS

1. The chapter stated that health inequities are avoidable. Do you agree or disagree? Why?
2. Do you believe the social constructs surrounding health inequities are also avoidable? Provide a specific example.

3. Community-based intervention programs do improve social environments and health. How can they be maintained and sustained beyond their initial effectiveness?

REFERENCES

Airhihenbuwa, C. O., & Liburd, L. C. (2006, August). Eliminating health disparities in the African American population: The interface of culture, gender, and power. *Health Education and Behavior, 33*, 488–501.

Bachar et al. (2006, July 5). Cherokee choices: A diabetes prevention program for American Indians. *Preventing Chronic Disease, 3*. Retrieved October 8, 2006, from http://www.cdc.gov/pcd/issues/2006/jul/05–0221.htm

Berkman, L. F., & Lochner, K. A. (2002). Social determinants of health: Meeting at the crossroads. *Health Affairs*, 21(2), 291–293.

Blum, H. L. (1981). Social perspective on risk reduction. *Family and Community Health, 3*, 41–50.

Braveman, P. A. (2006). Health disparities and health equality: Concepts and measurement. *Annual Review of Public Health, 27*, 167–194.

Braveman, P. A., & Gruskin, S. (2003). Defining equity in health. *Journal of Epidemiology and Community Health, 57*, 254–258.

Braveman, P. A., Krieger, N., & Lynch, J. (2000). Health inequities and social inequalities in health. *Bulletin of the World Health Organization, 78*, 232–233.

Braveman, P. A., & Tarimo, E. (2002). Social inequalities in health within countries: Not only an issue for affluent nations. *Social Science and Medicine, 54*, 1621–1635.

Centers for Disease Control and Prevention (CDC). (2007a). *The power to reduce health disparities: Voices from REACH communities*. Atlanta: U.S. Department of Health and Human Services, Centers for Disease Control and Prevention.

Centers for Disease Control and Prevention (CDC). (2007b). *REACHing across the divide: Finding solutions to health disparities*. Atlanta: U.S. Department of Health and Human Services, Centers for Disease Control and Prevention.

Cho, Y., & Hummer, R. A. (2000). Disability status differential across fifteen Asian and Pacific Islander groups and the effects of nativity and duration of residence in the U.S. *Social Biology, 48*, 171–195.

Commission on Social Determinants of Health. (2008). Closing the gap in a generation: Health equity through action on the social determinants of health. *Final report of the commission on social determinants of health*. Geneva: World Health Organization.

Cutler, D. M., Glaser, E. L., & Vigdor, J. L. (1997). Are ghettos good or bad? *Quarterly Journal of Economics, 112*, 827–872.

Dressler, W. W. (1993). Health in the African American community: Accounting for health inequalities. *Medical Anthropology Quarterly, 7*, 325–345.

Feinstein, J. S. (1993). The relationship between socioeconomic status and health: A review of the literature. *Milbank Quarterly, 71*, 279–322.

Freudenberg, N. & Ruglis, J. (2007). Reframing school dropout as a public health issue. *Preventing Chronic Disease, 4*(4). http://www.cdc.gov/pcd/issues/2007/oct/07_0063.htm

Gee, G. C. (2002). A multilevel analysis of the relationship between institutional and individual racial discrimination and health status. *American Journal of Public Health, 92*, 615–623.

Geronimus, A. T. (2000). To mitigate, resist, or undo: Addressing structural influences on the health of urban populations. *American Journal of Public Health, 90*, 867–872.

Geronimus, A. T., Hicken, M., Keene, D., & Bound, J. (2006). "Weathering" and age patterns of allostatic load scores among blacks and whites in the United States. *American Journal of Public Health, 96*(2), 1–7.

Giles, W. H., Anda, R. F., Casper, M. L., Escobedo, L. G., & Taylor, H. A. (1995). Race and sex differences in the rate of invasive cardiac procedures in U.S. hospitals: Data from the National Hospital Discharge Survey. *Archives of Internal Medicine, 155*, 318–324.

Giles, W. H., Kittner, S. J., Hebel, J. R., Losoconzy, K. G., & Sherwin, R. W. (1995). Determinants of black-white differences in the risk of cerebral infarction: The National Health and Nutrition Examination Survey Epidemiologic Follow-Up Study. *Archives of Internal Medicine, 155*, 1319–1324.

Giles, W. H., & Liburd, L. C. (2006). Reflections on the past, reaching for the future: REACH 2010—the first seven years. *Health Promotion Practice, 7*, S179–S180.

Institute of Medicine. (2001). *Promoting health: Intervention strategies from social and behavioral research.* B. D. Smedley & S. L. Syme (Eds.). Washington, DC: National Academies Press.

Institute of Medicine. (2002). *Unequal treatment: Confronting racial and ethnic disparities in health care.* B. D. Smedley, A. Y. Stith, & A. R. Nelson (Eds.). Washington, DC: National Academies Press.

Krieger, N., Williams, D. R., & Moss, N. E. (1997). Measuring social class in U.S. public health research: Concepts, methodologies, and guidelines. *Annual Review of Public Health, 18*, 341–378.

Leventhal, T., & Brooks-Gunn, J. (2003). Moving to opportunity: An experimental study of neighborhood effects on mental health. *American Journal of Public Health, 93*, 1576–1582.

Liburd, L. C. (2010). Diabetes and health disparities: community-based approaches for racial and ethnic populations. In L. Liburd, *Diabetes and health disparities: community-based approaches for racial and ethnic populations.* New York: Springer.

Liburd, L. C., Jack, L., Williams, S., & Tucker, P. (2005). Intervening on the social determinants of health. *American Journal of Preventive Medicine, 29*(5 Suppl. 1), 18–24.

Lin, C. Y., Rogot, E., Johnson, N. J., Sorlie, P., & Arias, E. (2003). A further study of life expectancy by socioeconomic factors in the National Longitudinal Mortality Study. *Ethnicity and Disease, 13*, 240–247.

Mays, V. M., Cochrane, S. D., & Barnes, N. W. (2007). Race, race-based discrimination, and health outcomes among African Americans. *Annual Reviews of Psychology, 58*, 201–225.

McGinnis, J. M., & Foege, W. H. (1993). Actual causes of death in the United States. *Journal of the American Medical Association, 270*, 2207–2212.

Myers, H. (2009). Ethnicity and socio-economic status-related stresses in context: An integrative review and conceptual model. *Journal of Behavioral Medicine, 32*, 9–19.

National Center for Health Statistics. (2009). *Health, United States, 2008, with chartbook.* Hyattsville, MD.

Nguyen et al. (2006). Papanicolaou testing among Vietnamese Americans: Results of a multifaceted intervention. *American Journal of Preventive Medicine, 31,* 1–9.

Oliver, M. L. (2006). *Black wealth, white wealth: A new perspective on racial inequality.* New York: Routledge.

O'Rourke, T., & Iammarino, N. (2006). The American mirage of equity: Is social justice myth or reality? *American Journal of Health Education, 37,* 58–62.

Politzer et al. (2001). Inequity in America: The contribution of health centers in reducing and eliminating disparities in access to care. *Medical Care Research and Review, 58,* 234–278.

Rose, G. (1985). Sick individuals and sick populations. *International Journal of Epidemiology, 14,* 32–38.

Wallace, R., & Wallace, D. (1997). Socioeconomic determinants of health: Community marginalization and the diffusion of disease and disorder in the United States. *British Medical Journal, 314,* 1341–1345.

Williams, D. R. (2003). The health of men: Structured inequities and opportunities. *American Journal of Public Health, 93,* 724–731.

World Health Organization. (1996). *Equity in health and health care: a WHO/SIDA initiative.* Geneva, World Health Organization, (unpublished document WHO/ARA/96.1; available on request from Division of Analysis, Research and Assessment, World Health Organization, 1211 Geneva 27, Switzerland).

ZaZa, S., Briss, P. A., & Harris, K. W. (2005). *The guide to community preventive services.* New York: Oxford University Press.

Zenk et al. (2005). Neighborhood racial composition, neighborhood poverty, and the spatial accessibility of supermarkets in metropolitan Detroit. *American Journal of Public Health, 95,* 660–667.

3

Individual, Family, and Community Resilience

Bonnie Benard

LEARNING OBJECTIVES

- Compare and contrast the strengths and limitations of risk-focused research with resilience-focused research.
- Identify protective factors and characteristics of resilient individuals, families, and communities.
- Understand a framework that connects resilience, community development, and youth development.
- Articulate the importance of a resilience perspective both in practice and in personal life.

A major breakthrough in prevention research and practice occurred in the late 1980s and early 1990s with a discovery that offers the *hope of prevention* to all who care about improving the lives of individuals, families, and communities. This hope lies in the growing field of resilience research and practice. This field has evolved from the study of how individuals, families, and communities facing multiple risks, challenges, and adversities have not only successfully adapted but have even grown stronger through overcoming these obstacles. A classic definition of *resilience* is "a class of phenomena characterized by patterns of positive adaptation in the context of significant adversity or risk" (Masten & Reed, 2002, p. 75; see also Luthar, 2003). Resilience research and practice provides the prevention field with nothing less than a fundamentally different knowledge base, one offering the promise of transforming interventions. The identification of the attributes of individuals who have succeeded despite early stress and trauma; the characteristics of families, schools, and communities that facilitated this success; and the factors that lead communities as a whole to overcome challenging circumstances create a new paradigm for both research and practice, a paradigm that is based on entirely different assumptions and that asks entirely different questions. Resilience research provides a powerful rationale for moving our focus in the social and behavioral sciences from risk to resilience and from a concern with individual deficit and pathology to an examination of the strengths individuals, families, and communities have brought to bear in promoting healing and health.

RISK-BASED APPROACHES

Initially, discussion and research examining the predictive impact of risks on individual lives was an important and exciting development. Risk-based approaches offer a way to identify social factors that are correlated with negative outcomes (for example, drug abuse, mental illness, and criminal behavior) and get away from blaming individuals for their poor life outcomes. The implications were great for public policies addressing the most pervasive risks, such as poverty and educational opportunity. The promise existed that through exploratory research, all of the risks for a given pathology could be identified and remedied, and the pathology itself could be eliminated.

To a field desperate to have a research base, risk-focused prevention has been hailed as a breakthrough. According to the Institute of Medicine, "The concept of risk reduction is at the heart of prevention research" (Mrazek & Haggerty, 1994, p. 6). In fact, the Institute's report, *Reducing Risks for Mental Disorders: Frontiers for Preventive Intervention Research*, is named "because of the power of the risk reduction model" (p. 6). However, to prevention practitioners and researchers concerned with digging deeper into causality and not just correlation, this risk-focused research base is sometimes problematic and harmful at worst.

Historically, the social and behavioral sciences have followed a problem-focused approach to studying human and social phenomena. This *pathology* model of research traditionally examines problems, disease, illness, maladaptation, incompetence, deviance, and so on. The emphasis has been placed on identifying the *risk factors* for individual problems, such as alcoholism and mental illness, family problems (for example, intimate partner violence and child abuse), and community problems (for example, poverty and violence). Most of the research has been retrospective in design involving a one-time historical assessment of individuals, families, and communities with these existing identified problems. This research design has perpetuated a problem perspective and has implicated an inevitability of negative outcomes. For example, researchers have found that among adults who have abused their children, a higher percentage experienced abuse in their childhoods than is found in the general population. Similarly, a higher percentage of adults who abuse alcohol have grown up in an alcoholic family themselves. In general, risk-focused research has usually found that the risk factors are cumulative: as the number of risk factors increases, so does the likelihood of negative outcomes. Similarly, the predictive power of risks is also influenced by the intensity and duration of the stressors and risk conditions (Rutter, 1989).

For prevention practitioners, this research base raises several concerns. First, the study and identification of risk factors for a condition, such as violence or mental illness, does not answer the key questions practitioners care about: "How does knowing that my student or client grew up with a mentally ill (or drug-using or criminal) mother or father help me help this person?" "What can I do Monday morning to improve the chances for this person?" In other words, risk-focused studies do not generally give us research-based answers or prevention strategies. According to Norman Garmezy, the "grandfather" of resilience research, this pathology model of research has "provided us with a false sense of security in erecting prevention models that are founded more on values than facts" (quoted in Werner & Smith, 1982, p. xix).

A second concern is that, although risk is a statistical concept applicable to the study of groups, it does not account for individual variation within the risk group. Risk research has been transferred to clinical and educational settings wherein individuals—even whole groups of people, such as adolescents, their families, and their communities—are identified and subsequently labeled according to their perceived deficit, be it hyperactive, emotionally unstable, dysfunctional, disadvantaged, at-risk, high-risk, or a plethora of others. Regardless of the original benevolent intention (for example, getting help to individuals, families, or communities who are hurting), the application of research focused on risk factors usually leads to the labeling and stigmatizing of youth, their families, and their communities as "at-risk" and "high-risk," as well as to the implementation of drastic public policy practices like zero tolerance in schools and incarceration in our communities.

Perhaps most deleterious of all, as you'll see later in the light of resilience practice, this deficit approach has encouraged prevention practitioners and other helping professionals to view, identify, and name children, families, and communities exclusively through a deficit lens. This *glass-is-half-empty* perspective blocks helpers' ability to see and engage the capacities and strengths of individuals, families, and communities; to see the whole person or environment; and to hear the whole story. Such a perspective creates stereotypes or myths about who people, families, and communities really are and promulgates the self-fulfilling prophecy of finding exactly what you're looking for. Ultimately, according to longtime prevention researcher Richard Jessor, our "univocal preoccupation with risk tends to homogenize and caricature those who are poor" (1993, p. 121).

In terms of risk-focused research, two problems predominate. First, the examination of the correlates of problems such as violence tend to focus on individual and family risk factors, which are easier to measure, and to ignore the larger societal or environmental risk factors such as poverty and racism. Policymakers, politicians, the media, and often researchers have personalized *at-riskness*, locating it in youth and their families, thereby avoiding difficult discussions about the impact of environmental conditions on community members. In fact, more than forty years of social science research has clearly identified poverty—the direct result of public abdication of responsibility for human welfare—as the factor most likely to put a person *at risk* for social ills, such as drug abuse, teen pregnancy, child abuse, violence, and school failure, not to mention being imprisoned, having no health care, attending poor schools, being unemployed, lacking recreational facilities, and having no housing (Currie, 1994; Males, 1996; Swadener & Lubeck, 1995).

A second concern is that even researchers doing retrospective or correlational studies of risk factors for the development of problem behaviors were stymied by the issue of whether risk factors in people already diagnosed as schizophrenic, criminal, violent, or alcoholic were the causes or the consequences of their condition. In other words, which came first, and which is the true risk? Is mental illness a risk factor for poverty, or vice versa? It is this research question that ultimately paved the way for what is now called resilience research.

THE GIFT OF RESILIENCE RESEARCH

With the exception of a few earlier studies, beginning in the 1950s and on into the 1960s and 1970s, a handful of researchers decided to circumvent the causality-correlation dilemma by studying individuals postulated to be at high risk for developing certain disorders. Researchers studied children growing up under conditions of great adversity that included neonatal stress, poverty, neglect, abuse, physical handicaps, war, and parental schizophrenia, depression, alcoholism, and criminality. This second wave of risk research used a prospective research design that is developmental and longitudinal; the research assesses children at various times during the course of their lives to better understand the nature of the risk factors that result in development of a disorder. Although much of the research on risk and resilience focuses on children (based on their ability to change, the perceived moral injustice of youth suffering, and the relative ease of studying youth over time and in settings such as schools), the frameworks and lessons learned can, in general, be applied to all individuals.

As the children studied in various longitudinal projects grew into adolescence and adulthood, a consistent and amazing finding emerged. Although a certain percentage of these high-risk children developed various problems (a higher percentage than in the normal population), a greater percentage of the children became "competent, confident, and caring" youths and adults (Werner & Smith, 1982, 1992, 2001). For example, one early study found that only 9 percent of children of schizophrenic parents became schizophrenic, while 75 percent developed into healthy adults (Watt, Anthony, Wynne, & Rolf, 1984). Similarly, whereas one out of four children of alcoholic parents develops alcohol problems (compared to one out of ten in the general population) three out of four do not. In fact, in most studies, the figure seems to hover at around 70 to 75 percent resilience when exposed to a significant risk factor. This includes children who were placed in foster care (Fanshel, 1975; Festinger, 1984), were members of gangs (Vigil, 1990), were born to teen mothers (Furstenberg, Cook, Eccles, Elder, & Sameroff, 1999), were sexually abused (Higgins, 1994; Wilkes, 2002; Zigler & Hall, 1989), had substance-abusing or mentally ill families (Beardslee & Podoresfky, 1988; Chess, 1989; Watt et al., 1984; Werner, 1986; Werner & Smith, 2001), and grew up in poverty (Clausen, 1993; Schweinhart, Barnes, & Wiekart, 1993; Vaillant, 2002). In absolute worst-case scenarios, when children experience multiple and persistent risks, still half of them overcome adversity and achieve good developmental outcomes (Rutter, 1989, 2000).

Researchers Emmy Werner and Ruth Smith, in their seminal community-wide epidemiological study of risk and individual resilience (1982, 1992, 2001), followed nearly seven hundred children growing up with risk factors (one-third of whom had multiple risk factors) from birth to adulthood. As the cohort of children aged, they grew increasingly more like their peers without risk factors. Werner and Smith report, "One of the most striking findings of our two follow-ups in adulthood, at ages thirty-two and forty, was that most of the high-risk youths who did develop serious coping problems in adolescence had staged a recovery by the time they reached midlife. . . . They were in stable marriages and jobs, were satisfied with their relationships with their spouses and teenage children, and were responsible citizens in their community" (2001, p. 167). In fact, only one out of six of the adult subjects at either age thirty-two or forty was doing poorly, "struggling with chronic financial problems, domestic conflict, violence, substance abuse, serious mental health problems, and/or low self-esteem" (p. 37).

Positive development and successful outcomes in any human system depend on the quality of the relationships, expectations, and opportunities for participation, as shown in Table 3.1. Keep in mind that these three protective *factors* are not separate entities; rather, they are three aspects or components of a dynamic protective *process* in which they work synergistically. For example, caring relationships without high expectations or opportunities for meaningful participation foster dependence and codependence, not positive human

Table 3.1   Protective factors and processes in families, schools, and communities

Caring Relationships	High Expectations	Opportunities for Participation or Contribution
Being there	Belief in people's resilience	People focus
Paying attention	People focus	Engaging, challenging, interesting experiences
Showing interest	Challenge using support messages	Active learning
Showing respect	Guidance without coercion	Cooperative and inclusive small group activities
Offering loving support	Freedom with structure and safety	Reflection and dialogue
Showing compassion	Rituals and rites of passage	Creative expression
Listening without judgment	Focus on strengths	Decision making and planning
Showing patience	Reframing	Responsibilities
Getting to know interests, strengths, and dreams	Demonstrating innate resilience	Leadership
Maintaining trust		Service (giving back)

system development. High expectations without caring relationships and support to help people meet them are a cruel "shape-up-or-ship-out" approach associated with negative outcomes. And caring relationships with high-expectation messages but no opportunities for active participation and contribution create a frustrating situation that blocks the natural process of human development in any system.

"Much of the task of prevention in this new century," predicts Martin Seligman (2002, p. 5), "will be to create a science of human strengths whose mission will be to understand and learn how to foster these virtues in young people"—and in their families, schools, and communities as well.

Resilience strengths are the characteristics, also called *internal assets* or *competencies*, associated with healthy individual, family, and community development. They are not the causes of resilience but rather are the positive developmental *outcomes* demonstrating that human systems are engaging their innate resilience. These strengths are what resilience looks like. Table 3.2 lists the four categories of often overlapping strengths that are consistently found in resilience and other related literature (Benard, 1991, 2004).

These findings challenge a core belief of many risk-focused social scientists that risk factors for the most part predict negative outcomes. Instead, individual resilience research suggests that risk factors are predictive of outcomes for only about 20 to 49 percent of a given high-risk population. In contrast, *protective factors* (supports and opportunities that buffer the effect of adversity and enable development to proceed) appear to predict positive

Table 3.2 How to recognize resilience in individuals, families, and communities

Social Competence	Problem Solving	Autonomy	Sense of Purpose
Responsiveness Communication	Planning Flexibility	Positive identity Internal locus of control	Goal direction Achievement motivation
Empathy	Resourcefulness	Initiative	Educational aspirations
Caring Compassion Forgiveness	Critical thinking Insight	Self-efficacy Mastery Adaptive distancing	Special interests Creativity Imagination
		Resistance	Optimism
		Self-awareness	Hope
		Mindfulness	Faith
		Humor	Spirituality Sense of meaning

outcomes in anywhere from 50 to 80 percent of a high-risk population. Werner and Smith have described the importance of protective factors:

> Our findings and those by other American and European investigators with a life-span perspective suggest that these buffers [that is, protective factors] make a more profound impact on the life course of children who grow up under adverse conditions than do specific risk factors or stressful life events. They [also] appear to transcend ethnic, social class, geographical, and historical boundaries. Most of all, they offer us a more optimistic outlook than the perspective that can be gleaned from the literature on the negative consequences of perinatal trauma, care-giving deficits, and chronic poverty [1992, p. 202].

In other words, the protective factors that foster resilience do indeed offer the *hope of prevention.*

The gift of resilience research to the prevention- and intervention-community is that in contrast to risk-focused prevention, it actually does provide a knowledge base for practice; it does answer the question, "What works to promote health and healing, even in the face of challenge and risk?" The protective factors or processes within individuals, families, and communities that support the resilience of individuals can be incorporated into the repertoires of prevention practitioners and also of parents, teachers, neighbors, child protective workers, youth workers, counselors, therapists, and anyone else at their work, home, or in their community. These protective factors encompass the critical developmental supports and opportunities of caring relationships, high-expectation messages, and opportunities for meaningful participation and contribution that are found in healthy families, effective schools, and competent and caring communities (Benard, 1991, 2004; see Table 3.1).

Similarly, the resilience strengths that are demonstrated by individuals in the face of challenges have also been clearly identified (Benard, 1991, 2004; see Table 3.2). Identification of these strengths provides us with a language for research and practice that motivates positive change by drawing the focus away from deficits, dysfunction, and problems and toward strengths, assets, and competencies present in all individuals, even those facing multiple challenges. For example, having a language of strengths helps practitioners and caregivers working with youth begin to look for and find strengths in the young people they serve—and then to name and reflect the strengths they have witnessed. This positive language helps practitioners and caregivers reframe how they see their clients and begin to shift from seeing only risk to seeing resilience, especially among those facing a range of challenges and adversity. For the research community, having a nomenclature helps legitimate the study of strengths, to empirically measure developmental outcomes from prevention and education interventions, and to better understand what works and what does not. The positive psychology movement, with leadership from Christopher Peterson and Martin Seligman, has compiled *Character Strengths and Virtues: A Handbook and Classification* (2004), which is intended to be psychology's positive response to psychiatry's *Diagnostic and Statistical Manual* of human *dysfunctions*.

Resilience strengths are not fixed personality traits that inevitably result in resilience. Research instead suggests that human beings are biologically driven to develop these strengths and to use them for survival. In fact, an elegantly simple definition of resilience is that of Robert J. Lifton (1993), who refers to resilience as the capacity of human systems to transform and change. What appears to be driving this process of adaptation is an internal force, an amazing developmental wisdom often referred to as intrinsic motivation. Human beings are intrinsically motivated to meet basic developmental needs, including needs for belonging and affiliation, competence, autonomy, safety, and meaning (Baumeister & Leary, 1995; Deci, 1995; Maslow, 1954). How these needs are expressed and met varies, of course, not only within a person and over time but from person to person and from culture to culture. The bottom line for resilience theory and practice is that these psychological needs are givens. These needs are increasingly referred to by developmentalists as "fundamental protective human adaptational systems" (Masten & Reed, 2002, p. 82). All human beings are compelled to meet these needs throughout their lives. For young people, whether these needs are allowed expression in positive, prosocial ways depends to a great extent on the people, places, and experiences they encounter in their families, schools, and communities.

A key point for prevention practitioners and researchers is that because these strengths are intrinsic, dynamic, contextual, and culturally expressed, they are not learned, for the most part or in a lasting way, through a social skills program or a life skills curriculum that attempts to teach strengths directly. A long history of prevention program evaluation (Kohn, 1997; Kreft & Brown, 1998) testifies to the short-lived effects of eight-week life skills programs. That this approach still predominates in both education and prevention speaks to the strong hold behaviorism has on our culture and institutions—in terms of focusing on individual behavior change and *kid fixing*.

Although researchers and writers often use differing names for these strengths, the categories have continued to hold up under the scrutiny of a decade and a half of research. In fact, as Masten states, "Recent studies continue to corroborate the importance of a relatively small set of global factors associated with resilience" that are both personal and environmental (2001, p. 234). These competencies and strengths appear to transcend ethnicity, culture, gender, geography, and time and apply at a deeply human level as essential skills needed to thrive. According to an Institute of Medicine report on youth development, "The little available evidence suggests that most of these characteristics are important in all cultural groups" (Eccles & Gootman, 2002, p. 81).

REASONS TO ADOPT A COMMUNITY RESILIENCE APPROACH

- For individuals to be healthy, they need healthy communities.
  Communities have strengths and assets that can provide an environment that promotes health and well-being.
- Health disparities by definition affect groups or whole populations of people, not individuals.
  A community resilience approach allows for community-level action that will benefit the population within the community.
- The absence of risk does not equal health; a community resilience approach goes beyond risk.
  Addressing risk factors results in the absence of factors that threaten health and safety; however, it does not necessarily achieve conditions that support health.
- A community approach minimizes *blaming the victim*.
  Behavior is typically constructed in individualist terms, leaving many to conclude that poor health is the result of poorly informed choices. However, researchers are increasingly recognizing the relationship between behavior and environment in determining health outcomes and acknowledging the limits of efforts that focus solely on individuals' behavior changes.

- A community approach means ensuring that fewer people get sick, not just that more people get well.

  Addressing the ways in which root factors play out at the community level creates opportunities to ensure that people do not get sick in the first place, thereby reducing disparities.
- A resilience approach is based on the unique culture of the community.
- Different ethnic and racial groups have unique values, perspectives, assets, and living styles. A resilience approach builds on what is already working within cultures and is tailored to the community's strengths.
- A community resilience approach is responsive to the range of people's developmental needs.
- Every community must address a range of developmental needs, from the very young to the elderly. A community resilience approach enables communities to develop solutions that benefit all.
- A community resilience approach meets community needs for well-being by strengthening the overall environment within a community.
- Such an approach identifies the needs within a community that support overall well-being. This approach acknowledges the direct impact of the environment on health and its impact on behavior, which in turn affects health outcomes.
- A community resilience approach changes conditions shaped by oppression, poverty, and economic disparity.

  The root factors of health disparities, such as oppression, discrimination, and poverty, play out at the community level, which results in the populations of some communities being at higher risk for a range of poor health and safety outcomes. By strengthening key community factors, communities can build their own capacity to effect change where they see a need. Empowering communities to take action will minimize the impact of these root factors.
- Multiple health and safety concerns are addressed simultaneously and before the onset of symptoms.

  By going *upstream* from injury and illness, a community resilience approach enables communities to design effective strategies that prevent multiple health and safety problems. Such an approach creates community norms that are focused on being healthy, not on protecting people from illness. These norms can therefore address the causes of multiple health issues. A focus before the onset of symptoms translates into more cost-effective interventions.

Source: Prevention Institute.

Table 3.3 Paradigms for prevention

	Risk	Resilience
Focus and language	Deficits	Assets and strengths
Goal	Problem prevention	Healthy development
Attitude toward people	People as problems	People as resources
Attitude toward diversity	Eurocentric	Multicultural
Attitude toward learning	Mechanistic	Constructivist
Strategic emphasis	Program and content	People and places
Locus of control	External	Internal
Philosophy	Control	Connectedness
Needs being met	Bureaucracies' despair	Hope and motivation
Feelings		

Resilience research provides a powerful rationale for moving our focus in the prevention field from a risk approach to a resilience approach, as shown in Table 3.3. This requires a different paradigm that ultimately changes what we believe, what we do, and how we do it. The good news is that the *resilience paradigm* gives all who work with despairing individuals, families, and communities the ultimate gift of dwelling in possibility and of working for change with hope in their hearts.

RESILIENCE, YOUTH DEVELOPMENT, AND COMMUNITY DEVELOPMENT

Resilience research has played a pivotal role in providing a research base for many of the strengths-based movements currently gaining momentum, including youth development, asset building, positive psychology, strengths-based social work practice, personalized learning environments (in high school reform), and social capital (for example, the amount and strength of associations and networks within communities that produce social cohesion, trust, and a willingness to engage in community activities), to name a few. Resilience research also validates the long-standing approach in public health known as health promotion and the interdisciplinary field of community development.

What all these approaches share is their focus on: a language of assets and strengths; healthy development of human systems as the goal; the viewing of people as resources and not problems; an embracing of diversity as a strength; the understanding that people are constructors of their own knowledge and *stories*; strategies that move beyond programs and curricula to the deep restructuring of the relationships, beliefs, and participation within a system; the development of internal *locus of control* or empowerment; and a philosophy not of control but of connectedness. It is ultimately this underlying philosophy that drives this developmental paradigm and unites the approaches that go by the names of resilience, youth development, and community development. This underlying philosophy acknowledges the interconnectedness of human and other living systems and their innate resilience and capacity to transform and change—and the developmental wisdom that motivates human behavior. Without this philosophy, approaches like youth development and community development result in new wine being poured into old bottles. That is, they evolve into the same old deficit-based programs.

RECOGNIZING RESILIENCE IN COMMUNITIES

Longitudinal studies conducted during the past two decades indicate that, although the absence of a strong community is devastating for young people, the reverse is also true; positive community contexts can be transformational (Carnegie Task Force, 1992; McLaughlin, 2000; McLaughlin, Irby, & Langman, 1994; Werner & Smith, 1992). As with the other two major settings in which children are socialized—the family and school—the community that supports the positive development of young people promotes the building of strengths and competencies (such as social competence, problem solving, autonomy, and a sense of purpose and future) that are associated with healthy development and resilience. Social scientists refer to the ability of a community to build resilience in its members as *community competence* or *capacity*.

Perhaps the most obvious manifestation of the protective factors at the community level is the availability of resources necessary for healthy human development, such as health care, child care, housing, education, job training, employment, and recreation. Resilient communities exert a direct influence on the lives of young people and, perhaps even more important, exert a profound influence on the lives of the families, schools, and neighborhood-based organizations that serve youth within their domain. Resilient communities are therefore indirectly—but powerfully—influencing outcomes for children and youth. According to most researchers, the greatest protection we could give children is ensuring that they and their families have access to these necessary resources (Coleman, 1987; Garmezy, 1991; Long & Vaillant, 1989; Sameroff, Barocas, & Seifer, 1984; Wilson, 1987). Conversely, the greatest risk factor for the development of nearly all problem behaviors is poverty, a condition characterized by the lack of these basic resources.

The fact that the rate of child poverty has remained hovering at around 25 percent for the past two decades clearly testifies to the lack of national political will to provide the opportunities for all children to succeed. In light of this national neglect of children and families, the imperative falls to local communities to fill the gap. And the only way communities can succeed—and have succeeded—in this endeavor is through the building of formal and informal social networks that reweave the social fabric by linking families and schools and agencies and organizations through the common purpose of collaborating to address the needs of children and families throughout the community (Coleman, 1987; Putnam, 2000; Putnam & Feldstein, 2003; Schorr, 1988, 1997). In a resilient community, community members and organizations support and work in partnership with families, youth, and schools. Families support youth, volunteer in their community, and work in partnership with schools. Schools not only support and work in partnership with their students but also support and work in partnership with families and with community groups, especially with their community-based organization partners.

A major finding of almost every successful youth-serving entity is that its success was enhanced by creating partnerships. For example, mentoring by a community organization is more successful when the family is also a partner and when schools are cooperative. After school programs run by community organizations (but located in schools) benefit from the commitment of the school and from involved parents. In contrast, the absence of partnerships and collaboration has the opposite effect. Eccles and Gootman's *Community Programs to Promote Youth Development* analyzes why programs fail:

> Quantitative and qualitative implementation data also tell us a great deal about why programs fail. These studies make it clear how the programs are nested into larger social systems that need to be taken into account. When adequate supports are not available in these larger systems, it is unlikely that specific programs will be able to be implemented well and sustained over time [2002, p. 221].

Formal community-building or change efforts are now recognizing the truth of White and Wehlage's argument that supporting a community's informal social networks and relationships is key to successful prevention efforts (1995). The Rockefeller Foundation's report on successful community initiatives concluded that although "community building is more an art than a science, research shows that relationships are key to turning lives around. . . . Building on this insight to develop networks of social support in low-income neighborhoods cannot help but yield positive change" (Walsh, 1997, p. vi).

The Project on Human Development in Chicago Neighborhoods led by Robert Sampson and his colleagues found that the informal networks in poor neighborhoods served as protective factors against youth crime and violence (Sampson, Raudenbush, & Earls, 1997). Sampson's team use the term *collective efficacy* to describe communities whose residents consistently interact in positive and cooperative ways. As Sampson explains, "It's a sense of shared expectations among neighbors. It's the social networks people have, the values that they share and whether or not they trust each other" (quoted in Owens, 2002, p. 5). When these characteristics exist, regardless of a community's poverty level, neighbors look out for the young people in the community, hold them to *orderly* behavior, and take collective action (for example, to get rid of a local drug hangout). The Chicago Neighborhoods researchers reported that rates of violence differed dramatically in poor communities with similar demographics, depending on the level of collective efficacy. "At the neighborhood level, the willingness of local residents to intervene for the common good depends in large part on conditions of mutual trust and solidarity among neighbors" (Sampson et al., 1997, p. 919).

MAPPING COMMUNITY ASSETS

In other words, the heart of community can be found at the relational level. Any attempt to rebuild a sense of community connection for young and old must begin with caring relationships that communicate high expectations through positive beliefs in the capacities of young people and their families and that focus on strengths and assets. In every model of successful community change, the initiatives start with a mapping of the community's assets and strengths rather than with an inventory of risks and problems. The following examples illustrate this high-expectations approach.

Roger Mills's Community Health Realization initiatives (1993) start with helping community members directly recognize their innate wisdom and resilience and develop a sense of self-efficacy, which in turn results in their feeling powerful and hopeful enough to take collaborative action to improve their community themselves. The approach of asset-based community development is to begin with a *community assets map*. John McKnight explains the asset-based community development approach as follows (1992):

> The starting point for any serious development effort is the opposite of an accounting of deficiencies. Instead there must be an opportunity for individuals to use their own abilities to produce. Identifying the variety and richness of skills, talents, knowledge, and experience of people in low-income neighborhoods provides a base upon which to build new approaches and enterprises [p. 10].

Creating a community assets map thus begins the process of neighborhood regeneration, which "locates all of the available local assets, begins connecting them with one another in ways that multiply their power and effectiveness, and begins harnessing those local institutions [and individuals] that are not yet available for local development" (Kretzmann & McKnight, 1993, p. 6).

The natural outcome of having high expectations for people, especially for expecting youth to be resources and not problems, is to create opportunities for people of all ages to contribute to their communities. Just as healthy human development involves the process of bonding to the family and school through the provision of opportunities to be involved in meaningful and valued ways in family and school life, developing a sense of belonging and attachment to one's community also requires opportunities to participate in the life of the community. Once again, resilience research has found that young people who have opportunities in their communities to be a part of clubs, teams, work apprenticeships, mentoring programs, neighborhood-based youth development organizations, and community service-learning programs are able to overcome other challenges in their lives and become healthy and successful adults (McLaughlin et al., 1994; Werner & Smith, 1992). An essential element in creating effective communitywide initiatives for all people, young and old, is engaging their active involvement. Youth, just like adults, need to have ownership and active roles in the life of their community if the community is to serve as a protective factor.

A FOCUS ON COMMUNITY RESILIENCE

In addition to the power that communities have to support individual resilience, communities themselves demonstrate resilience. Although it is vital to foster resilience in individuals, the opportunity for a broader impact is being missed. The range of health, safety, and social ills that afflict families, schools, and communities are too broad to be simply addressed one individual at a time. Rather, what is needed to complement individual work is a multifaceted approach that strengthens the overall environment. Communities have an enormous capacity to contribute to the resolution of their own problems and to build on strengths that may previously have been overlooked. In addition, in the same way that focusing on risk can lead to blaming the victim, focusing on community support for individual resilience can lead to blaming the community for not providing adequate opportunity for assets and strengths to emerge. By focusing on community resilience, the responsibility is placed even more broadly on all of us to create the conditions and policies that support the emergence of community assets and strengths.

According to the National Charrette Institute (2002), resilient communities that promote health and safety often work toward improving the social, economic, and physical well-being of their people, places, and natural environments. These communities work to enhance existing resilience factors, such as daily physical activity, social cohesion and trust, safe streets (including walking paths and trails for residents), and transportation options that reduce automobile congestion and encourage economic, social, environmental, and cultural sustainability.

A resilient community, like a resilient individual, can be described as having social competence, problem-solving capacity, a sense of identity, and hope for the future. A resilient community provides the same *triad* of protective factors as resilient families and schools: caring relationships, high expectations, and opportunities for participation. Sociologists have recently begun describing community protective factors in terms of the concept of *social capital*, that is, as "social networks, norms of reciprocity, mutual assistance, and trustworthiness" (Putnam & Feldstein, 2003, p. 2).

THE HEALTHY-IMMIGRANT PARADOX

First-generation immigrants tend to be healthier than U.S.-born populations of the same race and ethnicity (National Institutes of Health [NIH], 2003). This holds true even when the immigrant populations have characteristics that are associated with poorer health outcomes, such as low socioeconomic status. This phenomenon, known as the *healthy-immigrant paradox*, can be seen in U.S. immigrants and migrants. Significantly, the protective influence of immigration tends to dissipate with acculturation to mainstream U.S. culture; second-generation immigrant populations are less healthy than their elders.

Theories postulated to explain the healthy-immigrant paradox include the notions that immigrants are a self-selected group and that healthier people tend to immigrate. A study of infant health among Puerto Rican migrants provides some evidence for these theories. Puerto Ricans are not immigrants; they are native-born U.S. citizens, but they share many characteristics with immigrants. Despite their relatively low socioeconomic status, Puerto Rican migrants to the U.S. mainland have relatively low levels of infant mortality. In fact, infant mortality is lower among new migrants to the mainland than among families who remain in Puerto Rico, suggesting that selective migration is an important explanatory factor. But among migrants to the mainland, infant mortality rates rise as time on the mainland increases. The positive association between infant mortality and length of stay on the mainland increases when other behavioral, demographic, and socioeconomic factors are controlled (NIH, 2003).

Another theory posited for healthy immigrants is that they bring with them cultural practices from their home countries that are protective for some adverse health outcomes (Guendelman et al., 1999). Birth outcomes among Mexican-born women might provide evidence for this theory. Immigrant Mexican women tend to face significant challenges to their health during pregnancy, but their babies tend to be healthier on average than other babies in the United States. Immigrant Mexican women have high rates of fertility, low incomes, and delayed access to prenatal care—all significant contributors to infant mortality (Guendelman et al., 1999). However, rates of infant mortality are lower for babies born to Mexican-born women than for population groups that face fewer correlated risks (Guendelman, Thornton, Gould, & Hosang, 2005), and birth outcomes for second-generation Mexican American women are worse than for their mothers.

The explanation for these differences may lie in cultural practices. Although first-generation Mexican American women hold lower socioeconomic status than second-generation or non-Hispanic white women, they average a higher intake of protein, vitamins A and C, folic acid, and calcium than the other two groups.

In fact, intake of these nutrients was highest among first-generation Mexican women and lowest among their second-generation counterparts. Although low incomes correlate with less healthy diets for non-Hispanics, low incomes are associated with healthier diets for first-generation Mexicans (Guendelman & Abrams, 1995).

In addition, an NIH study shows that mothers of Mexican origin born in the United States are more than twice as likely to smoke during pregnancy than Mexican-born mothers. A review of related research shows that a higher level of U.S. cultural assimilation is associated with worse birth and prenatal outcomes (for example, prematurity, low birthweight, teen pregnancy, and neonatal mortality), as well as with undesirable prenatal and postnatal behaviors (for example, smoking and using drugs during pregnancy and decreased number of breastfeeding mothers) (Marielena, Gamboa, Kahramanian, Morales, & Bautista, 2005). Therefore, babies born to Mexican-born women are less likely to have adverse birth outcomes associated with cigarette smoking. Less quantifiable factors in the relative health of Latino babies may also include positive cultural attitudes toward pregnant women, strong family ties, kinship networks, religious faith, and cultures that promote the consumption of whole foods.

Public health practitioners can use this kind of information to build on the cultural strengths of Mexican-born women to prevent the development of health problems that may put their children at risk. Furthermore, by identifying populationwide characteristics that offset high risks, practitioners may be in a better position to direct their public health efforts in a way that would have the greatest impact. By shifting the focus of our public health approach from one that is centered around individuals to an approach that focuses on larger communities, it is possible to effectively promote the health and well-being of entire at-risk populations that face health disparities in the United States.

Source: Prevention Institute.

A resilient community is characterized by mutually caring relationships, high expectations in the form of shared positive beliefs, and respect for all citizens, especially for those on the margin, such as young people. A resilient community is also characterized by all members' active participation and contributions. It is a community in which young people, families, schools, and organizations work as partners to ensure that individuals receive the critical supports and opportunities necessary for healthy development—and that community strengths are supported and developed. Fostering the kind of community that supports individuals requires paying attention to a broad range of factors. Prevention Institute did an extensive examination of the literature and research and developed the Toolkit for Health and Resilience in Vulnerable Environments (THRIVE) for the U.S. Department of Health and Human Services' Office of Minority Health. THRIVE outlines four clusters of community factors that directly affect resilience: *built environment factors*, such as housing, environmental quality, and transportation; *social capital factors*, such as collective efficacy, social cohesion, and social norms; *structural factors*, such as economic capital, racial relations, and media and marketing; and *service and institution factors*, such as education, cultural opportunities, and public safety (http://preventioninstitute.org/component/jlibrary/article/id-96/127.html).

Evaluators of the New Futures venture, an ambitious communitywide initiative to benefit young people in five large communities, warn that we neglect the qualities of the immediate caregiving environment at our peril. On-site evaluators of the five-year initiative, which was funded by the Annie E. Casey Foundation, attribute the failure of these early communitywide collaborations to the finding that systems and organizations talked only to each other; they did not, for example, bring in the families or youth they served, nor did they invite teachers to the table. According to evaluators Julie White and Gary Wehlage (1995), "it is the strengthening of neighborhoods from the inside that is vital, something that traditional social services have not succeeded in doing" (p. 35). They elaborate further that if the goal is

> building social capital, the criteria for a successful collaborative would shift from delivering services more efficiently to success in fostering community. Social capital contributes to community by fostering networks of interdependency within and among families, neighborhoods, and the larger community [p. 35].

Furthermore, White and Wehlage argue, "the shift from delivering services to individual clients to investing in the social capital of whole groups of people appears to be essential if collaboratives are to ultimately improve the life chances of generations of at-risk children" (p. 35).

A FRAMEWORK FOR RESILIENCE AND COMMUNITY AND YOUTH DEVELOPMENT

Getting youth involved as partners to improve their conditions and opportunities is an important and powerful strategy. Community youth development (CYD), an emerging movement, places the emphasis on young people themselves becoming community change agents, fully capable of improving their communities for the young and also for families and other community members. For example, the California Wellness Foundation funds community-based initiatives in which, according to Foundation president Gary Yates, "young people work in leadership roles alongside of adults to determine what changes are needed in their physical, social and chemical environments to promote health and wellness in their communities" (California Wellness Foundation, 1999).

In contrast to other community development approaches, CYD holds that healthy communities cannot be built without a youth development approach that actively enlists young people in the change effort. The ultimate goal of the CYD approach is the creation of "safe, just, prosperous communities, countries, and world where young people are partners and contributors working with adults to positively influence the conditions affecting the security and quality of their lives" (Curnan & Hughes, 2002, p. 33). This approach is exemplified in the Ford Foundation's Community Youth Development Initiative (Cutler & Edwards, 2002), Stanford University's Gardner Center for Youth and Community (McLaughlin, 2000), the Annie E. Casey Foundation (Hyman, 1999), the Innovation Center for Community and Youth Development at the University of Wisconsin (2002), and the National 4-H Council (2002), to name just a few.

As illustrated in Figure 3.1, the CYD approach recognizes that youth participation and contribution (in the context of caring relationships and high-expectation messages) benefit young people by promoting positive developmental outcomes. The CYD approach also recognizes that youth participation and contribution are critical and necessary if we are to actually improve communities. CYD recognizes the web of interconnectedness that defines a resilient community, reminding prevention practitioners and supporters that besides taking "a whole village to raise a child," it also takes "a child to raise a whole village" (Kretzmann & Schmitz, 1999).

Figure 3.1   The community youth development process: Resilience in action

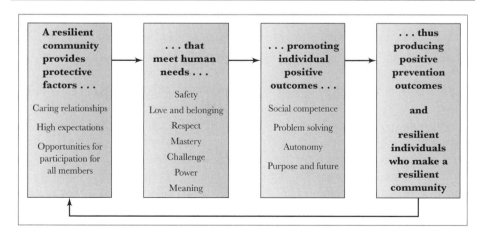

YOUTH DEVELOPMENT, RESILIENCE, AND PRIMARY PREVENTION

The framework in Figure 3.1 not only illustrates the interconnectedness of the fields of resilience, community development, and youth development but also presents a theory of change that postulates that prevention outcomes are best achieved by the community youth development process. This process starts by enhancing community support for resilience by helping communities provide the protective factors of caring relationships, high expectations, and opportunities for participation at the community level that meet youth needs both directly and indirectly through supporting families and schools. Protective factors promote young people's positive social, emotional, cognitive, and moral and spiritual development (individual resilience strengths) and help bring about positive prevention outcomes (for example, reductions in problem behaviors across the board). These healthy and successful young people feed right back into their communities, in turn strengthening the resilience of the community.

When communities fail to provide the critical protective factors needed to meet developmental needs, young people can be drawn to seek support elsewhere, often from groups that prey on youthful needs for affiliation and belonging, such as gangs. It is past time for the prevention field to move from its dominant risk-based paradigm, especially from the current focus on narrow *evidence-based programs* designed to fix *high-risk youth*, to embrace a community youth development approach that recognizes the resilience and other innate gifts every young person possesses.

CREATING A RESILIENCE PERSPECTIVE

Much progress has been made in bringing a strengths perspective to the table. Unfortunately, many human service professions (including education, criminal justice, social services, and even public health) often still reflect a deficit perspective. How do we influence caregivers (service providers) and, even more important, transform human service systems so they take a positive, community youth development or resilience approach to prevention?

This question is similar to the question that has been at the heart of the resilience movement. *How do we transform risk into resilience?* One important answer and starting point is to help caregivers recognize their own resilient nature. This allows them to reframe their experience and see themselves and their lives in new ways. More than a decade of research has shown that this reframing is facilitated by the protective factors of caring relationships, high expectations, and opportunities for participation and contribution. Providing organizational supports and opportunities to the caregivers of youth and others thus becomes the ultimate starting point for resilience-based efforts. A supportive and nurturing climate for youth and community development is exponentially enhanced when governments, communities, and schools support the *health of the helpers*. Healthy helpers model in their own lives and work the resilience strengths of social competence, problem solving, autonomy, and sense of purpose.

Other strategies include directly disseminating and teaching what we know about resilience to adult caregivers and to our children and youth. A resilience study group is a powerful tool for helping people learn about their resilience, that is, the power they have to see themselves and their lives in new ways. In these groups, service providers, youth, and community members learn about resilience research and about other people's successes and share their own histories. All of these stories of resilience create hope, as Werner and Smith explain (1992):

> The life stories of the resilient youngsters now grown into adulthood teach us that competence, confidence, and caring can flourish, even under adverse circumstances, if children encounter persons who provide them with the secure basis for the development of trust, autonomy, and initiative. From odds successfully overcome springs hope—a gift each of us can share with a child—at home, in the classroom, on the playground, or in the neighborhood [p. 209].

Directly teaching caregivers and youth about their personal resilience is also a major strategy for engendering a belief in resilience. For example, the Health Realization and Community Resilience work of Roger Mills (see Mills & Spittle, 2001) is being used in schools, communities, workplaces, and organizations nationally and internationally to help parents, teachers, managers, youth workers, and law enforcement officers recognize their own resilience so they can in turn see the resilience of the populations they serve. Resilience classes (Vasquez, 2000) and insight meditation (Lozoff, 2000) are becoming more commonplace in juvenile halls and prisons for both caregivers and inmates—with transformational results (Donnenfield, 2000; Menahemi & Ariel, 1997). The National Resilience Resource Center at the University of Minnesota is using this *health-of-the-helper model* of change in schools and communities around the country (Marshall, 1998). Meditation and mindfulness programs are also often critical components of programs focused on reducing the stress of caregivers—and even young people themselves—so they can see the health in themselves and others (Kabat-Zinn, 1995).

As Barrera and Prelow point out, caregivers who learn about and model their own resilience are also able to directly teach young people about their own resilient nature (2000):

> An important direction for future research would be to investigate how support provision affects the well-being of the support provider (e.g., mentor). . . . The well-known helper-therapy principle would suggest that the benefits for the support providers are at least as great as the benefits for the support recipients [p. 333].

Instead of burning out or developing a strong case of compassion fatigue, this research may just find that having a resilient attitude, that is, a belief in one's own innate capacity and in the capacities of one's children, students, or clients, is a protective factor support-ing caregiver self-efficacy, optimism, and hope—and, in turn, young people's resilience strengths.

CONCLUSION

The challenge to the research community is to focus more time and resources on the study of resilience in communities and individuals. According to Shannon, our goals will deter-mine our research priorities (1995):

> Our choices about what to research and how to go about it are conditioned by where we hope to go in the broadest sense. Our ideas about values, aesthetics, politics, and normal behavior and preferences are integral to educational [and public health] research, its interpretation, and its utilization. Science and research cannot determine or validate these values, visions, and ideas. Science and research can only be used to help us develop effective methods for working toward our values, visions, and ideas [p. 127].

The challenge to practitioners and caregivers is to get in touch with their own innate resilience and to understand it so they can model it and recognize it in the communities and people they serve. The *power of one* is clearly a major finding of four decades of resilience research. The *power of one* validates the influence each of us has in every interaction with others to nurture or block their innate resilience.

Yet as important as our individual relationships with people are, they are not enough, especially in the face of the barriers to change within the bureaucracies of the human serv-ices and public health. So a third challenge is to our human-serving systems and bureauc-racies. In *Common Purpose* (1997), Lisbeth Schorr analyzes and explains why half of the successful programs for children and families she had reported on in her previous book, *Within Our Reach* (1988), were defunct five years later and none had been expanded or replicated.

> When effective programs aiming to reach large numbers encounter the pressures exercised by prevailing attitudes and systems, the resulting collision is almost always lethal to the effective programs. Their demise can be prevented only by changing systems and public perceptions to make them more hospitable to effective efforts to change lives and communities [1997, p. 20].

What Schorr is ultimately advocating for is the importance of trusting local knowledge and capacity and building resilient communities. The final challenge requires the atten-tion of everyone, not just public health professionals. Farsighted economists and political scientists view the rebuilding of our communities as the key to our future survival as a nation, world, and even species. In his seminal book, *The End of Work* (1995), Jeremy

Rifkin writes that as we entered the twenty-first century, the world was in the throes of the third Industrial Revolution, a revolution transforming our industrial age into a "postmarket economy," a "new phase in world history," and "one in which fewer and fewer workers will be needed to produce the goods and services for the global population." Rifkin concludes that "only by building strong, self-sustaining local communities will people in every country be able to withstand the forces of technological displacement and market globalization that are threatening livelihoods and survival of much of the human family" (p. xvi).

Similarly, John Gardner writes prophetically about resilient communities in his classic essay *Building Community* (1991):

> Without the continuity of the shared values that community provides, freedom cannot survive. . . . [Only] strong and resilient communities can stand between the individual and any government that tries to impose dictatorial solutions from the right or left. Undifferentiated masses never have and never will preserve freedom against usurping power [p. 5].

Just as the resilience paradigm focuses on the *glass half full* versus the risk paradigm of the *glass half empty*, Gardner states that it is the generative rather than the disintegrative functions "that deserve our closest attention. . . . The regenerative powers of human society have not weakened. The capacity of humankind to create and re-create social coherence is always there—enduring and irrepressible" (1991, p. 9). As noted many times in this chapter, one of the major assumptions of resilience theory is that human systems are innately resilient. At the individual level, this means we are genetically wired with the capacities for social competence and caring, problem solving and change, autonomy and identity, and hope and meaning. At the community level, this translates into communities also having this inherent transformative capacity to adapt and change.

Explains Gardner, "Passive allegiance isn't enough today. The forces of disintegration have gained steadily and will prevail unless individuals see themselves as having a positive duty to nurture their community and continuously reweave the social fabric" (1991, p. 11). What has become apparent is that just as the degenerative forces at work today have grown, so has the importance of the intentional work done by public health practitioners in building or emerging community. What is at stake is not only the support provided to those in need but also the ability of all of us and our communities to grow and thrive.

DISCUSSION QUESTIONS

1. Suppose you were to design a community-based research study that focuses on resilience. How might you begin to measure community assets and resilience strength? What types of data and indicators would be useful for measuring outcomes of a resiliency-focused intervention program?

2. Our health system has traditionally focused on identifying and treating risk factors and health conditions, rather than on promoting overall health and well-being. What are some novel approaches to improving the health system that would provide for community, family, and individual resilience?

3. What can we learn from the experience of first-generation immigrants to the United States that may be useful when promoting resilience in other population sub-groups in the United States?

4. The text mentions "when communities fail to provide the critical protective factors needed to meet developmental needs, young people can be drawn to seek support elsewhere, often from groups that prey on youthful needs for affiliation and belonging, such as gangs." Do you think that developing healthy, resilient communities would prevent gangs and related groups from developing in the first place? Why or why not?

REFERENCES

Barrera, M., & Prelow, H. (2000). Interventions to promote social support in children and adolescents. In D. Cicchetti, J. Rappaport, I. Sandler, & R. P. Weissberg (Eds.), *The promotion of wellness in children and adolescents* (pp. 309–339). Washington, DC: Child Welfare League of America Press.

Baumeister, R., & Leary, M. (1995). The need to belong: Desire for interpersonal attachments as a fundamental human motivation. *Psychological Bulletin, 117*, 497–529.

Beardslee, W., & Podoresfky, D. (1988). Resilient adolescents whose parents have serious affective and other psychiatric disorders: The importance of self-understanding and relationships. *American Journal of Psychiatry, 145*, 63–69.

Benard, B. (1991). *Fostering resiliency in kids: Protective factors in the family, school, and community*. Portland, OR: Northwest Regional Educational Laboratory.

Benard, B. (2004). *Resiliency: What we have learned*. San Francisco: WestEd.

California Wellness Foundation. (1999, Summer). Youth lead the way to healthier communities. *TCWF Newsletter*, p. 1. This is available in hard copy by calling The California Wellness Foundation at (818) 702–1900.

Carnegie Task Force on Youth Development and Community Programs. (1992). *A matter of time: Risk and opportunity in the nonschool hours*. New York: Carnegie Corp.

Chess, S. (1989). Defying the voice of doom. In T. F. Dugan & R. Coles (Eds.), *The child in our time: Studies in the development of resiliency* (pp. 179–199). New York: Bruner/Mazel.

Clausen, J. A. (1993). *American lives: Looking back at the children of the Great Depression*. New York: Free Press.

Coleman, J. (1987). Families and schools. *Educational Researcher, 16*(6), 32–38.

Curnan, S., & Hughes, D. (2002). Towards shared prosperity: Change-making in the CYD movement. *CYD Journal, 3*, 25–33.

Currie, E. (1994). *Reckoning: Drugs, the cities, and the American future*. New York: Hill & Wang.

Cutler, I., & Edwards, S. (2002). Linking youth and community development: Ideas from the Community Youth Development Initiative. *CYD Journal, 3*, 17–23.

Deci, E. L. (with R. Flaste). (1995). *Why we do what we do: Understanding self-motivation*. New York: Putnam.

Donnenfield, D. (2000). Changing from the inside [Video]. San Francisco: David Donnenfield Productions.

Eccles, J. S., & Gootman, J. A. (Eds.). (2002). *Community programs to promote youth development*. Washington, DC: National Academy Press.

Fanshel, D. (1975). Status changes of children in foster care: Final results of the Columbia University Longitudinal Study. *Child Welfare, 555*, 143–177.

Festinger, T. (1984). *No one ever asked us: A postscript to the foster care system*. New York: Columbia University Press.

Furstenberg Jr., F. F., Cook, T. D., Eccles, J., Elder Jr., G. H., & Sameroff, A. (1999). *Managing to make it: Urban families and adolescent success*. Chicago: University of Chicago Press.

Gardner, J. (1991, September). *Building community*. Paper prepared for the Leadership Studies Program. Washington, DC: INDEPENDENT SECTOR.

Garmezy, N. (1991). Resiliency and vulnerability to adverse developmental outcomes associated with poverty. *American Behavioral Scientist, 34*, 416–430.

Guendelman, S., & Abrams, B. (1995). Dietary intake among Mexican-American women: Generational differences and a comparison with white non-Hispanic women. *American Journal of Public Health, 85*, 20–25.

Guendelman et al. (1999). Birth outcomes of immigrant women in the United States, France, and Belgium. *Maternal and Child Health Journal, 3*, 177–187.

Guendelman, S., Thornton, D., Gould, J., & Hosang, N. (2005). Social disparities in maternal morbidity during labor and delivery between Mexican-born and U.S.-born white Californians, 1996–1998. *American Journal of Public Health, 95*, 2218–2224.

Higgins, G. O. (1994). *Resilient adults: Overcoming a cruel past*. San Francisco: Jossey-Bass.

Hyman, J. (1999). *Spheres of influence: A strategic synthesis and framework for community youth development*. Baltimore: Annie E. Casey Foundation.

Innovation Center for Community and Youth Development. (2002). *Mission and goals*. Madison: University of Wisconsin.

Jessor, R. (1993). Successful adolescent development among youth in high-risk settings. *American Psychologist, 48*, 117–126.

Kabat-Zinn, J. (1995). *Wherever you go, there you are: Mindfulness meditation in everyday life*. New York: Hyperion.

Kohn, A. (1997, Summer). The limits of teaching skills. *Reaching Today's Youth*, pp. 14–16.

Kreft, I., & Brown, J. (Eds.). (1998). The zero effects of drug prevention programs: Issues and solutions. *Evaluation Review, 22*(Special issue), 3–14

Kretzmann, J. P., & McKnight, J. L. (1993). *Building communities from the inside out: A path toward finding and mobilizing a community's assets.* Evanston, IL: Northwestern University, Center for Urban Affairs and Policy Research.

Kretzmann, J. P., & Schmitz, P. H. (1999). It takes a child to raise a whole village. *Resiliency in Action, 4*(2), 1–4.

Lifton, R. J. (1993). *The protean self: Human resilience in an age of fragmentation.* New York: Basic Books.

Long, J. V., & Vaillant, G. E. (1989). Escape from the underclass. In T. F. Dugan & R. Coles (Eds.), *The child in our time: Studies in the development of resiliency* (pp. 200–213). New York: Brunner/Mazel.

Lozoff, B. (2000). *It's a Meaningful Life—It Just Takes Practice.* New York: Viking.

Luthar, S. S. (Ed.). (2003). *Resilience and vulnerability: Adaptation in the context of childhood adversities.* New York: Cambridge University Press.

Males, M. (1996). *The scapegoat generation: America's war on adolescence.* Monroe, ME: Common Courage Press.

Marielena, L., Gamboa, C., Kahramanian, M. I., Morales, L. S., & Bautista, D. E. (2005). Acculturation and Latino health in the United States: A review of the literature and its sociopolitical context. *Annual Review of Public Health, 26,* 367–397. Retrieved July 25, 2006, from http://www .rand.org/pubs/reprints/RP1177

Marshall, K. (1998). Reculturing systems with resilience/health realization. *Promoting positive and healthy behaviors in children: Fourteenth annual Rosalynn Carter Symposium on Mental Health Policy* (pp. 48–58). Atlanta: The Carter Center.

Maslow, A. (1954). *Motivation and personality.* New York: HarperCollins.

Masten, A. (2001). Ordinary magic: Resilience processes in development. *American Psychologist, 56,* 227–238.

Masten, A., & Reed, M. (2002). Resilience in development. In C. R. Snyder and S. J. Lopez (Eds.), *Handbook of positive psychology* (pp. 74–88). New York: Oxford University Press.

McKnight, J. L. (1992, Winter). Mapping community capacity. *New Designs for Youth Development,* pp. 9–15.

McLaughlin, M. W. (2000). *Community counts.* New York: Public Education Network.

McLaughlin, M. W., Irby, M. A., & Langman, J. (1994). *Urban sanctuaries: Neighborhood organizations in the lives and futures of inner-city youth.* San Francisco: Jossey-Bass.

Menahemi, A., & Ariel, E. (Dirs.). (1997). *Doing time, doing Vipassana* [Video]. Tel Aviv, Israel: Karuna Films.

Mills, R. (1993). *The Health Realization model: A community empowerment primer.* Alhambra: California School of Professional Psychology.

Mills, R., & Spittle, E. (2001). *Wisdom within.* Auburn, WA: Lone Pine Publishing.

Mrazek, P., & Haggerty, R. (Eds.). (1994). *Reducing risks for mental disorders: Frontiers for preventive intervention research.* Washington, DC: National Academy Press.

National 4-H Council. (2002). *The national conversation on youth development in the 21st century: Final report*. Chevy Chase, MD: National 4-H Council.

National Charrette Institute. (2002). *Healthy communities*. Retrieved October 4, 2002, from http://www.charretteinstitute.org/

National Institutes of Health (NIH), National Institute of Child Health and Human Development. (2003). Demographic and Behavioral Sciences Branch, NICHD: Report to the NACHHD Council, 2003. Retrieved October 10, 2006, from http://www.nichd.nih.gov/publications/pubs/upload/council_dbsb_2003.pdf

Owens, J. (2002, February 20). Breaking new ground: Two neighborhood studies on crime, children aim to change policy, improve lives. *Chicago Tribune*, p. 5.

Peterson, C., & Seligman, M.E.P. (2004). *Character strengths and virtues: A handbook and classification*. New York: Oxford University Press.

Putnam, R. D. (2000). *Bowling alone: The collapse and revival of American community*. New York: Simon & Schuster.

Putnam, R. D., & Feldstein, L. M. (2003). *Better together: Restoring the American community*. New York: Simon & Schuster.

Rifkin, J. (1995). *The end of work: The decline of the global labor force and the dawn of the post-market era*. New York: Tarcher.

Rutter, M. (1989). Pathways from childhood to adult life. *Journal Child Psychology and Psychiatry, 30*, 23–51.

Rutter, M. (2000). Resilience reconsidered: Conceptual considerations, empirical findings, and policy implications. In J. P. Shonkoff & S. J. Meisels (Eds.), *Handbook of early childhood intervention* (pp. 651–682). New York: Cambridge University Press.

Sameroff, A., Barocas, R., & Seifer, R. (1984). The early development of children born to mentally ill women. In N. F. Watt, E. J. Anthony, L. C. Wynne, & J. E. Rolf (Eds.), *Children at risk for schizophrenia: A longitudinal perspective* (pp. 482–514). New York: Cambridge University Press.

Sampson, R. J., Raudenbush, S. W., & Earls, F. (1997). Neighborhoods and violent crime: A multilevel study of collective efficacy. *Science, 277*, 918–924.

Schorr, L. B. (with D. Schorr). (1988). *Within our reach: Breaking the cycle of disadvantage*. New York: Doubleday.

Schorr, L. B. (1997). *Common purpose: Strengthening families and neighborhoods to rebuild America*. New York: Anchor Books.

Schweinhart, L. J., Barnes, H. V., & Wiekart, D. P. (1993). *Significant benefits: The High/Scope Perry Preschool Study through age 27*. Ypsilanti, MI: High/Scope Press.

Seligman, M. E. P. (2002). Positive psychology, positive prevention, and positive therapy. In C. R. Snyder & S. J. Lopez (Eds.), *Handbook of positive psychology* (pp. 3–9). New York: Oxford University Press.

Shannon, P. (1995). *Text, lies, and videotape: Stories about life, liberty, and learning*. Portsmouth, NH: Heinemann.

Swadener, B. B., & Lubeck, S. (Eds.). (1995). *Children and families "at promise": Deconstructing the discourse of risk*. Albany: State University of New York Press.

Vaillant, G. E. (2002). *Aging well: Surprising guideposts to a happier life from the landmark Harvard Study of Adult Development*. Boston: Little, Brown.

Vasquez, G. (2000). Resiliency: Juvenile offenders recognize their strengths to change their lives. *Corrections Today, 62*, 106–110, 125.

Vigil, J. D. (1990). Cholos and gangs: Culture change and street youth in Los Angeles. In R. Huff (Ed.), *Gangs in America: Diffusion, diversity, and public policy* (pp. 146–162). Thousand Oaks, CA: Sage.

Walsh, J. (1997). *Stories of renewal: Community building and the future of urban America*. New York: Rockefeller Foundation.

Watt, N. F., Anthony, E. J., Wynne, L. C., & Rolf, J. E. (Eds.). (1984). *Children at risk for schizophrenia: A longitudinal perspective*. New York: Cambridge University Press.

Werner, E. E. (1986). Resilient offspring of alcoholics: A longitudinal study from birth to age 18. *Journal of Studies on Alcohol, 14*, 34–40.

Werner, E. E., & Smith, R. S. (1982). *Vulnerable but invincible: A longitudinal study of resilient children and youth*. New York: Adams, Bannister, & Cox.

Werner, E. E., & Smith, R. S. (1992). *Overcoming the odds: High-risk children from birth to adulthood*. Ithaca, NY: Cornell University Press.

Werner, E. E., & Smith, R. S. (2001). *Journeys from childhood to the midlife: Risk, resilience, and recovery*. Ithaca, NY: Cornell University Press.

White, J. A., & Wehlage, G. G. (1995). Community collaboration: If it is such a good idea, why is it so hard to do? *Educational Evaluation and Policy Analysis, 17*, 23–28.

Wilkes, G. (2002). Abused child to nonabusive parent: Resilience and conceptual change. *Journal of Clinical Psychology, 58*, 261–278.

Wilson, W. J. (1987). *The truly disadvantaged: The inner city, the underclass, and public policy*. Chicago: University of Chicago Press.

Zigler, E., & Hall, N. W. (1989). Physical child abuse in America: Past, present, and future. In D. Cicchetti & V. Carlson (Eds.), *Child maltreatment: Theory and research on the causes and consequences of child abuse and neglect* (pp. 38–75). New York: Cambridge University Press.

PART TWO

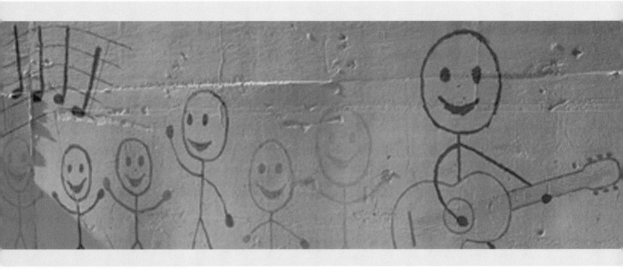

KEY ELEMENTS
OF EFFECTIVE
PREVENTION
EFFORTS

Part Two provides in-depth descriptions of strategies and methods for current and future practitioners of primary prevention. Each of its six chapters covers a skill set that, when effectively put to use, helps primary prevention efforts succeed.

People coming together and insisting on their community well-being is as important a factor in achieving well-being as any scientific or technical capacity. There is a rich history of community organizing for primary prevention, of people gathering to develop effective strategies that prevent a range of health and social issues, such as widespread youth violence; epidemic, acute, and chronic illnesses; and the ever-expanding gap between the powerful and the powerless that underlies so much illness and injury. In Chapter Four, "Community Organizing for Health and Social Justice," authors Vivian Chávez, Meredith Minkler, Nina Wallerstein, and Michael Spencer examine community organizing in local settings and its effect on building people's capacity, relationships, and ability to take action to change their communities. Chapter Four authors offer a historical context and a perspective on women's organizing and youth activism; they emphasize the notion of *cultural humility*, which advocates nonpaternalistic partnerships with self-reflection. The *wheel of community organizing*, a set of principles to create, put into practice, and evaluate prevention initiatives, is provided as a practical framework, along with a list of essential qualities for organizing.

There are numerous examples of collaborations achieving significant primary prevention outcomes that would not have been possible by one group alone. In fact, the formation of a coalition often marks the beginning of significant prevention efforts. At the same time, not everyone knows how to collaborate effectively; collaboration is a skill that should not be taken for granted.

Chapter Five, "Working Collaboratively to Advance Prevention," by Larry Cohen and Ashby Wolfe, focuses on *coalitions*, which are one particular form of collaboration. The authors detail the steps necessary to ensure coalitions are diverse and effective and that they add to, rather than risk detracting from, quality prevention efforts. A new sidebar by Ellen Wu describes how to effectively build and maintain multicultural coalitions. Deborah Balfanz and Soowon Kim describe the YMCA's efforts to convene a healthier communities collaborative. The information presented is applicable to both leaders and participants in all types of coalitions, whether newly initiated or already existing.

Public policy development is an important tool for primary prevention because policy shapes the environment in which we live, work, and play. Makani Themba-Nixon, author of Chapter Six, "The Power of Local Communities to Foster Policy," describes basic elements for developing policy initiatives and offers specific advice to overcome common challenges. The chapter focuses in particular on local policy development for historically disfranchised communities. Local policy development is ideal for primary prevention efforts because so many community efforts are organized locally, and it provides realistic and achievable means to address large-scale community health issues. In addition, decisions made at the local level are easier to monitor and evaluate and often act as a catalyst for statewide and national change.

Media are more than educational or public relations tools. Media advocacy provides the voice prevention advocates need to reach key decision makers and alter public opinion. Without effective approaches to working with media, primary prevention efforts will continually fall short of their potential. In Chapter Seven, "Using Media Advocacy to Influence Policy," Lori Dorfman describes the basic elements of developing a strategic plan for media advocacy, noting it is much more than a method for information dissemination. It is also a process of developing media literacy, effective messaging, and political and cultural savvy. From efforts seeking to eliminate tobacco advertising to those restricting the sale of handguns, media advocacy is a natural complement to community-organizing and coalition-building efforts aimed at primary prevention.

Chapter 8, "The Impact of Corporate Practices on Health and Health Policy," by Nicholas Freudenberg and Sandro Galea, is an important new contribution to this second edition. The authors reveal how large industries and corporations, including the food, automobile, and pharmaceutical industries, develop products and policies that don't just contribute to negative outcomes on public health, but also become part of the determinants of health in the United States. The authors argue that addressing the negative health influences of large corporations should be a key component of prevention policy. A sidebar written by Prevention Institute describes the pioneering work of Patti Rundall, Policy Director for United Kingdom-based Baby Milk Action, and the efforts to address the misleading global marketing practices of the infant formula industry.

A common yet unfounded criticism of primary prevention efforts is that they cannot be evaluated. The argument is based on a belief that primary prevention efforts are too diffuse and aren't applied to sufficiently discrete populations. Dan Perales, author of Chapter Nine, "Primary Prevention and Program Evaluation," dispels this notion, providing examples of primary prevention evaluation. Yet evaluation of primary prevention does have unique challenges. Prevention efforts are aimed at large populations, do involve collaborations, and are by definition long-term processes. Primary Prevention evaluators do need to have a clear strategy and the ability to see if it is being effectively followed. Evaluators of primary prevention must have the tools as well as the theoretical understanding of how preventive evaluations differ from traditional models. The author describes some of the most useful tools and principles (such as community-based participatory research) and emphasizes the importance of a respectful evaluation process in preventing illness and injury over the long-term.

4

Community Organizing for Health and Social Justice

Vivian Chávez

Meredith Minkler

Nina Wallerstein

Michael S. Spencer

LEARNING OBJECTIVES

- Identify key terms, historical context, and important aspects around community organizing.
- Understand how culture affects perceptions, relationships, and community building.
- Be able to describe the wheel of community organizing.
- Conceptualize the essential qualities of inclusion and empowerment.

C ommunity organizing—these two words, woven together, evoke vivid images and pro- voke an emotional response. The concept of community organizing is neither neutral nor easy to define. The term carries a deep history intricately tied to oppression, struggle, and resistance. The words community and organizing are contextualized with stories from people, places, and events that make up the diverse face of the United States. Community organizing includes persons of color demanding civil rights and claiming their equality through nonviolent marches, boycotts, and sit-ins. Community organizing is workers cre- ating unions and making agreements about their humanity and their labor. It is women speaking painful truths about their private lives so that violence is made into a public issue. Community organizing is about gay, lesbian, bisexual, and transgender people lifting the veil of secrecy and stigma around sexual identity and sexual health. It's young people marching and participating in protests, mobilizing to get tobacco ads targeting youth of color removed from their communities, and being civically engaged in efforts to promote change, despite being too young to vote.

The label *community organizing* has been attached to a variety of activities drawing on disparate traditions and historical periods. Community organizing is about primary prevention—people coming together to effectively ward off a range of health and social problems, including youth violence, chronic illness, skyrocketing medical costs, and the ever- expanding gap between rich and poor. Of course, community organizing can also be used to promote agendas that are not conducive to good health, as in the case of anti-immigrant organizing, or denial of civil rights on the basis of sexual orientation, or efforts to limit women's reproductive rights.

However, this chapter intentionally focuses on the positive, examining community organizing that occurs in local settings to empower individuals, build relationships, and create action for community change (Beckwith, 1997; Bobo, Kendall, & Max, 1991; Kahn, 1991; Minkler, 2004; Stall & Stoecker, 1998).

We limit our analysis primarily to the United States, although we recognize that com- munity organizing methods are used internationally to address health disparities, hunger, and poverty. We describe community organizing as a major primary prevention strategy linked to personal and community well-being. As the Canadian health promotion leader Ronald Labonte (1994) reminds us, we are careful not to romanticize community.

After providing background on definitions and terminology, the chapter offers a brief historical summary, a perspective on women's organizing and youth activism, and an overview of the notion of *cultural humility*. The *wheel of community organizing* is then explored as a conceptual framework and practical guide to the application of preven- tion methodologies. The chapter concludes with a list of essential qualities for organizing and a critique of empowerment as a key concept for future directions in the field.

Portions of this chapter are adapted from M. Minkler and N. Wallerstein, (2004), Improving health through community organization and community building: A health education perspective. In M. Minkler (Ed.), *Community Organizing and Community Building for Health*. New Brunswick, NJ: Rutgers University Press.

DEFINITIONS AND TERMINOLOGY

"Definitions," observes bell hooks (2000), "are vital starting points for the imagination. A good definition marks our starting point and lets us know where we want to end up. As we move toward our desired destination we chart the journey, creating a map" (p. 14).

COMMUNITY

Often we think of community in terms of homogeneous groups made up of people like ourselves, of similar background, from the same class, religion, race, ethnicity, and language. We define community, beyond exclusivity, as a group of people who have identified common interests and act together to achieve them. A community's ability to act together may have existed for centuries or may be triggered in a very short time by an urgent problem. The World Health Organization (WHO) defines community as a group of people, often living in a defined geographical area, who share a common culture, values, and norms (1998, p. 5). Although typically thought of in geographical terms, communities may also be identified with no particular locality and based instead on shared interests or characteristics, such as race or ethnicity, language, sexual orientation, age, or occupation (Fellin, 2001). Members of a community gain their personal and social identity by sharing common beliefs. They exhibit awareness of their identity as a group and share common needs and a commitment to meeting them. Communities sustain life and ensure human survival. Although each person is a unique individual, people need others not merely for sustenance or company but also to add meaning to their lives (Peck, 1987). A community is "a group that has learned to transcend its individual differences" (p. 62). Contrary to the myth of rugged individualism, a community recognizes and strives for interdependence. As Bellah and his associates (1985) noted, the tension between individualism and community is central to understanding social tensions in the United States. People need to be recognized as individuals as much as they need to unite with others for collective well-being.

COMMUNITY ORGANIZING

Community organizing is defined here as a dynamic process that encompasses a wide range of community engagement strategies. In its best practice, it is a long-term approach that includes people defining their community, identifying common problems or goals they wish to address, defining the solutions they wish to pursue and the methods they will use to mobilize resources, and implementing strategies for reaching the goals they have collectively set (Minkler & Wallerstein, 2004). Community organizing is a craft that requires building an enduring network of people who identify with common ideals and who can engage in social action (Stall & Stoecker, 1998). A critical dimension of community organizing is a power analysis of social change rooted in political economy and concerned with dynamics of oppression and privilege. Such an analysis carefully considers the role of factors such as race, class, gender, and sexual orientation that help determine how health and social problems are defined, treated, or ignored (Minkler & Wallerstein, 2004).

Community organizing involves advocacy and organized activism in direct favor of or in direct opposition to an issue. The term includes notions of community building and asset-based approaches (Kretzmann & McKnight, 1993; McKnight, 1995) that focus on solutions and resilience as opposed to strictly focusing on problems. Community building is concerned as much with interpersonal relationships as it is with the identification, nurturing, and celebration of community strengths (Walters, 2004) and the integration of personal experience (hooks, 1984). Although the terms *organizer, activist*, and *advocate* are often used loosely and interchangeably, some experts in the field differentiate between these terms in the following ways.

- Advocates tend to be professionals working on behalf of or for a community that may not be able to represent themselves (Stoecker, 2001).
- Activists tend to be people involved in militant actions, protests, and social movement; people tend to be proud of the label or to shy away from it (Prokosch & Raymond, 2002).
- Community organizer tends to describe a range of experiences, from working behind the scenes to support the community voice to serving as a campaign or program manager, a coordinator, or a prevention planner.

CIVIC ENGAGEMENT

Civic engagement encompasses a large range of activities such as working in a soup kitchen, writing a letter to an elected official, and voting (Putnam, 1996). Ehrlich (2000) defines civic engagement as working to make a difference in the civic life of the community and developing the combination of knowledge, skills, values, and motivation to make that difference through both political and non-political processes. With examples from college campuses, churches, and neighborhood associations, Ehrlich notes:

> [A] civically responsible individual recognizes himself or herself as a member of a larger social fabric and therefore considers social problems to be at least partly his or her own; such an individual is willing to see the moral and civic dimensions of issues, to make and justify informed moral and civic judgments, and to take action when appropriate [Ehrlich, 2000, p. xxvi].

The Coalition for Civic Engagement and Leadership (n.d.) uses the following working definition of civic engagement:

> A heightened sense of responsibility to one's communities, including developing civic sensitivity, participation in building civil society, and benefiting the common good. Civic engagement encompasses the notions of global citizenship and interdependence. Through

civic engagement, individuals—as citizens of their communities, their nations, and the world—are empowered as agents of positive social change for a more democratic world. Civic engagement involves one or more of the following:

Learning from others, self, and environment to develop informed perspectives on social issues

Recognizing and appreciating human diversity and commonality

Behaving, and working through controversy, with civility

Taking an active role in the political process

Participating actively in public life, public problem solving, and community service

Assuming leadership and membership roles in organizations

Developing empathy, ethics, values, and sense of social responsibility

Promoting social justice locally and globally

Campus Compact, a national coalition of more than a thousand colleges and universities dedicated to promoting civic engagement, defines civic engagement as:

More than just volunteering, although volunteering can be engagement. (Civic) engagement is more than just voting, although voting can be engagement. Engagement exists when individuals recognize that they have responsibilities not only to themselves and their families, but also to their communities—local, national, and global. It exists when they recognize that the health and well-being of these communities is essential to their own health and well-being. They act in order to fulfill those responsibilities and try to affect those communities for the better. Those actions, in turn, give them an even deeper understanding of their interdependence with communities.

A criticism of the language of civic engagement is that it is often used to promote individual volunteerism as a means of helping shore up the safety net sagging under the weight of government cutbacks in health and human services (Martinson & Minkler, 2006). Therefore, from a primary prevention context, we prefer the term community organizing, as it includes participation in the life of the community (following community issues, working on community solutions, collective engagement with government agencies) as well as fighting the politics of retrenchment that makes people dependent on services in the first place (Martinson & Minkler, 2006).

HISTORICAL CONTEXT

The expression community organizing was first used by American social workers in the late 1800s to describe their efforts to coordinate health and social services for European immigrants and the poor through the settlement house movement (Minkler & Wallerstein, 2004).

Garvin and Cox (2001) point out that, although community organizing is often described as having begun with the settlement house movement, several important milestones outside of social work must be included. Some examples of milestones are as follows:

- the post-Reconstruction period organizing by African Americans fighting white supremacy and Jim Crow segregation laws in the last two decades of the nineteenth century
- the Populist movement that started in the late nineteenth century among farmers and became a multisectoral coalition and a national political force
- direct social action organizing from the labor movement that taught the importance of forming coalitions around issues and the use of conflict as a means of bringing about change

Direct social action organizing was pioneered in Chicago's old stockyards neighborhood by Saul Alinsky in the late 1930s. A criminologist by training, Alinsky is often credited with leading strikes that led to better health and work conditions for all factory workers. Direct social action organizing emphasizes redressing power imbalances, building communitywide identification, and helping members devise winnable goals and nonviolent conflict strategies to bring about change. Although the Alinsky tradition was historically dominated by white male organizers, many of whom eschewed critical analyses of race and gender, the community organizing model was adapted throughout the 1960s and 1970s in communities of color (Pintado-Vertner, 2004).

DR. JACK GEIGER

So much milk, so much meat, so many vegetables, so many eggs.
—*H. Jack Geiger, The Unsteady March, p. 9*

We always need colleagues in other disciplines. Doctors aren't very good as community organizers. We are trained in hierarchical systems, and it's hard for us to get over that. We don't have the same skills that are necessary for activism, so we need to find ways to work with community organizers, health educators, nurses, clinical psychologists, social workers, labor leaders and others who have the skills to supplement the skills that we have.
—*H. Jack Geiger, The Unsteady March, p. 8*

In 1965, H. Jack Geiger, physician and civil rights activist, opened one of the first two community health centers in the United States in Mound Bayou, Mississippi (Geiger Gibson Program, n.d.). The invention of the double-row cotton picking machine had recently replaced the need for an entire population of sharecroppers, causing massive unemployment and exacerbating poverty (Caplan & Rodberg, 1994). Geiger's community health work has left a distinct imprint on the world of public health, changing acceptable methodologies for achieving health and eliminating health disparities by addressing poverty and racism directly.

To assess the needs of the community, the Mississippi health center began by holding a series of meetings in homes, churches, and schools. As a result of these meetings, residents created ten community health associations, each with its own perspective and priorities. Some communities needed clean drinking water without having to walk three miles; others needed child care or elder care.

Community participation played a central role in broadening traditional conceptions of health. In the beginning, the health center saw an enormous amount of malnutrition, stunted growth, and infection among infants and young children. Geiger and his colleagues linked hunger, a health issue, to acute poverty and linked poverty to the massive unemployment that had turned an entire population into squatters.

Instead of just treating individual cases, Geiger and his colleagues addressed the problem of malnutrition, first by writing prescriptions for food. Health center workers recruited local black-owned grocery stores to fill the prescriptions and reimbursed the stores out of the health center's pharmacy budget:

> Once we had the health center going, we started stocking food in the center pharmacy and distributing food—like drugs—to the people. A variety of officials got very nervous and said, "You can't do that." We said, "Why not?" They said, "It's a health center pharmacy, and it's supposed to carry drugs for the treatment of disease." And we said, "The last time we looked in the book, the specific therapy for malnutrition was food" [Geiger, 2005, p. 7].

The health center then sought to prevent hunger and began urging people to start vegetable gardens. The health center used a grant from a foundation to lease six hundred acres of land to start the North Bolivar County Cooperative Farm. By pooling their labor to grow vegetables instead of cotton, members of a thousand families owned a share in the crops. In the first two years, scores of tons of vegetables were grown. Health center workers also repaired housing, dug protected wells and sanitary privies (Geiger, 2005, pp. 7–8), and later even started a bookstore focused on black history and culture.

By addressing the roots of illness drawn from community concerns, these health centers pioneered an effective methodology for approaching health care in underserved communities. They explored environmental conditions, such as housing, food, income, education, employment, and exposure to environmental dangers, and linked them to health outcomes. Then, in an effort to prevent poor health outcomes, they moved *upstream* to change the conditions that led to those outcomes.

Some forty years later, Geiger told a graduating class of medical students that "You can do more than bail out these medical disasters after they have occurred . . . [You can] go upstream from medical care to forge instruments of social change that will prevent such disasters from occurring in the first place. One of those disasters is the combination of racism and poverty" (2005, p. 4).

Today there are almost a thousand community health centers in the United States, making health care accessible for more than 11.5 million patients each year (Fairchild, 2005).

Source: Prevention Institute.

Fisher and Romanofsky (1981) divide community organizing into four historical periods (see Table 4.1): organizing European immigrants through settlement houses, national-level organizing, direct social action, and local organizing. The sociologist Aldon Morris (1984) notes that the tactics of direct social action organizing were refined by the civil rights movement in the South through the mobilization of networks of local black churches, NAACP chapters, and black colleges. The legacy of social action traveled to California, where César Chávez and Dolores Huerta combined Saul Alinsky's and Mahatma Gandhi's strategies with their profound commitment to agricultural workers to found the United Farm Workers union, a network of organizations (Ferris & Sandoval, 1997). Communities of color found community organizing to be an especially powerful strategy for challenging racial oppression (Sen, 2003). As noted by Gary Delgado (1987), cofounder of Center for Third World Organizing, organizers in communities of color brought a new level of analytical sophistication, emphasizing issues of race, class, and gender—and development of indigenous leadership.

In the health field, a historical example of community organizing was the work of the Medical Committee for Human Rights in the Mississippi Delta in the 1960s when Jack Geiger and others linked health to the consequences of racism and poverty.

Another health-related illustration of community organizing efforts was WHO's adoption of a new approach to health promotion that stressed increasing people's control over the determinants of their health (1986). The WHO-initiated Healthy Cities/Healthy Communities movement now involves thousands of localities worldwide. It aims to create sustainable environments and processes in which governmental and nongovernmental sectors work in partnership to create healthy public policies, achieve high-level participation

Table 4.1 **Four historical periods in community organizing**

Period	Activities
1890–1920	Organizing European immigrant neighborhoods. Building community through settlement houses, service delivery, and social work.
1920–1940	Organizing on a national scale, especially during the Great Depression, because the nation's economic problems did not seem solvable at the community level.
1940–1960	Direct social action organizing. Federal involvement in reshaping communities through post–World War II urban renewal programs and the War on Poverty.
1960–1980	Local organizing. Thoughtful responses among activists and theorists in the early 1970s informing broader social change objectives through the civil rights, women's health, gay rights, antiwar, student, and disability rights movements.

Source: Adapted from Fisher and Romanofsky (1981).

in community-driven projects, and ultimately reduce health disparities (Norris & Pittman, 2000). More recently, as Makani Themba-Nixon notes in Chapter Six, prevention specialists and health advocates have organized against the alcohol and tobacco industries' irresponsible advertising and marketing to young people and communities of color.

In the past twenty years, the Internet has enhanced communication for community organizing efforts around the world (Hick & McNutt, 2002; Van de Donk, Loader, Nixon, & Rucht, 2004). Groups across the political spectrum go online to build community and to identify and organize supporters on a mass scale (Herbert, 2005). Prevention specialists, community organizers, and other advocates today must actively rely on their computers and other forms of media to research, learn skills, plan, solve problems, and connect with others (Fawcett, Schultz, Carson, Renault, & Francisco, 2003). Although community organizing continues to be based heavily on direct interaction among physically present people, direct interaction is complemented by media (billboards, newsletters, newspapers, television, and radio) and other communications technologies like computers and cell phones. (For specific information on community organizing through the media, see Chapter Seven.)

WOMEN'S HEALTH AND ORGANIZING

The women's health movement of the 1960s and 1970s in the United States was a grassroots movement that challenged medical authority in many aspects of women's health, health access, and health care delivery. Community organizing methods were used to transform women's health knowledge, health politics, and the health care service systems. Women's health organizing was based on interactive reflection linking health status, personal experience, and political processes (Evans, 1980). This type of organizing developed out of the consciousness-raising education genre with the explicit political agenda of reducing women's isolation, building community empowerment, and shifting the site of knowledge creation (Naples, 2002). Through community building, organizing, and education, the women's health movement has addressed many issues, including abortion, battering, rape, and contraception. Movement participants have developed self-help manuals such as *Our Bodies, Ourselves* (Boston Women's Health Book Collective, 1973, 2005) and founded birth centers run by midwives.

Women of color and working-class women have created and sustained numerous protest efforts and organizations to alter living conditions or policies that threaten their families and communities (Gutierrez & Lewis, 1992; Naples, 2002; Stall & Stoecker, 1998). Stall and Stoecker (1998) examine two strains of community organizing distinguished by philosophy (and often by gender) and influenced by the historical division of American society into public and private spheres. Stall and Stoecker compare the well-known Alinsky model, which focuses on communities organizing for power, with what they call the *women-centered model*, which focuses on organizing relationships to build community. The women-centered model cannot be attributed to a single person or movement. Although it has a long history, it has received attention from feminist researchers and organizers only in the past two decades (Barnett, 1993; Gutierrez & Lewis, 1992, Stall & Stoeker, 1998). The model can be traced back to African American women's efforts to sustain home and community under slavery (Davis, 1981) and to the women's health movement (Evans, 1980). In women-centered organizing, power is gained by bringing people together to resolve disputes and build relationships within their own community. The goal of women-centered organizing is empowerment through improvements in women's health, reproductive rights, body awareness, sexual and domestic violence prevention, legislation, and knowledge of their own bodies, and through changes in norms in relationships, sexuality, work, and family (Evans, 1980).

YOUTH ORGANIZING

> Since time immemorial, young people have often been on the front lines
> of social movements, bravely questioning what others merely accepted,
> and energetically demanding—if not always winning—justice, equality
> and freedom.
>
> *—Mohamed & Wheeler, 2001, p. 11*

Youth organizing is an innovative developmental and social justice strategy that trains young people in community organizing and assists them in employing these skills to alter power relations and create meaningful institutional change in their communities (Pintado-Vertner, 2004). Young people are and have long been innovative members of society who can create community change (Checkoway et al., 2003). Despite generally being politically disempowered and denied access to the decision-making process, youth are nevertheless protesting unfair laws, getting school clinics built, defeating curfew laws, changing school curricula to make them more reflective of diversity, and working on environmental justice campaigns (Maira & Soep, 2004). Engaging in social change helps to develop transferable skills, such as writing, public speaking, critical thinking, and improved group skills (Mohamed & Wheeler, 2001). The efforts of this burgeoning youth movement are slowly and systematically being knitted together with inclusive principles and strategies that view youth as producers, contributors, creators, and leaders.

The field of youth organizing is the outgrowth of three important elements: the legacy of traditional organizing models informed by Saul Alinsky, the progressive social movements of the 1960s and 1970s, and the rise of positive youth development (Pintado-Vertner, 2004). Youth organizing pays attention to culture and identity as it studies political systems and structures and values sustained relationships with caring adults and expanded opportunities for youth leadership. Community organizing strategies have particular promise for youth who are negatively affected by racism, sexism, classism, or discrimination based on immigrant status or sexual orientation. Youth from poor and working-class communities of color are particularly likely to conclude they are society's lowest priority; they need only look critically at the neighborhoods in which they live, the buses they ride, the parks they play in, and the schools they attend to draw this conclusion.

Youth can be among our greatest teachers in terms of primary prevention. The process through which youth critically analyze their circumstances and then develop both a personal and a collective response can be deeply empowering (Mohamed & Wheeler, 2001). For example, in Oakland, California, the Environmental Prevention in Communities (EPIC) program effectively involved youth in the process of educating businesses and community organizations to reduce crime and alcohol and tobacco use in Oakland's economically depressed communities. Youth from these affected communities identified an overconcentration of alcohol outlets and advertising in their neighborhoods as a major roadblock to their personal and academic success. EPIC youth organized with community residents, retailers, and city officials to make changes in their community to resolve and prevent alcohol problems (Environmental Prevention in Communities, 2006). Like other youth activists all over the country (Checkoway et al., 2003), they conducted surveys and facilitated workshops in the community. The skills and knowledge learned through activism prepared them to create a youth-initiated prevention campaign. Similarly, the Youth Leadership Institute program YO! Mateo is organizing to ban sale of products from subsidiaries of tobacco companies on high school campuses. These youth organizers want their school district to recognize that the same multinational corporations that sell tobacco products also make huge profits from subsidiaries that sell nontobacco products, including many food items available in high school cafeterias and vending machines (Youth

Leadership Institute, 2006). Such efforts are important not only for their tangible results in schools and communities but also for empowering youth participants, for whom community organizing for social change may become an important lifelong commitment.

CULTURE

Culture includes beliefs, values, attitudes, and behaviors shared by members of a social group or organization. It shapes and is shaped by language, relationships, religion, and material goods. Our perceptions are informed by the cultures we are born into, grow up around, and are socialized by.

Culture affects health, disease, and health care by encouraging certain health behaviors and discouraging others, by providing definitions for personal experience and prescribing idioms of distress, and by providing a social context. Cultural variations across communities are numerous and complex, even within the same ethnic group. To avoid misleading reductionism or stereotypes, it is important to recognize it is impossible to predict the beliefs and behaviors of individuals based on their race, ethnicity, or national origin. In fact, one can never become truly *"competent"* or *"proficient"* in another's culture.

BEYOND CULTURAL COMPETENCE AND CULTURAL PROFICIENCY

The United States is a nation of many cultures; it is a country of immigrants, forced migration, and extermination. It has had policies—responses to immediate needs or political pressures—that are often contradictory and inadequate to cope with the size and diversity of its racial and ethnic populations (Crawford, 2004). In the United States, there are *two languages of race* (Blauner, 2001), one in which members of communities of color see the centrality of race in history and everyday experience and another in which whites see race as a peripheral reality and do not perceive themselves as racist. Omi elaborates,

> Whites tend to locate racism in color consciousness and find its absence in color-blindness. In so doing, they see the affirmation of difference and racial identity among racially defined minority students as racist. Black students, by contrast, see racism as a system of power and correspondingly argue that they cannot be racist because they lack power [2000, p. 257].

In this increasingly multicultural society, issues of culture, race, ethnicity, racism, and privilege are vital to recognize and address when organizing for primary prevention in the community. The concept of cultural competence emphasizes the ability to function effectively with members of different groups through cultural awareness and sensitivity when delivering services to culturally diverse populations. *Competence* implies having the capacity to function effectively as an individual and an organization within the context of the cultural beliefs, behaviors, and needs presented by the community as well as having the ability to foster respectful and effective interactions with people of many cultures (Cross, 1989; Lynch & Hanson, 1998). Within the context of health care, cultural competence is the ability "to recognize and respond to health-related beliefs and cultural values, disease incidence and prevalence, and treatment efficacy" (U.S. Department of Health and Human Services, Office of Minority Health, 2001). Despite widespread interest, cultural competence remains a vaguely defined goal with no explicit criteria established for its accomplishment or assessment (Hunt, 2001). Lindsey, Nuri-Robins, and Terrell (2003) argue that educators and advocates must learn as much as possible about culture and go beyond cultural competence to become culturally *proficient* to meet the needs of our diverse population. They define cultural proficiency as "the policies and practices of an organization or the values and behaviors of an individual that enable the agency or person to interact effectively in a culturally diverse environment" (p. 21). They offer a *cultural proficiency continuum* to illustrate the major concepts (see Figure 4.1). This model has been infused with the notion of cultural humility.

CULTURAL HUMILITY

Whereas cultural proficiency is used to gain awareness of and sensitivity toward others, cultural *humility* emphasizes the need to gain a greater awareness of and sensitivity to one's own worldview and the cultural implications of one's own identity group membership. Cultural humility connotes a deference of one's own cultural beliefs and assumptions, which can be clouded by hegemony and racism. Cultural humility has been described by Tervalon and Murray-Garcia (1998) as a lifelong commitment to self-evaluation and self-critique that redresses power imbalances and develops and maintains mutually respectful, dynamic partnerships based on mutual trust. In this model, the most serious barrier to culturally appropriate care is not a lack of knowledge of the details of any given cultural orientation but the failure to develop self-awareness and a respectful attitude toward diverse points of view and ways of living. Following the principle of cultural humility, community organizers are open and flexible enough to be able to identify the presence and importance of differences between their own orientation and that of each community member—and to explore compromises and possibilities acceptable to both.

Central to cultural humility is the need to develop individual critical reflection skills involving awareness of self and others. Several important elements of critical reflection are necessary when working with diverse communities. The first is an awareness and value of people's strengths and their daily contributions. Rather than viewing people as problems or challenges to tolerate, we must take into account their contributions. These contributions may come in the form of caring for younger siblings, interpretation and translation skills for parents who are not literate or proficient in English, doing housework, mediating with public institutions, or working outside the home (Orellana, 2001).

Figure 4.1 The cultural proficiency continuum

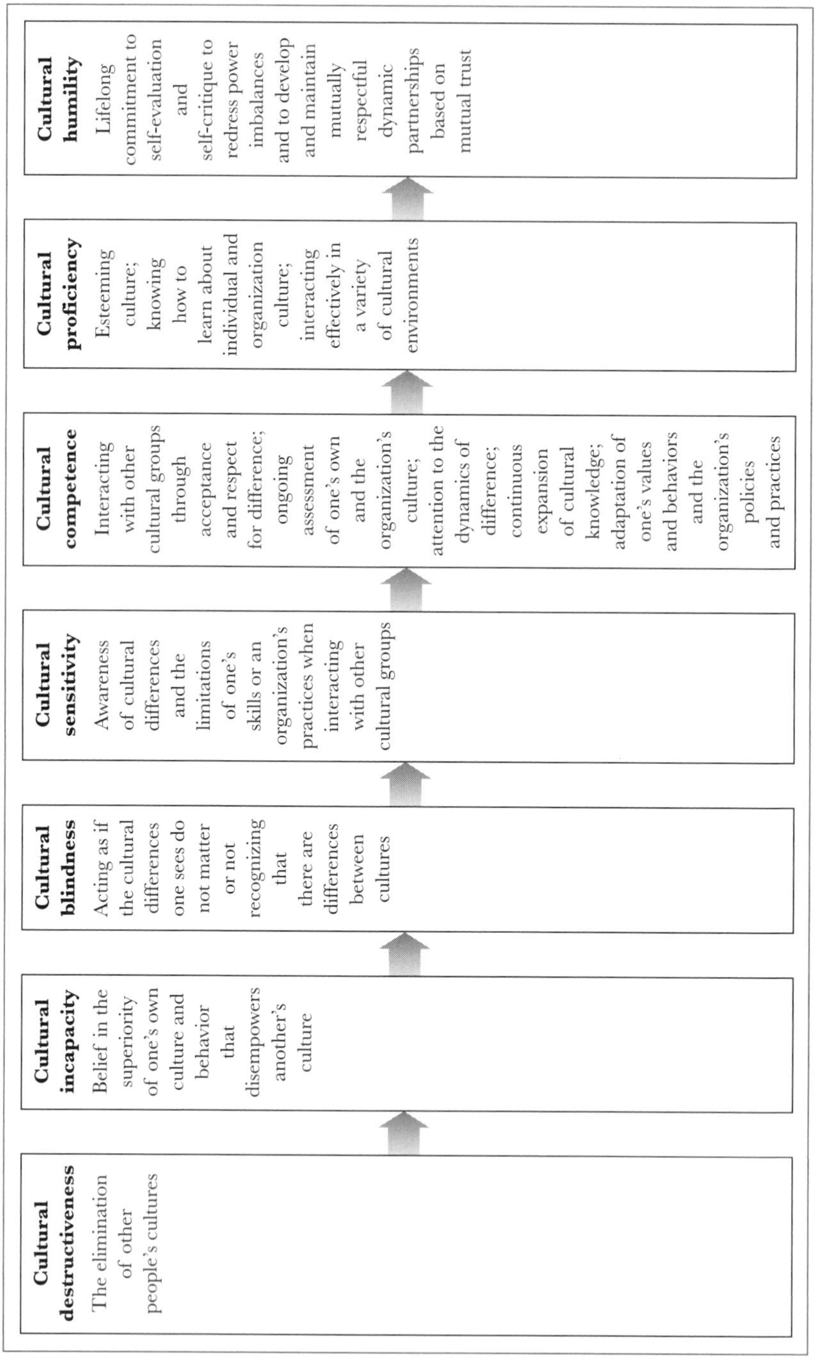

Cultural destructiveness	Cultural incapacity	Cultural blindness	Cultural sensitivity	Cultural competence	Cultural proficiency	Cultural humility
The elimination of other people's cultures	Belief in the superiority of one's own culture and behavior that disempowers another's culture	Acting as if the cultural differences one sees do not matter or not recognizing that there are differences between cultures	Awareness of cultural differences and the limitations of one's skills or an organization's practices when interacting with other cultural groups	Interacting with other cultural groups through acceptance and respect for difference; ongoing assessment of one's own and the organization's culture; attention to the dynamics of difference; continuous expansion of cultural knowledge; adaptation of one's values and behaviors and the organization's policies and practices	Esteeming culture; knowing how to learn about individual and organization culture; interacting effectively in a variety of cultural environments	Lifelong commitment to self-evaluation and self-critique to redress power imbalances and to develop and maintain mutually respectful dynamic partnerships based on mutual trust

Source: Adapted from Lindsey, Nuri-Robins, and Terrell (2003).

A second aspect of critical self-reflection is an understanding of our own diversity. Lum (2003) uses a framework of diversity developed by Schriver (2001) to explore our own understanding of diversity. He asks that organizers be able to articulate their own diversity perspective and worldview (for example, values and beliefs, culture, family, gender, sexual orientation, socioeconomic class, spirituality, ability status, and so on), the intersection between these perspectives (for example, the implications of our membership in multiple groups), and our interrelatedness and interconnectedness to other people (for example, our similarities and differences). Through the examination and exploration of our own multiple identities, we are able to situate ourselves within our world in relation to others and become more aware of our own biases and assumptions.

Finally, in the context of community organizing for social justice, cultural humility entails social transformation. It requires that we move beyond cultural competence toward social justice. Organizing racially and culturally diverse communities is certain to be a difficult task until we act within a framework of social justice. This requires a moral and ethical attitude toward equality and possibility and a belief in the capacity of people as agents who can transform their world. The Brazilian educator Paulo Freire (1970) notes that we must begin by examining the contradictions between our espoused social principles and our lived experience. If we are unable to perceive and resolve social, political, and economic contradictions in our own lives, we will have great difficulty organizing communities to take action toward social justice. In summary, cultural humility in community organizing for prevention and social justice promotes social transformation first through our work to transform ourselves and then through our work to educate and empower others.

THE WHEEL OF COMMUNITY ORGANIZING

The process of community organizing does not happen in predictable steps; nevertheless, the *wheel of community organizing* offers a set of cyclical principles an organizer can use to support the crafting, implementation, and evaluation of comprehensive prevention initiatives. It was developed from the Marin Institute publication *Community Organizing for the Prevention of Problems Related to Alcohol and Other Drugs* (Wechsler & Schnepp, 1993) and applied to teach community organizing and public health at San Francisco State University (Chávez & Turalba, 2006; Chávez, Turalba, & Malik, 2006). The model is based on seven organizing principles: listening, relationships, challenge, action, reflection, evaluation, and celebration. These principles are structured in beginning, middle, and ending phases (see Figure 4.2). They are cyclical in that they are repeated, each time building on assessments of earlier successes, errors, and lessons learned. The wheel provides a map to build an organized community where members are mutually invested in learning from one another. Its framework is not bottom-up, community-based, or grassroots in origin but aims at bottom-up, community-based, or grassroots strengthening as its goal; it promotes

Figure 4.2   The wheel of community organizing

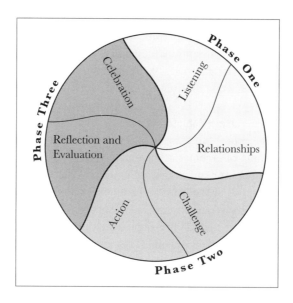

community participation in controlling the decision making for all actions affecting the community as a whole. The main steps are logically linked with each other and to the cycle as a whole. They are all needed. Absence of any one will seriously weaken the wheel's impact.

PHASE ONE

We are trained in a culture that values personal expression and speech more than *listening* (Rosenberg, 2003). Communities are made up of individuals who are often discouraged by a mainstream culture of individualism and mistrust. The strategy of community organizing requires listening not simply with one's ears but with one's heart. Listening with one's heart entails the use of empathy, genuineness, and sincerity. Listening is starting where the people are; it enables the organizer to become familiar with the community, its history, its demographics, its geography, and its political leadership. Entering a community requires listening and learning from norms of the community as well as developing personal relationships. An organizer meets first with people individually, rather than trying to meet everyone in a group to assess community goals. Conversations and information gathering are an important part of this phase of community organizing, as they lay the foundation for the work that comes after. The organizer must learn to hear what community concerns are and find out what community members identify as problems, not tell the community what the problems are. This phase is basic to building trust and promoting community involvement. Outreach includes asking questions, participating in formal community events, and engaging in many casual activities to demonstrate respect and cultural humility. A word of caution: even if organizers attempt to genuinely "start where the people are" (Nyswander, 1956), they may lack access to the *hidden discourse* in a community and misinterpret situations or conversations because of their own lack of cultural competence, lack of access to cultural translators, or lack of self-reflection on the problematic nature of power dynamics between themselves and community members (Chávez, Duran, Baker, Avila, & Wallerstein, 2003; Scott, 1990). Because hidden discourse exists as an inevitable reality between outsiders and insiders—even with the closest of relationships— we must remember to retain our humility in doing this work.

PHASE TWO

What are the challenges faced by the community? What are the root causes of community problems? *Phase Two* requires every organizer not just to answer these questions but to move beyond with action steps and realistic tasks that build on community strengths. Once the group has identified its goals, the organizer's responsibility is to keep the momentum of the group moving forward. One of the most important steps in community organizing practice involves the effective differentiation between *problems*, or things that are troubling, and *issues* the community feels strongly about (Miller, 1985). Once you have moved beyond identifying the problem to defining an issue, you are ready to take action. As Mike Miller (1985) suggests, a good issue must meet several important criteria. It must be winnable to ensure that working on the campaign doesn't simply reinforce fatalistic attitudes and beliefs. It must be simple and specific so that any member of the group can explain it clearly in a sentence or two. It must unite members of the group and involve them in a meaningful way in achieving resolution. It affects many people and is part of a larger plan or strategy that builds community capacity (Minkler & Wallerstein, 2004). An approach to issue selection that has proven especially helpful is the use of Freire's educational strategies to identify the core themes, which in turn generate social and emotional commitment for starting organizing efforts (Carroll & Minkler, 2000; Giroux, 1992; Hope & Timmel, 1984; Shor, 1993; Wallerstein & Auerbach, 2004). Key to this approach is being in touch with community *stakeholders* and operating in partnership with them. Stakeholders include any person or organization with an interest in the action, such as parents, children, customers, owners, employees, associates, and others who can affect or who are affected by achievement of a group's objectives.

PHASE THREE

As the action is designed and implemented, it is important to carefully review progress, ensure it is on track, and evaluate the community organizing efforts, limitations, and contributions. The goal is to understand what went right or wrong and to learn lessons for the future. Reflective questions include the following;

What was accomplished?
What still needs to be done?
What was done well?
What could have been done better?

Finally, every community organizing process ideally concludes with celebration. Celebration helps create a sustainable community. Phil Bartle (2005), in a series of training modules designed for community empowerment, suggests that celebration is more than a public party—it is a ceremony of completion that confirms the legitimacy and appropriateness of community participation and empowerment for social justice. Completion of a community project is an important element of community organizing and community building where the community is publicly recognized for successfully engaging in local action. Project completion also provides an opportunity to start another mobilization cycle. Si Kahn, in *How People Get Power* (1970), notes that as the organizing cycle is completed, the organizer must be sure folks in the community are ready and trained to sustain future efforts. Sustainability needs to be addressed at the start of the organizing effort, continue through capacity-building efforts, and be part of the reflective process.

ESSENTIAL QUALITIES

The cyclical principles at the heart of community organizing are enacted by individuals who possess essential qualities of inclusion, trustworthiness, leadership development, and self-reflection. Community organizers are required to clearly communicate their values, interests, and motivations. They "must constantly examine life, including [their] own, to get some idea of what it is all about, and [they] must challenge and test [their] own findings. Irreverence, essential to questioning, is a requisite. Curiosity becomes compulsive. The most frequent word is 'why?'" (Alinsky, 1971, p. 11). The Marin Institute (2006) notes that not all of us are well suited to be organizers. "Community organizers think strategically about their work while always keeping the final goal in mind and continually making contributions to the goal." The Institute suggests the following qualities go hand in hand with the practice of community organizing:

Imagination
Sense of humor
Organized personality
A free and open mind
A strong sense of self

Blurred vision of a better world
The ability to create something new out of the old

Furthermore, leadership development is a cornerstone of community organizing. As Beckwith (1997) notes, community organization "provides people with a lot of opportunities to practice, to try it out, to learn by doing. A broad team of folks who can lead is built by constantly bringing new people into leadership roles and supporting them in learning from this experience" (p. 8). After years of studying how to develop and sustain community organizations, the W. K. Kellogg Foundation (1995) found that a new kind of leadership is required. The "old structure that exalted control, order, and predictability has given way to a nonhierarchical order in which all individuals' contributions are solicited and acknowledged, and in which creativity is valued over blind loyalty." The Foundation's report identifies the qualities of collaborative leaders, noting they are global thinkers, multiculturally literate, creative and innovative, participative and inclusive, good communicators and networkers, encouraging and supportive, energetic, and adept at using conflict resolution skills.

EMPOWERMENT

As the great Chinese philosopher Lao-tzu noted some 2,600 years ago, "With the best leaders, when the work is done, the task is accomplished, the people will say, 'We have done it ourselves.'"

More than an essential quality of community organizing, *empowerment* is a core value and developmental process that includes building skills through repetitive cycles of action and reflection that evoke new skills and understandings, which in turn provoke new and more effective actions (Kieffer, 1984). Empowerment is a process in which people, organizations, and communities gain mastery over the issues that are important to them (Rappaport, 1987). Empowerment includes the development of self-confidence, a critical worldview, and the cultivation of individual and collective skills and resources for social and political action. Empowerment is a multilevel construct involving "participation, control, and critical awareness" at the individual, organizational, and community levels (Zimmerman, 2000). From a social justice perspective, empowerment has also been defined as having the capacity to identify problems and solutions (Cotrell, 1976), to encourage participatory self-competence in political life (Wandersman & Florin, 2000), and to embody both social change processes and outcomes of transformed conditions (Wallerstein, 2006).

Regrettably, the concept of empowerment has become common political rhetoric with a flexibility of meaning so broad it is in danger of losing its inherent activist roots. At the core of the concept of empowerment is the idea of power, resistance to domination, and social change. Power exists within the context of relationships between people and institutions. Because power is created in relationships, power and power relationships can change. Empowerment is thus a process of change. This is important to recognize when generalizing about what empowerment means cross-culturally. How empowerment translates into other languages raises the question of whether this concept is relevant, meaningful, and portable across cultures (Erzinger, 1994). A broad definition of empowerment highlights the ability to create change on the personal, interpersonal, and political levels. *Power from within* and *power with others* are moral, spiritual, and skill-based sources of power that can constantly expand as people empower themselves. Although empowerment includes the dimension of transferring power to others, the organizer cannot directly empower the community; empowerment is something people do for themselves. Furthermore, organizers must let go of their power and their need to control to make power more available to others.

Empowerment is strengthened by building critical consciousness, or *conscientization*, a concept that comes from Freire (1970). Darder, Baltodano, and Torres (2003) explain conscientization as a process that questions oppression and social privilege, builds empowerment, and works toward social change. They note that Freire developed conscientization to teach illiterate peasants to read by teaching them to "read" their political and social reality. Freire's theory and method of combining community organizing with popular education and community research is basic to the goal of empowerment. His methodology of listening, dialogue, and action strengthens the community organizing cycles of reflection and action (Wallerstein & Auerbach, 2004). Freire's work has been a catalyst worldwide for programs in adult education, health, and community development (Carroll & Minkler, 2000; Hope & Timmel, 1984; Tran et al., 2004; Wallerstein & Bernstein, 1994; Wallerstein & Weinger, 1992). Freire's theories are relevant to community organizers and prevention specialists in the United States as we experience health inequities among communities of color and a growing gap between the rich and poor.

CONCLUSION

The current system of power relations in the United States is unjust and challenging for most people in their quest to lead healthy and fulfilling lives. The problem is systemic, institutional, and also deeply personal. This chapter outlined broad themes of community organizing practice as well as the fundamental purpose of community organizing—to help discover and enable people's shared goals, as informed by values, knowledge, culture, and experience. Examples from women's health and youth organizing perspectives introduced community organizing as a strategy to change the balance of power and create new power bases at local, statewide, or national levels. Effective organizing leads to the levels of community engagement and empowerment that are vital for successful primary prevention efforts targeting environmental determinants of health. Community organizing is about resistance to domination, developing self-awareness and cultural humility, and meeting people where they are. It is activism bringing people together who want to work out common solutions that include the community every step of the way.

DISCUSSION QUESTIONS

1. The text identifies the attributes of community organizing, specifically mentioning Alinksy, who is often credited with leading strikes that led to better health and work conditions for all factory workers. In current events, we see organized community mobilization by students, baseball players, Hollywood writers, nurses, factory employees, and others. Provide a contemporary example that illustrates community organizing strategies to mobilize for healthier conditions.

2. Like Geiger in Mississippi, upstream thinkers are often told, "You can't do that" about a project or program. Can you think of other innovative health-promotion professionals—personal or public—who might have been similarly discouraged? How do you think they responded? How might you productively respond to being told "You can't do that"?

3. What community might you be able to motivate and organize around a health topic you have identified? Using the wheel of community organizing, how might you begin to organize and empower community members?

4. Culture is defined as "beliefs, values, attitudes and behavior shared by members of a social group or organization." The text mentions racial and ethnic populations. Professions can be cultural as well, causing *silos* of different education, language, backgrounds, beliefs, and objectives. Imagine you have been funded to promote health to a youth population through technology. How might you strive to increase your cultural proficiency to better interact with: (1) the technology developers, (2) the funders; and (3) the youth? What aspects of cultural humility might you find to be the most personally challenging?

REFERENCES

Alinsky, S. (1971). *Rules for radicals*. New York: Vintage Books.

Barnett, B. (1993). Invisible southern black women leaders in the civil rights movement: The triple constraints of gender, race, and class. *Gender and Society, 7*, 162–182.

Bartle, P. (2005). *Community empowerment training modules*. Retrieved September 20, 2005, from http://www.scn.org/cmp

Beckwith, D. (with Lopez, C.). (1997). *Community organizing: People power from the grassroots*. Retrieved October 11, 2006, from http://comm-org.wisc.edu/papers97/beckwith.htm

Bellah, R. N., Madsen, R., Sullivan, W. M., Swidler, A., & Tipton, S. M. (1985). *Habits of the heart: Individualism and commitment in American life*. Berkeley: University of California Press.

Blauner, B. (2001). *Still the big news: Racial oppression in America*. Philadelphia: Temple University Press.

Bobo, K., Kendall, J., & Max, S. (1991). *Organizing for social change: A manual for activists in the 1990s*. Santa Ana, CA: Seven Locks Press.

Boston Women's Health Book Collective. (1973) *Our bodies, ourselves: A book by and for women*. New York: Simon & Schuster.

Boston Women's Health Book Collective. (2005) *Our bodies, ourselves: A new edition for a new era*. New York: Simon & Schuster.

Campus Compact. (n.d.). Retrieved May 1, 2010 from http://www.terpimpact.umd.edu/content2 .asp?cid=2&sid=1

Caplan, R., & Rodberg, L. (1994, Fall). Rx: Federal support for community health: An innovative community-based approach to preventive health. *In Context*, p. 58. Retrieved July 25, 2006, from http://www.context.org/ICLIB/IC39/Caplan.htm

Carroll, J., & Minkler, M. (2000). Freire's message for social workers: Looking back, looking ahead. *Journal of Community Practice, 8*, 21–36.

Chávez, V., Duran, B., Baker, Q. E., Avila, M. M., & Wallerstein, N. (2003). The dance of race and privilege in community-based participatory research. In M. Minkler & N. Wallerstein (Eds.), *Community-based participatory research for health* (pp. 81–97). San Francisco: Jossey-Bass.

Chávez, V., & Turalba, R.-A. N. (2006). Pedagogy of collegiality. In J. L. Perry & S. G. Jones (Eds.), *Quick hits for educating citizens* (pp. 26–27). Bloomington: Indiana University Press.

Chávez, V., Turalba, R.-A. N., & Malik, S. (2006). Teaching public health through a pedagogy of collegiality. *American Journal of Public Health, 96*, 1175–1180.

Checkoway et al. (2003). Young people as competent citizens. *Community Development Journal, 38*, 298–309.

Coalition for Civic Engagement and Leadership. (n.d.). Working Definition of Civic Engagement. Retrieved May 1, 2010, from http://www.terpimpact.umd.edu/content2.asp?cid=7&sid=41

Cotrell, L. S. (1976). The competent community. In B. H. Kaplan, R. N. Wilson, & A. Leighton (Eds.), *Further explorations in community psychiatry*. New York: Basic Books.

Crawford, J. (2004). *Educating English learners: Language diversity in the classroom* (5th ed.). Los Angeles: Bilingual Educational Services.

Cross, T. L. (1989). Towards a culturally competent system of care. *A monograph of effective services for children who are severely emotionally disturbed* (Vol. I). Washington, DC: Georgetown University Child Development Center.

Darder, A., Baltodano, M., & Torres, R. (2003). *The critical pedagogy reader*. New York: Routledge.

Davis, A. (1981). *Women, race, and class*. New York: Random House.

Delgado, G. (1987). *Organizing the movement: The roots and growth of ACORN*. Philadelphia: Temple University Press.

Ehrlich, T. (2000). *Civic engagement, civic responsibility, and higher education*. Westport, CT: Oryx Press.

Environmental Prevention in Communities. (2006). Retrieved November 1, 2006, from http://www .marininstitute.org/take_action/epic.htm

Erzinger, S. (1994). Empowerment in Spanish: Words can get in the way. *Health Education Quarterly, 21*(3), 417–419.

Evans, S. (1980). *Personal politics: The roots of women's liberation in the civil rights movement and the New Left*. New York: Vintage Press.

Fairchild, P. (2005). *Community health centers in the United States: Expanding the power of community health centers in rural Indiana*. Retrieved July 25, 2006, from http://www.jsi.com/JSIInternet/ DITL/US/Community_Health_Centers_in_the_United_States.cfm

Fawcett, S. B., Schultz, J. A., Carson, V. L., Renault, V. A., & Francisco, V. T. (2003). Using Internet-based tools to build capacity for community-based participatory research and other efforts to promote community health and development. In M. Minkler & N. Wallerstein (Eds.), *Community-based participatory research for health* (pp. 155–178). San Francisco: Jossey-Bass.

Fellin, P. (2001). Understanding American communities. In J. Rothman, J. L. Erlich, & J. E. Tropman (Eds.), *Strategies of community intervention* (6th ed., pp. 118–133). Belmont, CA: Wadsworth.

Ferris, S., & Sandoval, R. (1997). *The fight in the fields: Cesar Chavez and the farmworkers movement*. Orlando, FL: Harcourt.

Fisher, R., & Romanofsky, P. (1981). Introduction. In R. Fisher & P. Romanofsky (Eds.), *Community organization for social change* (pp. xi–xviii). Westport, CT: Greenwood Press.

Freire, P. (1970). *Pedagogy of the oppressed*. New York: Seabury Press.

Garvin, C. D., & Cox, F. M. (2001). A history of community organizing since the Civil War with special reference to oppressed communities. In J. Rothman, J. L. Erlich, & J. E. Tropman (Eds.), *Strategies of community intervention* (6th ed., pp. 65–100). Belmont, CA: Wadsworth.

Geiger Gibson Program in Community Health Policy. (n.d.). Dr. H. Jack Geiger. Washington, DC: George Washington University, School of Public Health and Health Services, Department of Health Policy. Retrieved October 11, 2006, from http://www.gwumc.edu/sphhs/healthpolicy/ggprogram/ geiger.html

Geiger, H. J. (2005). The unsteady march. *Perspectives in Biology and Medicine, 48*, 1–9.

Giroux, H. *Border crossings*. New York: Routledge, 1992.

Gutierrez, L. M., & Lewis, E. (1992). A feminist perspective on organizing with women of color. In F. G. Rivera & J. L. Erlich (Eds.), *Community organizing in a diverse society*. Boston: Allyn & Bacon.

Herbert, S. (2005). Harnessing the power of the Internet for advocacy and organizing. In M. Minkler (Ed.), *Community organizing and community building for health* (2nd ed.). New Brunswick, NJ: Rutgers University Press.

Hick, S., & McNutt, J. G. (2002). *Advocacy, activism, and the Internet: Community organization and social policy*. Chicago: Lyceum Books.

hooks, b. (1984). *Feminist theory from margin to center*. Boston: South End Press.

hooks, b. (2000). *All about love: New visions*. New York: Perennial.

Hope, A., & Timmel, S. (1984). *Training for transformation: A handbook for community workers*. Gweru, Zimbabwe: Mambo.

Hunt, L. M. (2001, November–December). Beyond cultural competence: Applying humility to clinical settings. *Park Ridge Center Bulletin, 24*, 3–4.

Kahn, S. (1970). *How people get power: Organizing oppressed communities for action.* New York: McGraw-Hill.

Kahn, S. (1991). *Organizing: A guide for grassroots leaders.* Silver Springs, MD: NASW Press.

Kieffer, C. H. (1984). Citizen empowerment: A development perspective. *Prevention in Human Services, 3*, 9–36.

Kretzmann, J. P., & McKnight, J. L. (1993). *Building communities from the inside out.* Evanston, IL: Northwestern University, Center for Urban Affairs and Policy Research.

Labonte, R. (1994). Health promotion and empowerment: Reflections on professional practice. *Health Education Quarterly, 21*, 253–268.

Lindsey, R., Nuri-Robins, K., & Terrell, R. (2003). *Cultural proficiency: A manual for school leaders* (2nd Ed.). Thousand Oaks, CA: Sage Publications.

Lum, D. (2003). *Social work practice and people of color: A process-stage approach* (4th ed.). Belmont, CA: Wadsworth.

Lynch, E., & Hanson, M. (1998). *Developing cross-cultural competence: A guide for working with children and their families.* Baltimore: Brooks.

Maira, S., & Soep, E. (2004). *Youthscapes: The popular, the national, the global.* Philadelphia: University of Pennsylvania Press.

Marin Institute. (2006). *Take action: Community organizing action packs.* Retrieved October 11, 2006, from http://www.marininstitute.org/action_packs/community_org.htm

Martinson, M., & Minkler, M. (2006). Civic engagement and older adults: A critique. *The Gerontologist, 46*, 318–324.

McKnight, J. L. (1995). Regenerating community. In J. L. McKnight, *The careless society: Community and its counterfeits* (pp. 161–172). New York: Basic Books.

Miller, M. (1985). *Turning problems into actionable issues.* San Francisco: Organize Training Center.

Minkler, M. (Ed.). (2004). *Community organizing and community building for health* (2nd ed.). New Brunswick, NJ: Rutgers University Press.

Minkler, M., & Wallerstein, N. (2004). Improving health through community organization and community building: A health education perspective. In M. Minkler (Ed.), *Community organizing and community building for health* (2nd ed., pp. 30–52). New Brunswick, NJ: Rutgers University Press.

Mohamed, I., & Wheeler, W. (2001). *Broadening the bounds of youth development: Youth as engaged citizens.* New York: Ford Foundation & Innovation Center for Community and Youth Development.

Morris, A. D. (1984). *Origins of the civil rights movement: Black communities organizing for change.* New York: Free Press.

Naples, N. A. (2002). The dynamics of critical pedagogy, experiential learning, and feminist praxis. In N. A. Naples & K. Bojar (Eds.), *Teaching feminist activism: Strategies from the field* (pp. 9–21). New York: Routledge.

Norris, T., & Pittman, M. (2000). The healthy communities movement and the Coalition for Healthier Cities and Communities. *Public Health Reports, 113*, 118–124.

Nyswander, D. B. (1956). Education for health: Some principles and their application. *Health Education Monographs, 13*, 65–70.

Omi, M. A. (2000). The changing meaning of race. In N. J. Smelser, W. J. Wilson, & F. Mitchell (Eds.), *America becoming: Racial trends and their consequences* (Vol. 1, pp. 243–263). Washington, DC: National Academy Press.

Orellana, M. F. (2001). The work kids do: Mexican and Central American immigrant children's contributions to households and schools in California. *Harvard Educational Review, 71*(3), 366–389.

Peck, M. S. (1987). *The different drum: Community making and peace.* New York: Simon & Schuster.

Pintado-Vertner, R. (2004). *The West Coast story: The emergence of youth organizing in California.* New York: Funders Collaborative on Youth Organizing.

Prokosch, M., & Raymond, L. (2002). *The global activist's manual: Local ways to change the world.* New York: Thunder's Mouth Press/Nation Books.

Putnam, R. D. (1996). The strange disappearance of civic America. *The American Prospect, 24,* 34–48.

Rappaport, J. (1987). Terms of empowerment/exemplars of prevention: Toward a theory for community psychology. *American Journal of Community Psychology, 15,* 121–148.

Rosenberg, M. B. (2003). *Nonviolent communication: A language of life* (2nd ed.). Encinitas, CA: PuddleDancer Press.

Schriver, J. M. (2001). *Human behavior and the social environment: Shifting paradigms in essential knowledge for social work practice.* Boston: Allyn & Bacon.

Scott, J. C. (1990). *Domination and the arts of resistance: Hidden transcripts.* New Haven, CT: Yale University Press, 1990.

Sen, R. (2003). *Stir it up.* San Francisco: Jossey-Bass.

Shor, I. (1993). Education is politics: Paulo Freire's critical pedagogy. In P. McLaren & P. Leonard (Eds.), *Paolo Freire: A critical encounter* (pp. 25–35). New York: Routledge.

Stall, S., & Stoecker, R. (1998). Community organizing or organizing community? Gender and the crafts of empowerment. *Gender and Society, 12,* 729–756.

Stoecker, R. (2001). Community Development and Community Organizing: Apples and Oranges? Chicken and Egg? In R. Hayduk and B. Shepard (Eds.), *From ACT UP to the WTO: Urban Protest and Community Building in the Era of Globalization.* New York: Verso.

Tervalon, M., & Murray-Garcia, J. (1998). Cultural humility versus cultural competence: A critical distinction in defining physician training outcomes in multicultural education. *Journal of Health Care for the Poor and Underserved, 9,* 17–25.

Tran et al. (2004). Empowering communication: A community-based intervention for patients. *Patient Education and Counseling, 52,* 113–121.

U.S. Department of Health and Human Services, Office of Minority Health. (2001). *National standards for culturally and linguistically appropriate services in health care.* Washington, DC: Author.

Van de Donk, W., Loader, B. D., Nixon, P. G., & Rucht, D. (Eds.). (2004). *Cyberprotest: New media, citizens, and social movements.* New York: Routledge.

Wallerstein, N. (2006). *The effectiveness of empowerment strategies to improve health.* Copenhagen: World Health Organization. Available from http://www.euro.who.int/HEN/Syntheses/empowerment/20060119_10

Wallerstein, N., & Auerbach, E. (2004). *Problem posing at work: Popular educators' guide.* Edmonton: Grassroots Press.

Wallerstein, N., & Bernstein, E. (Eds.). (1994). Community empowerment, participatory education, and health. *Health Education Quarterly, 21,* 141–148.

Wallerstein, N., & Weinger, M. (Eds.). (1992). Special issue: Empowerment approaches to worker health and safety education. *American Journal of Industrial Medicine, 22*(5).

Walters, C. L. (2004) Community building practice: A conceptual framework. In M. Minkler (Ed.), *Community organizing and community building for health* (2nd ed., pp. 66–81). New Brunswick, NJ: Rutgers University Press.

Wandersman, A. H., & Florin, P. (2000). Citizen participation and community organizing. In J. Rappaport & E. Seidman (Eds.), *Handbook of community psychology* (pp. 247–272). New York: Plenum.

Wechsler, R., & Schnepp, T. (1993). *Community organizing for the prevention of problems related to alcohol and other drugs.* San Rafael, CA: Marin Institute.

W. K. Kellogg Foundation. (1995). *Sustaining community-based initiatives: Developing community capacity.* In partnership with The Healthcare Forum. Retrieved November 1, 2006, from http://www.community-wealth.org/_pdfs/tools/cdcs/tool-kellogg-cmty-cap.pdf

World Health Organization (WHO). (1986). *Ottawa charter for health promotion.* Retrieved November 1, 2006, from http://www.euro.who.int/aboutwho/policy/20010827_2

World Health Organization (WHO). (1998). *Health promotion glossary.* Geneva: WHO.

Youth Leadership Institute. (2006). *Prevention.* Retrieved July 28, 2006, from http://www.yli.org/prevention

Zimmerman, M. (2000). Empowerment theory: Psychological, organizational, and community levels of analysis. In J. Rappaport & E. Seidman (Eds.), *Handbook of community psychology* (pp. 43–63). New York: Plenum.

5

Working Collaboratively to Advance Prevention

Larry Cohen
Ashby Wolfe

Sidebar contributors:
Deborah Balfanz,
Soowon Kim, and Ellen Wu

LEARNING OBJECTIVES

- Gain an understanding of the importance of working collaboratively to achieve prevention outcomes.
- Become familiar with the eight steps required to build and maintain an effective coalition.
- Conceptualize each step of the process of coalition building, including how to resolve issues that may cause the coalition to be ineffective.

From the civil rights movement to women's health organizing to environmental justice advances, history is full of examples of the power of collaboration. Collaboration is useful for accomplishing a broad range of goals that reach beyond the capacity of any one individual or organization. This chapter focuses on coalition building, one of the more common forms of collaborative work for achieving preventive health success. A *coalition* is a union of people and organizations working to influence outcomes on a specific issue (see Exhibit 5.1).

EXHIBIT 5.1   COLLABORATIVES AND COALITIONS

Coalitions are affiliations of people or groups with a shared purpose. They are one of various types of group processes. People often use terms like coalition that describe collaborative efforts interchangeably. In this article, the word *coalition* is used in a general sense to represent a broad variety of organizational forms that might be adopted, including any of the following.

- **Advisory committees** generally provide suggestions and technical assistance to an individual or institution but do not make final decisions.
- **Alliances and consortia** tend to be semiofficial membership organizations. They typically have broad policy-oriented goals and may span large geographical areas. They usually consist of organizations and coalitions as opposed to individuals.
- **Commissions** usually consist of citizens appointed by official bodies.
- **Networks** are generally loose-knit groups formed primarily for the purpose of sharing resources and information.
- **Task forces** most often come together to accomplish a specific series of activities, often at the request of an overseeing body.
- **Associations** tend to have a formal structure and are generally formed by professionals or people who have common interests.

As noted by Butterfoss and Francisco (2004), "The pooling of resources and the mobilization of talents and diverse approaches inherent in a successful coalition approach make it a logical strategy for . . . prevention" (p. 108). Sometimes people assume it's *natural* to lead coalitions and take for granted they have the skills needed. But even though coalitions

Portions of this chapter are adapted from *Developing Effective Coalitions: An Eight-Step Guide* by Larry Cohen, Nancy Baer, and Pam Satterwhite, available at http://www.preventioninstitute.org/eightstep.html

are a common and a logical approach to solving a problem, creating a successful coalition can be much more difficult than it might seem. Often groups fail or, perhaps worse, flounder, because of challenges inherent in alliances between organizations and individuals. To avoid this type of experience, which only erodes faith in collaborative efforts, advocates need to sharpen the skills needed to make partnership building more efficient and purposeful.

This chapter addresses ways to build and maintain an effective partnership and common challenges of working in coalitions, including how to engage a diverse and effective membership, how to focus joint efforts on accomplishments, how to create an effective structure, how to develop and strengthen interdisciplinary partnerships, and how to resolve problems, including turf struggles, that can make coalitions ineffective. The information presented here is equally applicable to practitioners and organizations considering initiating and leading a coalition and to anyone participating in—and eager to strengthen—an established coalition.

SMOKING EDUCATION COALITION ACHIEVES A MULTI-CITY POLICY

In 1984, the Contra Costa County, California, board of supervisors and all eighteen city councils in the county adopted uniform multi-city tobacco laws—and became the first multijurisdictional region in the nation to do so. The legislation, which restricted smoking in restaurants, workplaces, and public spaces, represented a powerful victory against the tobacco industry and set the stage for other antismoking milestones. The victory was achieved through an intricate web of resources that only a powerful coalition could secure. Larry Cohen walks us through the process.

While working as director of prevention for the Contra Costa County Health Services Department, I was involved in forming a coalition that brought together local chapters of the American Cancer Society, the American Heart Association, and the American Lung Association, as well as the county health department. In creating the coalition, it became clear there was a lot to learn about how collaboration could be most effective in improving community health.

Since smoking contributes significantly to cancer and to heart and lung diseases, I assumed the aforementioned organizations would be eager to collaborate with one another. I also assumed they would identify policy as a key arena for changing tobacco norms and thus improving health. However, the organizations were not at first the natural partners I imagined they would be. Instead of seeing potential partners and a common goal, each organization viewed the others as competition for the donations it depended on to maintain its staff and services. And when it came to prevention approaches, most of the organizations' notions of prevention were limited to information and education.

Fortunately, organization leaders, reminding one another of the values that brought them to careers in health, were able to set competition aside and find common ground. The basis for our alliance was the need to support a policy proposal that would confront smoking and its deadly health effects. In addition to the policy goal, part of what enabled member organizations to set their competitive fundraising hats aside was the notion that promoting a powerful policy agenda could expand the financial pie instead of leaving only crumbs to fight over. By understanding the objectives of each coalition member organization and by appealing to the organizations' fundraising goals and interest in addressing an alarming health problem, we were able to create sustainably shared interests. Because the county was not interested in fundraising, it was seen as impartial in that sense and thus could credibly play a neutral facilitative role.

We formed the Contra Costa County Smoking Education Coalition. Together we proposed legislation that addressed the dangers of secondhand smoke exposure. One of the first challenges we faced was that a countywide policy doesn't have standing within the boundaries of the cities in that county. Contra Costa County had eighteen cities, some near one another, some contiguous, with many businesses operating in more than one city. We agreed that without a multijurisdictional policy, smoking laws would become hard for both consumers and business owners to comply with. Different policies, or a patchwork with some cities having policies and some not, wouldn't work; countywide success was the key to creating a policy that could be successfully implemented. We began to strategize ways to build support for our initiative.

My naïveté was again revealed by my belief that as a county health official, I would be able to call on city managers to influence their city councils to pass our proposed legislation. I did not know, however, that the apparently common friction between cities and counties over issues like property tax allocations was thriving in Contra Costa County. Furthermore, most cities in the United States (except those that also make up counties) do not see health as a key issue for them. They don't have staff with responsibility for health and are apt to say, "That's the county's responsibility—talk to the county health department." People involved with policy development in the county advised me that my calls to city managers would not have been returned, and even calls from the directors of the cancer, heart, and lung associations might well have been ignored, as such organizations have little influence on city government.

We set out in search of leverage and found that we already had it within our coalition. Board members of the Cancer Society, the Heart Association, and the Lung

Association included influential and involved community members who in many cases also contributed to local politicians' campaigns. Doctors involved in the associations treated local politicians and their families and knew other local politicians through social networks. By taking an inventory of board members and volunteers and their contacts, we were able to widen our support network.

Rather than looking at cities as a whole, the coalition began looking one by one at every member of each city council and considering who would most likely influence them. We identified who on each city council would be most likely to sympathize with our legislation and approached that member first. We figured that a city council member might ignore a call from me, but a call from his or her number-one contributor or his or her father's heart surgeon would almost certainly be returned. And when local media received op-ed pieces and letters to the editor written by local health practitioners, the media were apt to print their ideas.

Also, we identified the relevant skills and resources of each member organization. One was particularly adept at working with the media, another had strong ties to the business community, and some were able to rally their members and volunteers to show up at city halls and support the proposed legislation. As the initiative attracted attention, we received offers of funds and of volunteers, and these were funneled to the three nonprofits. In this way, we maximized our resources and quickly broadened our coalition to include business members, government officers, and other influential members of the community who would have seemed unlikely partners had we not fully appreciated the potential of our member organizations.

Media attention in the cities where legislation was proposed resulted in far more community education than might have been achieved through the use of brochures and also helped perpetuate volunteer involvement. Coordinators dispersed volunteers to various cities. They recruited citizens to sign petitions in support of the legislation or attend their local city council meetings in support of it. Involved community members, including members of the business community who helped counteract the notion that tobacco legislation was anti-business and would damage bottom-line revenues, bolstered our argument. Our coalition was able to garner widespread support. Each city became an impromptu strategy group. Coalition participants in each city figured out what the most important elements for success were in order to garner support and marshal those forces.

Such momentum did not go unnoticed by the tobacco industry. In fact, shortly after our coalition's first meeting, the tobacco industry approached me through its lobbying arm, the Tobacco Institute. The institute's lead lobbyist for the state tried to persuade me over lunch that our coalition should use an educational instead of a policy approach. "We're not opposed to prevention," he said. "Just prevention . . . policy." In fact, the lobbyist offered a lot (for example, resources for other prevention issues and educational materials with my name as the author) and implied that the Tobacco Institute would be happy to give me another job if we stayed away from policy. This was evidence we were on the right track.

As we continued to pursue legislation, the Tobacco Institute opposed it in every jurisdiction, attempting to organize business owners against it, questioning the veracity of our concerns about secondhand smoke, and flying in experts from across the country for media appearances and testimony. We identified clients who lived in the local communities and could speak about the impact of secondhand smoke to them. The industry efforts to parry our coalition failed.

Following the 1984 success, the local cancer, heart, and lung associations brought the collaborative approach to each organization's national offices. The national offices then joined with Americans for Non-Smokers' Rights to end smoking on airlines. Local coalitions prospered across the country, gradually upping their policy goals. In retrospect, it's clear these ordinances had a ripple effect that led to an increase in smoking regulations by all levels of government, a change in smoking norms, and ultimately an improvement in health.

To hear Larry Cohen describe his initial work on tobacco control, please visit YouTube and search for "From Kools to Cancer Sticks: How Quality Prevention Changed Tobacco Norms."

ADVANTAGES OF COALITIONS

Coalitions provide the opportunity to generate broad-based support to improve prevention efforts. They can serve as a forum to share information and resources, to consider a problem from different angles, and to combine forces to resolve it. By bringing together people who may be struggling to achieve the same solution, coalitions minimize duplication of effort and can accomplish objectives beyond the scope of any single organization. They are particularly useful for resolving complex problems. In fact, as the prevention strategist Marshall Kreuter and his colleagues point out, in attempting to solve complex community problems, prevention researchers and public health practitioners must understand that the process involves social, environmental, political, and scientific collaboration (Kreuter, De Rosa, Howze, & Baldwin, 2004). Policy victories (that no group could achieve alone) affect communities and systems and can be made by working together. This unique ability of coalitions to create system-wide changes is of particular importance.

Coalitions can be very beneficial for neighborhood groups when asking for community services or a change in government or corporate practices. Because coalitions are made up of a number of organizations, they tend to be taken more seriously and are often viewed as more credible than individuals. For example, if a city were to slate a local bicycle path for removal, a neighborhood association would be more successful than a lone individual in getting politicians' attention and preventing the path from being removed.

Coalitions can be particularly helpful for disenfranchised communities, which too often have no voice in decisions that affect them. In cases where these communities face the financial and lobbying power of corporations or address government institutions that maintain a bureaucratic *business as usual* approach and ignore neighborhoods with the least clout, collaboration is essential in securing change. As has been shown through environmental justice organizing, collaborations can bring to light the inequities of environmental health decisions, such as the siting of toxic wastes and the placement of factories in neighborhoods where, without organizing, residents would have neither the wealth nor the clout to stop them.

One of the most powerful differences coalitions have made for disenfranchised communities has been to encourage community-based participatory research. Community-based participatory research is built upon the belief the community should have input into the conditions of how research is conducted and shared—and that the community should also benefit from having allowed the research to be done. Traditionally, academic research institutions and government agencies perform studies in low-income communities, eliciting the support of grassroots organizations and other community members. Until residents organized effectively, these opportunities tended to benefit the institutions far more than the communities. Once communities organized into coalitions and began working together, they ensured that community needs were considered and that research done in a community would benefit it.

Coalitions can be valuable to government agencies. Coalitions between agencies allow governmental efforts to be aligned. Different departments of government tend to work in *silos* and have differing backgrounds, beliefs, and objectives. Sometimes this means government agencies can be duplicating efforts or working at cross purposes. But from the broader community perspective, we expect and need our government agencies to operate as one entity working toward a common goal. For example, in violence prevention, health education and justice agencies need to work together. For nutrition-related chronic disease, health education and agriculture must combine efforts. And traffic safety improvements require input from health education, justice, zoning, and planning agencies. The tool known as Collaboration Math (Prevention Institute, 2002) can be particularly helpful in understanding how to meld the objectives and approaches of different disciplines. Partnerships with community groups can help agencies, especially health and human service organizations, better understand community needs and more effectively achieve them.

EIGHT STEPS TO BUILDING AND MAINTAINING AN EFFECTIVE COALITION

Although collaboration is a strategic and beneficial method for prevention efforts, successfully achieving it is a challenge. The eight-step guide presented in Figure 5.1 provides a framework for acknowledging and addressing difficult issues.

These steps are not necessarily meant to be undertaken consecutively or sequentially. Sometimes a situation necessitates that steps be conducted in a different order or even simultaneously. And there isn't always one right direction at each step. The key to an effective approach to coalition design lies in considering each step and having clear reasoning related to each decision.

Most coalitions are developed by, or in any case require, a lead agency to work effectively. This paper is written from the perspective of the lead agency, although every member of a collaborative has responsibility for leadership in helping shape its success. The lead agency convenes the coalition and assumes significant responsibility for its operation. However, the lead agency does not control the coalition. A lead agency should consider carefully the responsibilities of developing and coordinating a coalition, including recognizing the amount of resources necessary to initiate and maintain it and the importance of respecting the differences between the coalition's and the lead agency's perspectives.

Figure 5.1   Developing effective coalitions with the eight-step process

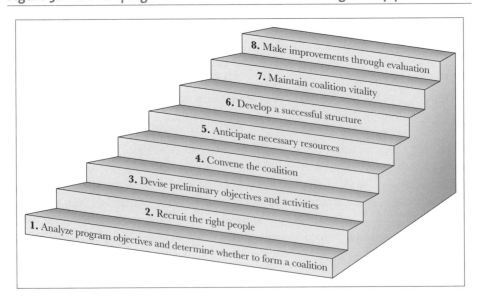

STEP 1: ANALYZE PROGRAM OBJECTIVES AND DETERMINE WHETHER TO FORM A COALITION

Typically, three different situations may cause an organization to consider forming a coalition: (1) the organization recognizes a community need or responds to community leaders' requests to facilitate an effort, (2) the organization recognizes that a coalition will help it fulfill its own goals, or (3) the process of building a coalition is required, for example, by a grant mandate. When deciding whether to form a coalition, a lead agency must first consider whether a coalition is the appropriate tool to serve the organization's needs and if the agency has the resources necessary to support the coalition.

First, the lead agency must clarify the objectives and appropriate activities. A coalition is one of a number of potential tools to get things done. Some tasks are inappropriate for coalitions because they may require a quicker response or an intensity of focus that is difficult to attain with a large group. Coalitions are best used when broad support is needed, a diversity of views is beneficial, or multiple activities are needed to achieve a solution. If improving well-being requires changes in organizational practice, policies, or norms, a coalition is probably essential.

Obviously, it is important to clarify a coalition's purpose, directions, and general methods before approaching potential members. One tool for doing so is the *Spectrum of Prevention*, described in Chapter One. The *Spectrum* is particularly useful for delineating the elements of broad-scale change.

Also, the agency should assess community strengths. In determining the coalition's efforts, it is important to fully assess current activities within the community. This clarifies the viability of the approach. It also generates knowledge about other groups working in similar arenas and locates crossovers or commonalities among interest groups (Action for Healthy Kids, 2003). Before initiating a coalition, it is important to determine if related partnerships already exist within the community. There are times when it will be far more effective to participate in an existing group with compatible goals than to form a new coalition.

It is valuable to determine the costs and benefits to the lead agency. Lead agencies tend to underestimate the requirements needed to keep coalitions functioning well, especially the commitment of substantial staff time. Coalitions also require significant commitment from the members, who must frequently weigh coalition membership against other important work.

STEP 2: RECRUIT THE RIGHT PEOPLE

"The main factor in unproductive business meetings is . . . having the wrong people present," says Lynn Oppenheim (as cited in Goleman, 1988). The makeup of a coalition's membership should be determined on the basis of its overall goals. Most coalitions should have members representing multiple sectors and points of view; however, coalitions with less diverse membership may communicate and work more quickly because members' objectives may be more alike. Less diverse coalitions may be weaker in their ability to comprehend factors that contribute to the problem that lies beyond the purview of their member organizations. When coalitions are performing community-oriented work, it is important that the coalition's membership reflect the community it serves. "Meaningful local-level engagement ensures the greatest relevance and appropriateness of programs for people affected and establishes essential ingredients for sustained collaboration" (Kreuter et al., 2004, p. 448). Those with the greatest stake in the community outcomes are likely to be highly effective in ensuring that collaboration serves the goals of the community, rather than the interests of one discipline or constituency.

As discussed previously, coalitions are one of the premier ways that disfranchised groups, largely ignored by interest groups and elected officials, can have a voice. Not only is the input of these groups valuable to advocates outside of their communities it provides group members with a sense of ownership and involvement.

Of course, not all coalitions are community-focused. For example, a statewide or national group might come together to develop a plan to address inequities in health. But if a coalition isn't diverse in every way (for example, ethnicity, class, and types of discipline) it should at minimum have considered the value of such diversity and be clear about the reasons it is taking another path.

The following are matters a lead agency should consider in recruiting coalition members.

Organizations
Start by identifying organizations that already work on the identified issue and look broadly for other organizations that should be involved. Consider those who have influence, those who will be supportive, and even those who may put obstacles in the coalition's path.

Individual Members
Many coalitions welcome individuals who aren't affiliated with organizations. These individuals may be community members, community leaders, or people who have directly experienced the problem. It is a good idea to include individual members (unless there is a reason not to) because they can perform functions other coalition members may not easily be able to perform. Since they are speaking for themselves and not for a larger organization, individual members may be perceived by the media as having less of a vested interest and therefore more credibility. In addition, individual members can provide advice and outreach from a different and perhaps more personal perspective. In one adolescent health coalition, a woman who had herself become pregnant as a teen was an effective spokesperson for legislative hearings and meetings with the press.

Competitors and Adversaries
Whether to include potential competitors and adversaries should be based on the sincerity of their commitment to the coalition's goals, how willing they might be to reconsider some of their positions, and whether they would be more of an impediment to the coalition if

excluded. For example, one violence prevention coalition did not allow a gun manufacturing company to join its coalition because the work of the company directly opposed the objectives of the coalition to reduce firearm use. However, the coalition did allow a toy company to join the coalition in the hopes the coalition's efforts would encourage the company to produce alternatives to toy guns.

Keep in mind that a coalition must get things done; it isn't just a forum for discussion. Although engaging adversaries seems appealing, it can result in a very rapid drop-off of current members.

Representatives of Organizations

Having identified key organizations, consider who will best represent each organization on the coalition. Agency directors are often more effective than line staff at making policy decisions and establishing credibility as coalition representatives. On the other hand, line staff might be more committed, enthusiastic, and available than top leaders and are often more in touch with the issues related to *hands-on* service delivery. Often participation by a mix of top leadership and line staff is best for achieving coalition goals. Of course, organizations must make their own decisions about who represents them but are often responsive to suggestions.

Membership Size

Consider the desired number of organizations and the diversity of membership when selecting organizations to approach about joining the coalition. The coalition's goals and objectives are an important consideration in deciding membership size. As size gets larger (beyond about fourteen members), approaches to the work need to become more structured (as through the creation of subcommittees), less formalized, and facilitation of meetings requires greater skill.

BUILDING MULTICULTURAL COALITIONS

Ellen Wu

Building coalitions with a diverse membership, particularly among varying racial and ethnic populations, poses unique challenges. These coalitions are faced with issues intrinsic to coalition building and additionally charged with bringing together individuals and organizations with divergent histories, a legacy of being resource poor and disenfranchised, and a greater potential for interracial tension. Therefore, building multicultural coalitions should be given care, time, and transparency.

The cornerstone of multicultural coalition building is developing and maintaining relationships. Although prioritizing relationships can be challenging, it establishes a culture for the coalition that affirms the value of collective work.

A foundation of trust and transparency allows coalitions to weather hardships and effectively catalyze social change.

The California Pan-Ethnic Health Network (CPEHN) is a direct example of the power behind inclusive, cross-cultural partnerships. Formed in the aftermath of the riots in response to the Rodney King verdict, four ethnic organizations came together to form CPEHN with the shared vision of creating a unified voice to advocate for the health of communities of color. Currently the only multicultural health advocacy organization in California, much of CPEHN's success rests on creating and working with coalitions. A recent and most notable example, Having Our Say, co-founded by CPEHN in 2007, has a membership of over fifty communities of color organizations advocating for health care reform that works for everyone. It is from this wealth of experience that we present strategies for building effective multicultural coalitions.

Build Relationships

Although you might want to jump right into work, it is vital you carve out time for relationship building. For example, open each meeting with an icebreaker to foster cross-cultural understanding and help members connect with each other. During the lifespan of a coalition, there will be confounding issues, conflicting agendas, and difficult decisions to be made. A coalition can overcome these obstacles if it ensures a safe space where members can openly disagree, discuss, and process. For productive, honest conversations, create a space where people feel safe and are heard. This is especially crucial for supporting cross-cultural dialogues.

Build Capacity

A coalition is only as strong as its weakest members. Communities of color organizations that have been traditionally underfunded and understaffed may lack the capacity to do the work the coalition needs of them. If lead organizations and other coalition members reach out and help build their partner's capacity by assisting with events and activities or by identifying funding opportunities and providing trainings, these partnerships can help bring more strength and diversity to your movement. In addition to increasing the breadth of organizations able to participate, capacity building and active partnering between coalition members will benefit the coalition as a whole and create cohesion.

Share Resources

As a coalition, consider who will receive the majority of funding for the work and identify opportunities to share resources. For example, the Having Our Say coalition provides subcontracts to members to recognize the value of their participation and spends money on shared outreach efforts to advance the coalition's policy goals.

Remaining funds support the coalition overall, such as to cover meeting expenses. Creating a structure that shares resources can diffuse tensions and validate the value of each member's contributions.

Create Consensus

Too often communities of color do not feel their voices are heard. It is important that these feelings are not perpetuated in the coalition's work. Coalitions need to move forward in making decisions and taking policy positions, but not at the expense of members who are uncomfortable with doing so. A successful coalition invests the time to talk with individual members and thoroughly understand each other's perspectives. With adequate engagement and discourse, coalitions can often reach consensus on how to proceed.

Conduct Purposeful Recruitment

When recruiting representatives from various racial and ethnic organizations, be cautious that representatives do not become *tokens*. During recruitment, assess the interest, availability, and capacity of organizations to participate in the coalition. Have an honest conversation about what they can offer the coalition, and about what the coalition has to offer them.

Honor Diverse Communication Styles and Languages

Honoring different communication styles is key to the success of diverse coalitions. For example, consider the needs of members for whom English is their second language. Address their needs by adding extra time to the agenda, providing an interpreter, and translating documents. The coalitions should explicitly commit resources to address these needs.

STEP 3: DEVISE PRELIMINARY OBJECTIVES AND ACTIVITIES

In Step 1, the lead agency's objectives were examined in determining whether a collaborative was needed. It is important to meld these objectives with the objectives of other members and with the interests of stakeholders in the community whose goals generally fit with coalition objectives. Defining coalition goals and objectives and determining how to implement them requires the inclusion of all coalition members in discussions. Therefore, the lead agency will need to broaden and modify its objectives. A written mission statement can be a useful tool to achieve clarity about coalition goals. However, it is important to avoid getting too bogged down in semantics early in the life of a coalition.

In some cases, coalition objectives or activities may be at cross purposes with those of an individual organization. Based on these cross purposes, one or another organization may elect not to participate in the coalition. It is important to anticipate these issues before they arise and try to design win-win situations.

Melding Objectives of Member Groups

Although some coalitions arise with a number of commonalities among the member organizations, each member organization usually has its own varying goals. It is important to create options that satisfy the goals of other coalition members and community partners and to structure both objectives and activities in such a way that other coalition members feel included in the decision-making process. The central mission of the coalition must fit both its own primary objectives and the overall community goals (Action for Healthy Kids, 2003). An example of this is the Harm Reduction Coalition, a group of individuals and agencies concerned with the lack of effective and respectful services for active drug users, particularly those underserved by traditional social and medical services: youth, women, people of color, and people living in poverty. Although members may vary in their ultimate goals, they share a belief in harm reduction, a set of practical strategies that reduce the negative consequences of drug use and that range from safer use to managed use to abstinence.

Coalition Goals, Objectives, and Activities

When dealing with long-term objectives over time, it is important to identify some objectives and activities that can be addressed by all member organizations more immediately. Activities that parallel stakeholder interests will reinforce commitment to the coalition and may garner further community support. These activities increase members' motivation and pride and also enhance coalition visibility and credibility. However, always keep the long-range objectives clearly in mind. "Far too often . . . the effectiveness of a coalition decreases as the breadth of its agenda increases" (Black, 1983, p. 266). Activities should be well-defined, should meet the needs of participating organizations, and should make use of the skills of coalition representatives.

In some cases, broad goals can be accomplished best by joint activities with other coalitions rather than by a single coalition. For example, a traffic safety coalition, a sexual violence prevention coalition, and an alcoholism prevention forum could join together on a media campaign focusing on the norms promoted through alcohol billboards. Although regular meetings of all of the coalitions in one broad group might prove unwieldy to the members, it can be in everyone's interest to work cooperatively on a specific issue.

Bear in mind that what keeps a coalition going is the commitment of the individual representatives and the support of the organizations they represent. Coalition members come to meetings with their own perspectives, interests, and approaches. In general, the more directly coalition activities relate to and resonate with the specific values and objectives of the participants—and the more each member is able to enjoy and be proud of his or her individual participation and contributions—the more the coalition will flourish.

STEP 4: CONVENE THE COALITION

Before convening the coalition for the first time, carefully select and talk with potential members to determine their individual goals and goals for the coalition. This way, conveners will have a good idea beforehand of how the first meeting will turn out. At the first meeting, the lead agency should clearly define the purpose of the coalition. In addition, the invited organizations and their representatives should have a chance to introduce themselves, state what they see as their role in the coalition, and consider what their organization's interest is in participating in the coalition. Potential members should be given an opportunity to define what they perceive as the purpose and goals of the coalition and to recommend others they think should be involved. Of course, not all potential members will find the coalition worth their time and energy. Two determinants will be the specific activities the coalition chooses to undertake and the worth of the coalition as seen by the management of the member organizations.

STEP 5: ANTICIPATE NECESSARY RESOURCES

Effective collaboratives generally require minimal financial outlay for materials and supplies but substantial time commitments from people. The most successful coalitions "take the time to build relationships, mobilize the community and personally visit the key players." (Wolff, 2001, p. 176). The ability to allocate considerable staffing to these and additional pursuits is one of the most important considerations for organizations providing coalition leadership.

Some of the specific resources coalition leaders should anticipate include clerical needs; meeting planning, preparation, and facilitation; member recruitment, orientation, and encouragement; research and data collection; and participation in activities and projects.

It is important to recognize that coalition members' time is their most valuable contribution. Commitments are sometimes made in response to the enthusiasm of the meeting and seem less realistic when members return to their regular jobs. At other times, coalition members will fulfill their commitments but may resent the extra work. Periodic discussions about members' resources, support, and time limitations can minimize potential problems. Members should never be pressured to do more than they are comfortable doing. The more the coalition's objectives complement those of its member agencies, the less member time will seem like *extra* work.

STEP 6: DEVELOP A SUCCESSFUL STRUCTURE

The technical details, or *anatomy*, of the coalition's structure are vital to achieving success. As with other coalition considerations, it is important to have well-developed ideas and the flexibility to allow for input and modifications by coalition members. Six key structural issues are coalition life expectancy; meeting location, frequency, and length; membership parameters; decision-making processes; meeting agendas; and participation between meetings. There are no set rules about how a coalition should be structured, but each of these six elements should be implemented thoughtfully. In all areas of coalition anatomy the same rules apply: minimize complications, maximize relevance to the objectives of the group, and encourage participation.

Coalition Life Expectancy

The coalition's goals should dictate its longevity. Although an open-ended time frame may seem attractive to the lead agency, member organizations and their representatives often prefer coalitions with a specific life expectancy; such coalitions achieve more, more quickly. When long-standing credibility is a vital goal, an ongoing coalition might be needed.

Meeting Location, Frequency, and Length

To promote an atmosphere of equal contribution, consider holding coalition meetings on neutral territory, such as in the local library. Rotating the meeting to different members' sites can add interest, although meetings may be delayed if people get lost or confused by ever-changing locations. Setting up conditions for thoughtful discussion and comfort and ensuring that people face one another (in other words, being attentive to the geography of the room) is essential to achieving success.

TENSION OVER TURF

Turf struggles are a common threat to coalition vitality and success. Peck and Hague (2003) have defined *turfism* as noncooperation or conflict between organizations with seemingly common goals or interests. There are three types of turf struggles.

Coalition member versus coalition member. Conflict between coalition members can reflect historical tensions between their organizations.

Coalition member versus coalition. As a coalition gains visibility and starts to apply for funding, conflict can develop between individual coalition members and the coalition as a whole because of the increased competition for resources.

Members versus lead agency. Lead agencies can sometimes benefit most from the work of the coalition, leading to tension among the members who see the lead agency acquiring the resources and recognition that result from the contribution of all coalition members.

Too often we expect self-sacrifice from individuals and organizations as they move toward coalition solutions. Instead of instructing members to "leave turf at the door," a more realistic approach acknowledges that turf issues will challenge the group and blends the pursuit of individual interests with the greater goals of the coalition. Coalition leadership can sometimes anticipate turf battles and make preemptive moves to avoid them. Following are techniques that coalition leaders can use to illuminate turf struggles by bringing attention to some of the problems with the coalition and to limit the negative impact of turf squabbles:

Acknowledge potential turf issues. Choose coalition representatives whose job descriptions and personalities make them less influenced by the past.

Talk details. Encourage coalition members to openly discuss their reasons for being at the table and share information about their respective organizations at the initial coalition meeting.

Shape collective identity. Develop opportunities to fulfill the needs for recognition among members and foster a sense of collectivity.

Make fair decisions. Create a clearly stated decision-making policy in conjunction with coalition members to develop consensus when possible and ensure fairness.

Seek funding for coalition coordination. Secure outside funding to help alleviate internal pressure for resources and develop a plan for how resourced needs will be shared, acquired, and distributed.

Reward members and celebrate successes. Acknowledge the accomplishments of the coalition to inspire and motivate members.

Build bridges. Maintain an environment that fosters trust, respect, and amicability among coalition members through a friendly tone, small workgroups, and after-meeting socializing.

Remind participants of the big picture. If turf issues arise, make space in a meeting where an objective coalition member dedicated to the coalition's cause, such as a survivor, youth, or faith leader, can reinvigorate coalition members.

Make struggles overt. Acknowledge that conflict exists and discuss potential causes so that it does not fester and drain the vitality of a coalition.

Encourage flexibility. Create an open environment where members feel comfortable with diverse perspectives and with conflict.

Source: Adapted from Cohen & Gould (2003).

Meeting frequency can affect the commitment of the membership as well. Other than an impromptu emergency situation—such as a legislative deadline—coalitions typically should not meet more frequently than once a month.

Membership Parameters

Coalition members must play a role in decisions about the extent to which new members will be invited and how defined or open the membership should be. In many cases, a compromise solution in which certain people are recruited and encouraged but virtually no one is excluded is best. More formalized membership procedures may become an issue when and if the coalition wishes to make public statements or endorse policy measures; otherwise, less formal procedures are preferable.

Decision-Making Processes

Miller (1983) identifies good decision-making procedures as key to coalition success. He recommends establishing a specific decision-making process before problems occur. "You cannot count on stamina," he writes. "Make clear early in the life of the coalition . . . how decisions are going to be made" (p. 49). Decisions can be made by consensus. Research on community-based coalitions has suggested that this process reduces impulsive decision making and improves stakeholder participation (Snell-Johns, Imm, & Wandersman, 2003). However, this process can become unmanageable. To avoid this, define consensus as an approach the majority supports and others can live with. Health-based coalitions are usually happy to relinquish some of the detailed decision making in exchange for simplicity and reasonable results. There will be cases in which consensus cannot be reached and the group must either vote or accept there will be no action on a certain issue. Sometimes having the group clarify in advance the kinds of issues that are charged (grants, turf, or legislation, for example) will help avoid problems later.

Meeting Agendas

One of the most important ingredients for an effective coalition is a good meeting agenda. It gives participants, especially new ones, a road map and lets them know where they can best fit in. A clear and reasonably consistent agenda, which may be modified by those present at the beginning of the meeting, can reinforce the coalition's purpose and foster collaboration. The skill of keeping to the agenda but being flexible and open to new ideas is a vital one in maximizing meeting success.

Participation Between Meetings

Successful coalitions often have subcommittees that carry out coalition activities. Unless coalition objectives are closely related to the objectives of the membership, it is not wise to expect more than a few hours of additional commitment between meetings. It may be helpful to encourage the most active and strategic participants in the coalition to form a steering committee, which provides leadership by discussing long-range goals and the tactics to achieve them. A steering committee often works well as an informal open body.

STEP 7: MAINTAIN COALITION VITALITY

Building an effective coalition includes articulating a vision, establishing adequate structure, developing leadership opportunities, and making significant commitment to community diversity (Bandeh, Kaye, Wolff, Trasolini, & Cassidy, 2003). Leadership in coalition building requires knowing not only how to create a coalition structure but also how to recognize the warning signs of problems that may arise. It is important for leaders to work hard at maintaining the vitality and enthusiasm of the coalition. By responding to potential problems as they emerge, however, the vitality of the coalition can be maintained. The following activities are important for maximizing coalition vitality.

Addressing Coalition Difficulties

One clear indication a coalition is having difficulties is a decline in coalition membership. This may be due to multiple factors, including conflicts of interest, overlapping efforts, and role confusion, all of which may lead to the loss of collective voice within a coalition (Weed, n.d.). Although earlier warning signs are less obvious, they might appear as repetitious meetings or as meetings that consist primarily of announcements and reports, meetings that become bogged down in procedures, significant failures in follow-through, ongoing challenges of authority or battles between members, lack of member enthusiasm, or an unacceptable drain on lead agency resources. Turf struggles are perhaps the most commonly identified explanation when vitality sags.

Kreuter and colleagues note that a high failure rate of coalitions suggests that problems are not well anticipated, nor are they skillfully resolved once they occur (Kreuter, Lezin, & Young, 2000). Therefore, it is crucial to maintain open communication among the members so that problems surface quickly. Although the lead agency will not always be able to overcome coalition challenges, effective management of the problem is an essential first step. In fact, all that may be needed is a breaking down of current activities into smaller, more achievable tasks. It may be necessary to revisit the original objectives of the coalition and modify them to more accurately reflect the current atmosphere (Action for Healthy Kids, 2003). It is the lead agency's responsibility to bring identified problems to the attention of coalition members and to encourage collaborative solutions. The most valuable source of information about negative coalition conditions is input from the coalition members themselves. People who are no longer attending or who have left the coalition are important sources of input as well.

Sharing Power and Leadership

Many coalition members will readily defer power to the lead agency to facilitate smooth functioning. However, if the coalition solidifies as an independent entity and develops a body of work it performs or creates collectively, members will expect greater involvement in decision making. It is at this point the coalition becomes a more independent group and requires less guidance from the lead agency. Ironically, the characteristics that indicate a strong coalition—a heightened sense of collective identity and a high degree of interest in and commitment to work that is developed collaboratively—can also exacerbate tensions in defining the direction of the coalition. It is important to deal with these issues directly. Negotiating issues of a power imbalance in decision making, especially when a coalition has achieved this state of maturity, calls for sensitivity and may require setting aside extra time to clarify.

New energy is often needed to restore a coalition. One way to achieve this is to recruit new members. Membership changes are to be expected. New members add energy and enthusiasm to the coalition's ongoing activities. Attention must be paid to ensure they are welcomed and oriented to fulfill vital coalition functions. Other ways to promote renewal include to provide training and to bring challenging, new ideas to a group.

Celebrating and sharing successes may be the most important step in maintaining morale. Everyone needs a sense—and reminders—that the coalition is playing a vital role in addressing the problem. Acknowledgment of success, however small, is a key to maintaining the vitality and motivation of the coalition (Action for Healthy Kids, 2003). Keys to boosting coalition morale can include implementing effective activities that result in tangible outcomes, giving coalition members credit for coalition successes, and celebrating short-term successes with publicity or awards.

STEP 8: MAKE IMPROVEMENTS THROUGH EVALUATION

Evaluation should be an ongoing process throughout the life of a coalition. Indeed, the success of the coalition can hinge on the evaluation process. According to Butterfoss and Francisco, "evaluation must be performed [to demonstrate] a sustainable infrastructure and purpose, programs that accomplish their goals, and measurable community impacts" (2004, p. 113). Evaluating a coalition can lead to changes in the coalition's approach. In addition, evaluation can increase the coalition's effectiveness and can ensure the community and participants benefit from the coalition's activities. Taking the time to evaluate the effectiveness of coalition efforts is a way of acknowledging that the skills and contributions of coalition members are important. Honest reflection also ensures that the coalition grows from its experiences, regardless of the programmatic outcome. The results, if positive, can also help the coalition improve its reputation in the community and can be included in future resource development proposals. Furthermore, when a coalition modifies its efforts to eliminate problems pinpointed by an evaluation, the coalition's credibility can improve significantly.

Coalitions can employ two basic types of evaluations, formative and summative. *Formative evaluations* focus specifically on the coalition's process objectives. For example, a coalition may want to encourage the media to promote a particular goal. A formative evaluation would analyze the process by which the coalition attempted to achieve this goal. The results of formative evaluations help staff and members improve the functioning of the coalition.

Summative evaluations help coalition members determine whether or not the coalition's strategies resulted in the desired consequences. The answers to summative evaluation questions help coalition members make strategic decisions about strengthening promising interventions and discontinuing ineffective ones. Coalitions often move in unexpected directions, and it is important to recognize that what may at first have been unintended consequences are in fact significant outcomes. Also, there is a tendency to just evaluate what the coalition as a whole has accomplished, but often new initiatives and new partnerships emerge from different dyads and triads whose relationships become more solidified through the coalition.

Coalition evaluation is an emerging field and is much more demanding than simply determining if a program is effective. Because coalitions aim in many cases to achieve multifaceted environmental change, changes are harder to see and the coalition's role in them is difficult to measure. To ensure that evaluators advance the important work collaboratives are engaged in requires melding existing evaluation skills with a new way of thinking.

YMCA AS A CONVENER IN HEALTHIER COMMUNITIES INITIATIVES

Soowon Kim and Deborah R. Balfanz

To combat the growing obesity and chronic disease epidemics, communities have taken strides to make healthier lifestyles more attainable. Unfortunately, the full potential of these changes often is not reached, as the various sectors of the communities lack a mechanism through which they can combine their separate efforts.

In an effort to bring existing community efforts together and to launch new efforts, the YMCA of the USA (Y-USA) embarked on a community initiative in 2004 called Pioneering Healthier Communities (PHC), as part of its larger "Activate America" initiative. PHC focuses on environmental and policy changes to implement prevention efforts at the community level and is supported by the Centers for Disease Control and Prevention (CDC) and corporate and foundation donors. By 2009, approximately 100 communities were participating in PHC.

Given YMCA's wide reach of 10,000 communities and 21 million members, local YMCAs are positioned to play a key role as a convener in community initiatives. PHC involves high-level community leaders at every step, capitalizing on their diverse assets, resources and skills, and leveraging their positions and influence to make changes within their organization and within the greater community.

PHC convenes leaders from sectors that include public health departments, city and state governments, transportation officials, educational leaders, local businesses, charitable foundations, hospitals, health insurers, faith-based organizations, and academics. Together, these leaders promote the planning and implementation of evidence-based strategies that influence policies and environmental changes to support healthy living.

PHC engages communities of various sizes and settings (urban, suburban, rural) and geographic diversity; special effort is made to reach low-income, underserved, racial and ethnic minority populations. To sustain a long-term commitment and to broaden impact, the initiative emphasizes policy and environmental changes more than programming. Although YMCAs serve as conveners, efforts are made for local initiatives to grow organically with strategies specific to their own particular needs.

Some communities are using the innovative Community Healthy Living Index (CHLI) to assess and improve their community's environment and policies. CHLI covers five major venues where people live, work, learn, and play: schools, after-school child care sites, work sites, neighborhoods, and the community-at-large. The assessment, convened by a local YMCA, guides community-driven and community-focused efforts to improve opportunities for healthy living. It not only assesses the environment, it provides mechanisms to mobilize all sectors and implement community plans for sustainable changes.

If working in isolation, a community's efforts might have been overwhelmed by its unique challenges. Because PHC draws upon the experience of leaders from multiple sectors, community efforts have improved chances for success. Achievements in environmental and policy changes as a result of the initiative are abundant and include the following:

- Providing all students adequate opportunities for physical activity before, during, and after school
- Influencing worksite policies
- Increasing healthy food choices in restaurants, grocery stores, work sites, schools and other community settings
- Increasing the locations and hours of farmers' markets
- Making fresh vegetables, fruits, and community gardens more accessible for community members
- Influencing complete street policies, such as those that impact the availability of sidewalks and countdown cross signals
- Reducing disparities in health and increasing opportunities for physical activity and healthy eating in low-income communities

Following the successful implementation of PHC, two new community initiatives have been launched: (1) Action Communities for Health, Innovation and EnVironmental ChangE (ACHIEVE), launched in 2008 and funded by the CDC; and (2) Statewide PHC, launched in 2009 and funded by the Robert Wood Johnson Foundation. YMCAs in nearly 50 states are facilitating community health improvements through collective collaborative efforts called the Healthier Communities Initiatives.

These initiatives not only provide opportunities for residents to engage in a healthier lifestyle but also strengthen the bonds between community residents and organizations as they come together to improve health. This process allows for coalition building and attracts a new set of volunteers to the effort to build healthy communities, thus increasing the community's ability to influence policy and environmental changes that prevent illness and encourage healthy living. These local communities, empowered with proven strategies and models, have been successful in making positive and sustainable changes that support healthy living in their community environments.

CONCLUSION

Widespread and lasting change is difficult for any organization to achieve alone. Major improvements require a variety of resources and perspectives, and health leaders increasingly recognize that improving community health requires a new way of working that not only gives direction but also engages in and facilitates partnership.

Virtually every carefully crafted coalition will have an impact. "An effort may fail, then partially succeed, then falter, and so on," explains Brown. "Since mutual trust is built up over a period of time, coalition organizers should avoid getting so caught up in any one effort as to view it as 'make or break.' Every effort (at cooperation among groups) prepares the way for greater and more sustained efforts in the future" (1984).

DISCUSSION QUESTIONS

1. What elements are important to consider in recruiting members to a new or existing coalition? How can you ensure the right players are at the table?
2. How might you apply the eight-step process to a coalition you are currently involved in?

3. If you became the lead in an existing coalition that seemed unproductive and if it seemed the current members were not collaborating, what would you do? Why?

4. Once mission, goals, and objectives are identified for a coalition, can they be changed? Why or why not.

REFERENCES

Action for Healthy Kids. (2003). *Coalition building: Tips and techniques*. Skokie, IL: Action for Healthy Kids. Available in hard copy from Action for Healthy Kids at (800) 416–5736.

Bandeh, J. G., Kaye, T., Wolff, S., Trasolini, A., & Cassidy, A. (2003). *Developing community capacity. Module 1: Sustaining community-based initiatives*. Battle Creek, MI: W. K. Kellogg Foundation and The Healthcare Forum.

Black, T. R. (1983). Coalition building: Some suggestions. *Child Welfare, 62*, 263–268.

Brown, C. R. (1984). The art of coalition building: A guide for community leaders. New York: American Jewish Committee.

Butterfoss, F. D., & Francisco, V. T. (2004). Evaluating community partnerships and coalitions with practitioners in mind. *Health Promotion Practice, 5*, 108–114.

Cohen, L., & Gould, J. (2003). *The tension of turf: Making it work for the coalition*. Oakland, CA: Prevention Institute. Retrieved October 12, 2006, from http://www.preventioninstitute v.org/pdf/TURF_1S.pdf

Goleman, D. (1988, June 7). Why meetings sometimes don't work. *The New York Times*, p. B1.

Kreuter, M. W., De Rosa, C., Howze, E. H., & Baldwin, G. T. (2004). Understanding wicked problems: A key to advancing environmental health promotion. *Health Education and Behavior, 31*, 441–454.

Kreuter, M. W., Lezin, N. A., & Young, L. A. (2000). Evaluating community-based collaborative mechanisms: Implications for practitioners. *Health Promotion Practice, 1*, 49–63.

Miller, S. M. (1983). Coalition etiquette: Ground rules for building unity. *Social Policy, 4*(2), 47–49.

Peck, G. P., & Hague, C. E. (2003). *Ohio State fact sheet: turf issues*. Retrieved April 13, 2003, from http://ohioline.osu.edu/bc-fact/0012.html

Prevention Institute. (2002). *Collaboration math*. Oakland, CA: Author. Retrieved October 12, 2006, from http://www.preventioninstitute.org/collmath.html

Snell-Johns, J., Imm, P., & Wandersman, A. (2003). Roles assumed by a community coalition when creating environmental and policy-level changes. *Journal of Community Psychology, 31*, 661–670.

Weed, D. (n.d.). *When coalitions collide: Managing multiple coalitions*. Amherst, MA: AEHC/Community Partners. Retrieved October 12, 2006, from http://www.compartners.org/stacks/archive/hcm/cb_collide.pdf

Wolff, T. (2001). A practitioner's guide to successful coalitions. *American Journal of Community Psychology, 29*, 173–191.

6

The Power of Local Communities to Foster Policy

Makani Themba-Nixon

LEARNING OBJECTIVES

- Learn the importance of policy as a tool for primary prevention.
- Be able to explain the policymaking framework at the local level from the perspective of historically disfranchised communities.
- Be able to identify strategies of policymaking that can be used when government or industry is either unsupportive of or opposed to proposed policies.

Prevention advocates increasingly find if they are interested in shifting norms, traditional health education approaches are not enough. More and more, advocates are looking to the domain of law and other forms of social policy where many norms are forged. In tobacco control, for example, policies that raised the price of tobacco products and prohibited smoking in certain public spaces contributed significantly to the drop in youth smoking. Such policies also contributed to increases in the total number of smokers who quit (Chaloupka & Wechsler, 1997). Policies that regulate gun safety have contributed to decreasing gun-related death and injury (Sugarmann & Rand, 1998), and laws mandating seat belt use have contributed significantly to decreasing death and injury as a result of auto crashes (National Highway Traffic Safety Administration [NHTSA], 1997). These are some of the many examples of the importance of policy as a tool for primary prevention.

Policy is more than law. It is any agreement (formal or informal) about how an institution, governing body, or community will address shared problems or attain shared goals. It spells out the terms and the consequences of these agreements and codifies the governing body's values as represented by those present in the policymaking process.

Prevention advocates need to be present in the policymaking process as policy formation can be an effective tool for prevention. *Policy initiatives* (concerted campaigns to advance specific policies) can affect a community in at least two ways. First, enactment of the policy itself can address problems that put communities at risk and can help improve quality of life. For example, policies to reduce access to tobacco have resulted in decreased tobacco use and mortality. Successful campaigns to raise local wages and benefits have resulted in increased access to health care and in stabilized nutrition for affected families. Second, the act of organizing a community to engage in the policy initiative can increase social networks and reduce isolation and alienation, which can be as effective in reducing problems as the policy itself. For example, research shows that participation in local community institutions and organizations is considered vital for effective crime and drug abuse prevention. Efforts that engage community residents and give them a sense of their own power can make a real difference in residents' ability to solve problems and can also strengthen individual members' sense of community. Community-based efforts to change policy not only address problems through the policy changes they achieve but also aid communities in addressing the factors that put them at risk in the first place (Curtis, 1987; Florin, 1989; Mayer, 1984; McMillan & Chavis, 1986).

The best kind of policy initiative engages the community that shares the problem and ensures the initiative is a part of the solution. These initiatives take into account the kind of advocacy efforts required to make policy changes and look to expand the base of support for public policy for future efforts. This chapter discusses policymaking strategies on the local level from the perspective of historically disfranchised communities. Many times these communities have had experiences leading to a well-deserved mistrust of government and industry. Therefore, this chapter includes policymaking strategies that can be used when government or industry is either unsupportive of or opposed to proposed policies.

MANDATORY CHILD SAFETY RESTRAINTS

"I walked out on the balcony alone and had a few tears well up. I said, 'By golly, it's happened, and if this works, it may happen all over the United States!'" That is how Dr. Robert Sanders, a soft-spoken Tennessee pediatrician and catalyst for groundbreaking injury prevention legislation, described his victory after a historic 1978 vote in the Tennessee senate about mandatory car seat use.

Today, few parents question the benefits of using child safety seats in cars. In fact, 99 percent of infants and 94 percent of toddlers nationally are restrained using child safety seats when riding in automobiles (NHTSA, 2004). Yet behaviors that are now norms were once anomalies. During the early 1970s, car crash injuries were the leading cause of death among children in Tennessee and in many other states, and car seat use was less than 15 percent nationally (Kahane, 2001). At that time, many legislators and citizens saw car seat use as an issue of personal freedom and civil liberties rather than as a matter of injury prevention (Solomon, Leaf, & Nissen, 2001).

When Sanders became chair of the Tennessee chapter of the Accident Prevention Committee of the American Academy of Pediatrics, he realized he had an opportunity and responsibility to address this easily preventable cause of morbidity and mortality through state legislation. In 1976, he proposed that Tennessee enact the nation's first mandatory child restraint law, but the bill was stopped in committee. Opponents vehemently attacked the bill and Sanders, even going so far as to falsely accuse him of owning stock in a safety seat manufacturing company.

The following year, Sanders redoubled his efforts. He, his wife, and the opposing lawmakers' own family physicians began to call legislators' homes on weekends to enlist their support. An impressive cadre of health professionals distributed fact sheets throughout the state. The bill was finally approved by two votes in 1978. By 1985, all fifty states had adopted similar legislation (NHTSA, 2002).

Between 1975 and 2004, approximately 7,472 lives were saved by child safety restraint systems, such as safety seats or seat belts (National Center for Statistics and Analysis, 2004). During that same time, risk of injury to children was reduced by 59 percent when compared to children who used only safety belts (New York State Department of Health, 2006). Sanders's efforts not only saved children's lives in Tennessee and beyond but also established a precedent for using policy to effect broad norm and behavior change. One person's willingness to see beyond current trends in thinking, to take on the often uncomfortable job of changing norms, and to recognize the power of legislation in altering behaviors resulted in sweeping national change and set a precedent for similar initiatives. Arguably, the successful enactment of similar policies (such as helmet laws, drinking age statutes, and tobacco control regulations) was, at least in part, due to Dr. Robert Sanders's success.

Source: Prevention Institute.

COMMON STAGES IN POLICY INITIATIVE DEVELOPMENT

Most initiatives go through a development process characterized by seven stages (see Figure 6.1). Initiatives usually begin with some kind of testing the waters to help identify key issues and concerns to shape the second stage. During the second stage advocates take the relevant issues and form them into a clear policy initiative. In the third stage, advocates engage in strategy and analysis to assess public and policymaker support as well as mechanisms for building support and influence to advance the initiative. Implementing the strategy takes place throughout stages 4 and 5 as advocates engage in direct issue organizing to build support around the specific initiative as a way to effectively address issues of concern. Organizing to build support often occurs while simultaneously working *in the belly of the beast* to steer the initiative through the appropriate policymaking channels. If successful, advocates will move on to stage 6, victory and defense, to help solidify their policy victory and ensure that no subsequent legislation or litigation occurs to undermine the initiative. In the final stage, advocates are focused on effective enforcement and implementation of the policy so that it works as intended.

These stages are not strictly sequential but tend to overlap (more like a spectrum than a staircase). Often groups are working at more than one stage at a time once an initiative is under way. For example, groups will *test the waters* throughout the life of an initiative and use that feedback to refine and improve their work. Effective initiatives rarely miss any of these stages in development. Weaker initiatives often do. Sometimes groups will go ahead without much preparation because of some unique opportunity that *just wouldn't wait*. It is true the right timing can aid an initiative's success, but it is more often the case that groups wish they had waited and become better prepared. In any case, good preparation and solid organizing invariably help a group take better advantage of existing opportunities as well as create new ones.

Initiatives concerned primarily with the enactment of policy necessarily involve considerations and assessments of power. Advocates must consider what body has the power to enact the policy, where each individual member stands, and what influence members may have to help build support for the initiative. Even seemingly *win-win* initiatives such

Figure 6.1 Stages in the development of a policy initiative

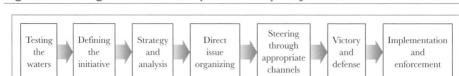

as seat belt mandates or lowering speed limits may face tough and at times unexpected opposition. Opposition can come from people who oppose the specific regulations, from people intrinsically concerned about regulations, or from people who feel this regulation might become a stepping-stone or precedent for other regulations they don't want to see developed. Those who oppose an initiative might even believe it will provide a distraction from other efforts they regard as more important. Consequently, prevention advocates must pay attention to issues of power and take care to undertake the research, strategy development, and analysis necessary to ensure they not only have evidence-based policy initiatives but community-based support as well.

A coalition in a small college town in Nebraska provides a poignant example of what can happen when groups try to skip the strategy development and organizing phases in the process. The group of alcohol policy advocates knew that alcohol abuse and consumption was involved in a large number of the hospital visits in their county, but the hospital did not keep track of alcohol involvement in admissions. The process of *external coding* or *E-coding* for alcohol-related injuries was beginning to catch on in hospitals in larger cities around the country, tracking additional factors in a hospital admission. The coalition surveyed the research and found clear evidence that developing a system for E-coding local data on alcohol-related admissions would be helpful in their efforts to better regulate alcohol in their town.

The chief hospital administrator, the policymaker with the power to enact the initiative, was a good friend of coalition leaders and a coalition supporter. The group took its initiative directly to the administrator without analysis or community organizing efforts because the leaders believed the request would be swiftly granted. They were caught completely by surprise when the hospital administrator would not agree to enact the policy and in fact expressed strong opposition. The coalition partners had banked on their relationship with a decision maker without thinking through how the administrator might perceive the impact of such a policy on his institution or the risks in implementation. Without public support for the issue, the proposal was easy to dismiss.

It is a common mistake to launch policy initiatives without any preparation or prior analysis (as required in the first three stages of development) before beginning direct advocacy. Numerous policy initiatives skip stage 4 and therefore suffer from inadequate grassroots support because not enough attention was paid to community organizing. Advocates often go directly to stage 5, working with policymakers, without grassroots support or even public awareness of their efforts, in hopes policymakers will be swayed by how sensible their initiative is. However, policy is not as much about acting sensibly as it is about negotiating interests. Advocates must never assume support based on the logic of their argument or on the strength of a personal relationship.

It is also important to recognize that policy is a process of negotiation and compromise. When working on a policy for which there is little or no precedent, keep in mind that local governments are often afraid to be the first jurisdiction to adopt a new and untested ordinance. First ordinances are usually more conservatively written and less comprehensive than those that follow. It is always helpful to know about similar policy initiatives that have been enacted without legal challenge or that have been upheld in court. Without some precedent, making a case for a new policy can be tough but not impossible. In any case, it helps to decide early on what can be given up and what is nonnegotiable.

STAGE 1: TESTING THE WATERS

In the initial stage, most groups are focused on the problem and are just beginning to develop ideas for solutions. People sense that something concrete can be done about an issue, but no one is sure exactly what. It is important for a group to spend time defining the specific problem or set of problems it would like to address through policy. Too often policy-related solutions to community issues are hard to find because the problems are too broadly defined. For example, a community with high rates of diet-related chronic diseases of children in local schools may need first to identify the problem it needs to address (for example, the food being served in schools, the lack of parks and open spaces in the neighborhood where children can exercise, the prevalence of junk food advertising in the neighborhood, or something else). Once the problem is clearly and specifically defined, suitable approaches are easier to propose. Often a number of approaches are tested and screened for community support, legality, and likelihood of success. When a San Diego community group organized in the wake of the shooting death of a local youth, its first target was gun regulation. After conducting research on the legislative remedies available, the group focused on a ban on junk guns and local regulation of bullets. A key lesson here was that the coalition was flexible and moved in the direction residents wanted to go.

Where to Focus

Policy development should not always focus on community problems. Sociologist John McKnight and his colleagues at Northwestern University pioneered a method of community mapping that enables neighborhoods to chart their assets and develop strategies for addressing issues based on their strengths. Used primarily in public health and community development efforts, asset mapping is a valuable tool for any group seeking to organize around any issue. The process includes detailed surveys of institutions and individuals, building networks that help leverage individual and institutional assets, and case studies and project ideas for implementing the project (see Kretzmann & McKnight, 1993).

Some of the best policies address a community's vision of what it would like to become instead of focusing on community problems or deficits. Usually, when a community works from a vision of itself, it manages to address a number of problems simultaneously. One example is found in the growing number of local policies to increase the number of open parks and amount of green space or unpaved natural areas for recreation and rest. Although these policies are a result of the residents' vision of their community as a beautiful place to live, increasing the number of parks in the community also helps address issues of blight, youth development, increasing physical activity, and negative land uses.

Community Context

Traditionally, advocates are individuals who speak on behalf of others. Advocates can be from a community affected by a particular issue or from outside the community but committed to working on the issue. Sometimes advocates who are not fully familiar with a community play an important role in helping community members shape policy; it is important for these advocates to get to know the community. Advocates often identify issues by spending time talking with neighbors, walking around observing their neighborhoods *with fresh eyes*, and identifying the assets (or protective factors) and factors that put neighbors at risk.

Any behavior or activity operates within a context or an environment that shapes it. Defining problems in a *social change* context means shifting the focus from individual problems to the social and environmental context in which these problems occur. Identifying risk and protective factors requires attention to a community's environment, the context in which these factors exist. This shift is important because environmental factors can play a major role in proliferation and prevention of problems in a community. This shift from an individual to an environmental perspective is much like shifting a camera lens away from a simple portrait to capture the *big picture* or landscape that surrounds it. Different levels and dimensions of a community landscape include the following:

- *Physical or land use factors.* Buildings, roads, open space, institutions, and businesses (or lack of them) are all a part of the physical infrastructure that forms the foundation of a community.
- *Availability of goods and services.* What we eat, wear, and read is largely determined by what is available to us. Goods and services are more than what we can buy; they include public services like schools, hospitals, water, and recreational facilities.
- *Institutional factors.* Institutional behaviors impact the community.
- *Human factors.* The people who live in a place affect the community, as do their affiliations to organizations.

Techniques for Community Assessment

Identifying risk and protective factors is important, but equally critical is knowing which factors are most important to address. As noted earlier, collecting data and conducting research are important activities that can help. Another equally important way to gather information is to listen to people in the community. Both outside advocates and locals need to have ways to deepen their understanding of the community that rely upon and further develop their *gut instincts*. Every coalition should have systems for collecting community input and feedback. Here are a few examples of community-focused methods of *listening*.

Surveys

Whether completed over the phone, online, or at the door, surveys provide a structured method for obtaining community input, for identifying issues, and for assessing the prevalence of problems or attitudes. One should take care not to develop long, complicated survey instruments or instruments that focus only on a community's problems. Well-done surveys enable groups to collect data in standardized form on a wide variety of issues and at the same time encourage residents to participate in the process of developing policies.

Canvassing

Going door to door unannounced can be a good way to reach new people who aren't on anyone's list, to raise public awareness, and to build name recognition in a neighborhood. Input gathered will be limited, however, because it is difficult to carry on an extensive conversation with a stranger, especially when time is limited and the list of neighbors to contact is long.

Focus Groups

One can gather solid, qualitative input from a small group, especially from a group of people who have something in common or are in some way demographically similar. Just listening to the exchange between participants can be very enlightening and can reveal more about the interests and concerns in a community than a survey. Of course, information collected from focus groups is harder (although not impossible) to quantify.

One-on-One Interviews with Key Players

Listening is one of the most important tools there is for building relationships. Listen actively with your whole body facing the speaker. Ask questions and probe more deeply. After offering a guiding question or two, go wherever the conversation leads you. Suspend your expectations and your agenda for the time being. Just listen to learn more about the other person and his or her concerns. Take notes if you need to and if it is not too obtrusive.

Walkabout

Map out a route in an affected or representative neighborhood. The route should provide a mix of things to observe (businesses, institutions, homes, parks, and so on) and take no more than sixty minutes to walk. If much of the business district is abandoned, that is worth observing, too. It is best to do a walkabout in a small group. Encourage participants to take notes and to pay attention to both assets and challenges; debrief the group's observations upon return.

THE IMPORTANCE OF RESEARCH

Prevention policy should have a strong research foundation that supports the initiative's particular strategy or approach toward addressing the problem. This is of particular importance in the case of progressive, regulatory policies, as they usually receive greater scrutiny than policies perceived to be probusiness. The extra scrutiny can be a good thing, as it forces proponents to make sure their policies have an effect on real-life issues that are of concern to communities.

Initiatives should start with a carefully structured data gathering effort. This can be done without starting from scratch or conducting new studies. Many studies are available that support prevention initiatives, although they may not be widely disseminated. The Internet is a good source for many of these documents and so are community-based groups or think tanks. In the area of child and family services, for example, there are literally hundreds of well-crafted studies that examine the impact of poverty on children and hundreds more that examine drug policy, employment, race relations, and many other topics.

Data can guide the development of an initiative in at least three ways. Data can (1) direct how the policy should be targeted by providing detailed information about the problem; (2) indicate the impact and severity of the problem; and (3) justify social action. Finally, by showing that some groups are disproportionately affected by the problem, the data establish the problem is not random but is linked to specific social and environmental factors.

Practically speaking, research should provide a clear analysis of the issues the policy initiative seeks to address. It is one thing to say, "We have a problem with teen pregnancy." It is quite another to say, "We have a problem with unsafe sex among teens" or "We have a problem with predatory sex between teen girls and men in their twenties and thirties." Community-based research helps us understand the difference and points to policies that are more effective. For example, we might want to insist on more accountability and punishment for adult fathers or to ensure better access to preventive health care. We might want to mandate counseling services and classes to bolster teen girls' sense of power in relationships or increase alternative activities for youth. Given the many ways one can define the issue, it is important to gather reports, surveys, personal observations, and other resources that accurately describe the problems and the protective factors in play.

Another reason to have detailed information to substantiate policy recommendations is that all legislation must be based on findings or facts that provide a clear rationale for enacting the law. These findings are important because they constitute much of the legal case if the law is challenged in court. In addition, policymakers are more likely to support issues that have data to back them up. Well-done research can legitimize an issue in the eyes of politicians, their constituents, and the media. Above all, you must have information that clearly describes the problem and your proposed solution in ways that policymakers, the community, the coalition, and the media can understand.

STAGE 2: DEFINING THE INITIATIVE

Once the primary issue or set of concerns is defined, it must be refined into a clear, practical policy initiative. The best initiatives emerge when residents articulate their *ideal* policy and then look for the best mechanisms to help bring their vision into reality. In Oakland, California, the Coalition on Alcohol Outlet Issues wanted fewer liquor stores and better regulation of those remaining. In its ideal policy, the group wanted store owners, not public funds, to pay for enforcement. Coalition members took their idea to the city council, which then instructed staff to find a solution. The resulting ordinance requires merchants to pay higher conditional use permit fees to support an augmented regulatory structure.

The process of defining an initiative is also tied to the needs and aspirations of coalition partners. As a result, diverse representation in the process is key to ensure the initiative defined is relevant to as many communities as possible, particularly to communities most affected by the issues the group is hoping to address. Expanding a coalition can bring significant changes to how a coalition is defined, as in the case of a statewide coalition working to increase the tobacco excise tax in Colorado. When the coalition expanded to include Padres Unidos, a group organizing in Denver-area Latino communities, Padres Unidos's accountability to its base would not allow the group to simply bring Latinos to the tax initiative. The organization had to negotiate with the coalition about the language, impact, and reach of the ballot initiative to ensure the initiative would be relevant to the group's base. Padres Unidos's extensive research on the impact of funding cuts to undocumented residents in Colorado helped expand the tax initiative to include the restoration of funding for health services for undocumented residents. When the ballot initiative passed in November 2004, a diverse group of Coloradans celebrated what was a victory for primary prevention and immigrant rights.

STAGE 3: STRATEGY AND ANALYSIS

After gathering information and identifying assets and challenges, it is time to analyze all of that information and develop approaches to building policymaker and public support for the initiative. The process of developing strategy in this regard is informed by an understanding of the values and interests that undergird how decisions are made on a daily basis.

Community values and interests are the ideal visions and the down-to-earth concerns we carry in our daily lives. They range from dreams of a safe, green world for all families to fears that the *wrong kind* of neighbors will move in. Advocates must factor in community sentiment from all across the spectrum to determine how to make the initiative meaningful for the people with whom they will be working.

A power analysis is an assessment to identify targets or decision makers, allies, opponents, and other important actors in the campaign. It is wise to conduct a power analysis early on, as the initiative can be refined further in light of this information. For example, a coalition in favor of living-wage legislation intentionally omitted construction work from its initiative as a strategic and political consideration. By omitting construction work, much of which already paid a living wage, the group was able to neutralize potential opposition and make allies out of building trade unions and other key players in the construction industry.

Every policy, no matter how benign it may seem, benefits some people more than others. A good organizer carefully dissects how key constituencies will perceive their self-interests as they relate to the proposed policy. Key questions include these:

- How much power do constituencies have over decision makers on this issue?
- How strongly will they support or oppose the initiative?
- What are the challenges or barriers to joining us?
- What do they risk by being involved? By not being involved?
- What is our relationship to each of these players?
- How might we shape the initiative differently to maximize allies and divide opponents without undermining our objectives?

STAGE 4: DIRECT ISSUE ORGANIZING

Informed by the power analysis and strategic planning, organizing begins in earnest. In citywide or countywide campaigns without a neighborhood focus, organizing is usually done through outreach to other organizations. For example, much of the organizing for living-wage campaigns focused on unions, advocacy organizations, and nonunionized employees.

Neighborhood-oriented campaigns tend to conduct more block-by-block canvassing operations. In Los Angeles, the Community Coalition for Substance Abuse Prevention and Treatment has organizers go door to door and holds house parties as neighborhood meetings. The group focuses on neighborhoods with problem liquor stores in order to build a solid base of support among the people most affected by the issue.

Community organizing and mobilization are, in the main, communication strategies. They are about reaching people directly and inviting them to get involved because it is in their interest to do so. Organizers must understand and appreciate that people have many issues to contend with and that although our policy initiatives are important, community involvement almost always clashes with real-life obligations. The venerable organizer Fred Ross Sr. used to say that to organize, you had to find someone "who had to do something about it." Often people with many issues to contend with are the hardest to reach because they are dealing with a range of social problems. As professionals, many of us feel safer working with *leaders* who have much less stake in the issue and who run a certain risk (of reputation, time, and so on) in being involved with us. This impulse to want to work with leaders can wreak havoc on efforts to build a strong, committed coalition with an authentic stake in the issue.

Even with the best analysis and outreach, potential allies can still be unresponsive. History can play a critical role in how groups respond to overtures for collaboration. It helps to do a *collaboration scan* by asking a few key residents about the history of relationships between your agency and similar agencies and targeted communities. Here are some guiding questions:

- How are resources allocated to support the various groups or communities with whom I want to work? Have there been tensions in regard to resources? How did these tensions evolve, and who were the key players?
- What is the group's experience with previous collaborations? Were they satisfying? Were their needs met? Was it a positive or negative experience overall? Why?
- What are the prevailing attitudes about collaboration? Are there issues (in professional training or culture, mistrust, and so on) that make collaboration difficult? Easier? What concerns the group most about getting involved with a collaborative project? How can those concerns be allayed?
- Who are the key opinion leaders in the group? Who is most open to collaborating? Who is least open? Do we (or does someone we know) have a relationship with any opinion leaders? List names.
- What would the group need to benefit from collaborating with others? What can we offer? What would the group be willing to contribute? What does it risk in joining us?
- What interests do we both share? Will this collaboration offer a vehicle for mutual benefit?

The answers to these questions will frame an initial recruitment plan. A recruitment plan identifies prospective partners, their probable interests, and background information to help begin the work of building relationships. It is important to choose candidates carefully because the first groups to join the coalition will send a strong signal to the rest of the community.

Candidates need not be the most prominent community members, but they must be trusted in their community, share common ground, and be concerned enough about the core issues to make a solid commitment. Although big-name affiliations can bring media attention to a cause, big names alone without any commitment will not build working relationships. They just breed resentment and reinforce the existing state of affairs. In addition, famous people have more to risk when they do get involved. Authentic collaborations require partners who are deeply concerned, have a strong personal interest in the initiative, and risk relatively little by getting involved.

When recruiting candidates to a policy initiative, identify any shared friends or colleagues who may consent to serve as go-betweens to initiate contact with the candidate. If possible, discuss any outreach with a colleague who knows the candidate well. Try role playing certain approaches and discussing the candidate's potential responses. A good recruitment pitch comes from detailed background information and plenty of practice.

Of course, recruitment is only the beginning. Building and sustaining public support for a policy initiative requires retaining partners for the long haul by integrating them into the team. This is not a blending process where everyone ends up acting and talking the same. It's more of a salad approach whereby every partner is tossed lightly until the new partner has blended in. Some organizations develop a new-partner orientation system and assign a partner to the new member to help with the transition. That partner makes the introductions, brings the new member up to speed, and works with the newcomer to identify potential areas for participation. When possible, it helps to recruit at least two partners from a community to minimize feelings of isolation.

Review your organizational structure. How are decisions made? Who holds the information and resources? Will there be room for new partners to make a meaningful contribution to the initiative's direction? What steps do you have in place to make new partners feel at home with the group? What language, or level of language, is spoken at meetings and gatherings? Will it alienate or welcome new partners?

Media Advocacy

It is also during stage 4 that media work moves into full swing. Media advocacy involves strategic use of mass media to support community organizing to advance a social or public policy initiative. Most media advocacy is focused on the initiative's target (or decision-making body) because it is the target that has the power to enact the desired change. In some cases, groups use media advocacy to mobilize supporters before they target policymakers. It's important to note that although the media can support organizing goals, the media can never be a substitute for organizing. That's why most groups shape their media strategy to target policymakers.

Spend time researching how targets get their information. Most elected officials and other gatekeepers read the editorial pages of local newspapers to gauge community concerns. Television news also helps set the public agenda and affects the *public conversation* on a particular issue. In any case, identifying the target will help shape a more effective and efficient strategy.

Developing a Message

A message is not a sound bite or a slogan (although it can help shape those things). It is the overarching theme that neatly frames the initiative for key target audiences. Messages should be relatively short, easy to understand, emotive, and visual. The message should be supportive of the overall strategy.

It is best to test messages on friends and coworkers, especially if they are not familiar with the issue. Colleagues working on similar issues are another good resource. Listen carefully to feedback. Did the message convey the importance of your issue? Did the recipient of the message *get* it? Keeping key targets in mind, use the input to help shape and refine the message.

STAGE 5: STEERING THROUGH APPROPRIATE CHANNELS

At some point in every initiative, advocates must meet with policymakers and begin the long process of getting the policy enacted. This stage is characterized by intensive work with government staff, negotiations, and accountability sessions. It is important to stay focused on the group's initial goals during this phase, as it is easy to become caught up in the politics of bureaucracy. Working with policymakers is an *inside* game, but it need not mean getting disconnected from grassroots support. As the veteran organizer Greg Akili often says, "Stay connected to your base. Always go in groups and rotate the people who attend the meetings so that you build leadership and confidence."

For prevention policy initiatives, this stage is a crucial one, as prevention-focused initiatives can be technical and complicated. Having a legislative champion (or several) can be important in negotiating this phase. At the very least, it will be critical that involved staffers understand key provisions and issues in the proposed policy. Staffers are an incredibly valuable resource because most policymakers depend heavily on their staff for making key decisions. Some technical understanding is important also because policy revisions that may seem inconsequential to a layperson can undermine the intent of the initiative. For example, ventilation options for restaurants facing clean indoor air policies might seem a reasonable compromise to address secondhand smoke. However, ventilation does not effectively address the health risks because it does not *eliminate* secondhand smoke. Advocates must be vigilant to ensure the final policy draft reflects their intentions for the initiative and at least does no harm.

It is also valuable to understand the political process and the decision-making bodies of the locale in which the policy is to be implemented. Policies are implemented by different bodies, from city councils to boards of supervisors. And some political strategies allow community groups to rely on voters, rather than policymakers, for organizing ballot initiatives or propositions. Understanding the options available is crucial.

Administrative Rule Making

Most regulatory agencies have the power to make rules and regulations without much oversight or input from elected officials or the public at large. In fact, agency rule making (not legislation) constitutes the bulk of the policies that regulate and shape our lives. Thus agency rule making is a supplement and at times an alternative to new policy creation. How public benefits are accessed and distributed, how data are gathered and made public, how jobs are created, and how most trade policies and other matters are determined is up to a small number of people as part of their daily job. The lack of formality and access that characterizes most rule making requires that advocates get a clear sense of who has the power to make what rules in which areas of concern to their efforts. This means conducting a power analysis to assess how decisions are made and where best to affect these decisions.

Once these *power points* are identified, it all becomes a classic organizing campaign to leverage additional scrutiny (including press) to raise the level of accountability in the process. Many of these agencies are rarely exposed to direct action. As a result, organizers who have focused on the rule-making process have met with a great deal of success.

Should the policy process break down so it becomes clear the policy cannot be won in the short term, other actions are needed to lay the groundwork for regulation down the line. The three most common policy actions at this stage are moratoriums, mandated studies, and lawsuits.

Moratoriums

Sometimes it is important to stop a policy activity until there can be further study of its impact and any possible alternatives. Common moratoriums include bans on new alcohol outlets, billboards, dump sites, or office construction. It is not enough to enact a time-limited ban; moratorium time should be used to gather more information and assess policy options.

Mandated Studies

Research can be costly and time-consuming. If time and support allow, why not get local government to do the research? Through policy that mandates a study or data collection, resources can be set aside to do a thorough job of information gathering. The policy can set parameters for: the kind of group or institution that can conduct the study, key questions framing the study, resident involvement and monitoring of the study, and the plan for dissemination and use of the results. A Los Angeles coalition convinced the city to conduct a study on the topic of a living wage. When it came time to discuss whether a living-wage law was needed, the data were beyond dispute because they were the city's own data.

Lawsuits and Other Complaints

Lawsuits and other court actions can be tedious and expensive. Therefore, groups should carefully consider all options before deciding to take on a lawsuit. If an organization has the resources (in staff, money, or pro bono legal support), a well-framed legal intervention can accomplish much in both the short term and the long term. At the very least a legal intervention may get the other side to the table or to negotiate in better faith. Other strategies include requests for information and documents from the opponents, injunctions against the implementation of laws before they have had a chance to take effect, organizing victims with standing to sue polluters or other institutions causing damage to a community, and civil suits when an institutional action has a pattern of discrimination or damage to certain populations (such as people of color, women, or people with disabilities).

In addition to lawsuits, it also helps to file complaints about bad or illegal practices with the appropriate regulatory agencies. For example, alcohol ads that appeal to children are violations in many states. Violations of pollution, labor, and fair trade laws are other avenues that can be pursued. If one regulatory agency is notoriously slow to act, try redefining the issue so it falls under the purview of a more active regulator. For example, redefining a violation from a bad business practice to a health issue often brings a whole new set of actors into play. In any case, find out who enforces what relevant regulations and work accordingly.

STAGE 6: VICTORY AND DEFENSE

Once an initiative is enacted, celebration is definitely in order. However, for most ordinances, as soon as the partying is over, the litigation begins. Prepare for the possibility of litigation at the beginning of the initiative and be ready to play an active role in any legal action, even if the local government (and not the advocating coalition or group) is the defendant. Some organizations, like the Community Coalition and the Coalition on Alcohol Outlet Issues, got intervenor status in litigation directed toward their city's government. Baltimore's Citywide Liquor Coalition made sure its attorney worked closely with the city attorney throughout the process, carefully crafting public testimony with an eye toward building a strong public record in preparation for the inevitable litigation against the ordinance it was promoting to regulate alcohol and tobacco billboards.

Media advocacy and framing are also important in this phase of the work. Framing the victory on a group's terms can help consolidate public support and build a base for future initiatives. Strong support for an initiative after its enactment can also help prevent lawsuits that challenge the policy's implementation.

STAGE 7: IMPLEMENTATION AND ENFORCEMENT

After the policy is enacted, it sometimes also needs to clear court hurdles. Then the work begins to get the new law properly implemented and enforced. One of the biggest mistakes in policy development is failing to consider implementation thoroughly, including mechanisms of funding and enforcement, before the policy is advanced. For initiatives with powerful opposition, negotiation continues around issues like the timeline for implementing the policy, interpretation of particular clauses, and fitting the new policy in with other government priorities.

Ensure there are adequate resources for monitoring and enforcement. Build in funding, excise tax, license fee increases, and other relevant resource allocation formulas that tie the amount of the enforcement budget to the scope and objectives of enforcement. For example, tying alcohol outlet licensing fees and penalties to the cost of enforcement helps ensure enforcement resources keep up with problems at the expense of those making a profit from the product. Such an approach does not force residents to shoulder the burden.

Develop an interagency oversight body that brings the partners together for comprehensive enforcement and monitoring. Such a body could include community members, school and youth-serving agencies, supportive business representatives, researchers, planners, and law enforcement and health department professionals to ensure compliance and oversight of monitoring and enforcement. Clear criteria for board membership, including independence from regulated industry funding or limits on the number of representatives with industry ties, must be established in advance. The body should hold the group accountable to open meeting and documentation requirements as outlined in municipal and state law.

Ensure enforcement of the policy in areas where underserved communities are most targeted. Communities of color and the lesbian, gay, bisexual, and transgender (LGBT) community are directly targeted by key industries on which prevention regulation is focused, such as tobacco and alcohol. As a result, care must be taken to ensure enforcement resources are equitably allocated. Some enforcement activities related to reducing disparities may include the following:

- Ensuring compliance with youth access laws
- Regular surveillance and research to monitor targeting
- Hiring enforcement staff with the appropriate cultural, language, and community competencies
- Advertising restrictions in specific neighborhoods

California-based *smoke-free bars* campaigns that promote the health interests of Asian American communities exemplify the promise and proven success of backing culturally specific enforcement activities. The Asian Pacific Islander Tobacco Control Network pushed a smoke-free campaign that focused on Asian American venues and cultural nights. After local bars went smoke-free, campaign activities shifted to enforcement as network members joined with local BREATH advocates (the California Smoke-Free Bars, Workplaces, and Communities Program) to monitor compliance at locales catering to Asian American patrons. This effort also provided a valuable opportunity to appraise the community impact of smoke-free laws while raising general awareness of the perils of tobacco use in these communities (Asian and Pacific Islander American Health Forum, 2004).

Work with business owners. On some issues, businesses are likely targets for prevention policy interventions. Many of the outlets (tobacco vendors, liquor stores, corner grocers, and so on) are heavily concentrated in low-income areas with large communities of color. Many business owners in these areas are themselves immigrants and racial minorities who have not received adequate training on policy enforcement or ways their businesses can be better community citizens. When ensuring compliance with newly enacted laws, it is imperative to use culturally sensitive approaches that embrace building relationships with business owners. Having outreach workers who can communicate in the appropriate ethnic or cultural language can facilitate constructive dialogue around enforcement. These outreach workers can offer on-site general education on policy enforcement. The working partnerships between community organizations and business owners can be the basis for future prevention efforts.

Ensure equitable application of enforcement activities. It is important to demonstrate even-handed application of enforcement activities, given the historically strained relationships between the criminal justice systems and diverse communities that are already over-represented in many areas of the criminal justice system. Although higher rates of violations in a specific community may be an indicator that law enforcement officers enforce policies differently in different communities, it may also reflect the greater concentration and impact of the problem in that community. Such a situation may be addressed most effectively through policy initiatives that decrease outlet concentration in communities saturated with negative uses; policy initiatives may be combined with culturally competent efforts to promote compliance with prevention policies.

CONCLUSION

Policy is a powerful tool for prevention, especially when used in concert with community organizing and media advocacy. The evidence of its efficacy is mounting as prevention-focused policies like mandatory seat belt laws, clean indoor air ordinances, and responsible beverage service regulations are literally saving tens of thousands of lives each year. However, there is much more to be done. There is a need for better, more strategic budget policies that ensure a fair allocation of resources to communities at greater risk. Some areas of prevention policymaking, such as family planning, face extraordinarily tough opposition, although organized opposition to public health interventions is on the rise overall (Woolley & Benjamin, 2004; Yañez, 2002).

Advocates face highly organized, well-funded media attacks that frame prevention-focused policies as government interference in people's private lives. The good news is that polls continue to show widespread support for much of the prevention policy agenda, including increases in certain taxes. Our challenge is to build a broad base of active supporters committed to moving these policy initiatives forward from the bottom up. As previous work has shown, when prevention advocates help build broad-based movements focused on concrete policy change, we can help create healthier environments that engage communities in ways traditional health education and health promotion approaches cannot.

DISCUSSION QUESTIONS

1. You are in charge of leading a community coalition that seeks to address the issue of intense alcohol advertising on large billboards and local bus shelters to which many school-aged children are exposed. Identify how you would effectively *test the waters* and *define the initiative*.

2. In the Discussion Question one scenario, what type of data might you access and analyze? Why? Where would you find it?

3. In the Discussion Question one scenario, what appropriate policymaking channels do you think you will use? Why? What resistance do you think you might encounter in your initiative? How might you overcome that resistance?

REFERENCES

Asian and Pacific Islander American Health Forum. (2004). Asian and Pacific Islander Tobacco Education Network. Retrieved October 13, 2006, from http://www.apiahf.org/programs/apiten

Chaloupka, F. J., & Wechsler, H. (1997). Price, tobacco control policies, and smoking among young adults. *Journal of Health Economics, 16*, 359–373.

Curtis, L. A. (1987). *Policies to prevent crime: Neighborhood, family, and employment strategies.* Thousand Oaks, CA: Sage.

Florin, P. (1989). *Nurturing the grassroots: Neighborhood volunteer organizations and America's cities.* New York: Citizens Committee for New York City.

Kahane, C. J. (2001). *An evaluation of child passenger safety: The effectiveness and benefits of safety seats.* Washington, DC: National Highway Traffic Safety Administration.

Kretzmann, J. P., & McKnight, J. L. (1993). *Building communities from the inside out: A path toward finding and mobilizing a community's assets.* Evanston, IL: Northwestern University, Center for Urban Affairs and Policy Research.

Mayer, N. S. (1984). *Neighborhood organizations and community development.* Washington, DC: Urban Institute Press.

McMillan, D. W., & Chavis, D. M. (1986). Sense of community: A definition and theory. *Journal of Community Psychology, 14*, 6–23.

National Center for Statistics and Analysis. (2004). Children. In *Traffic safety facts, 2004* (p. 5). Washington, DC: National Highway Traffic Safety Administration.

National Highway Traffic Safety Administration. (1997). *Traffic safety facts, 1997: Occupant protection.* Washington, DC: Author.

National Highway Traffic Safety Administration. (2002). *Traffic safety facts, 2001.* Washington, DC: Author.

National Highway Traffic Safety Administration. (2004, June). *Sixth report to Congress, fourth report to the president: The national initiative for increasing safety belt use*. Washington, DC: Author.

New York State Department of Health. (2006). *Child passenger safety*. Albany: New York State Department of Health.

Solomon, M. G., Leaf, W. A., & Nissen, W. J. (2001). *Process and outcome evaluation: The Buckle Up America initiative*. Washington, DC: National Highway Traffic Safety Administration.

Sugarmann, J., & Rand, K. (1998). *Cease fire: A comprehensive strategy to reduce firearms violence*. Washington, DC: Violence Policy Center.

Woolley, M., & Benjamin, G. (2004, November 9). *Research! America/APHA national poll on Americans' attitudes toward public health*. Paper presented at the 132nd annual meeting of the American Public Health Association, Washington, DC. Retrieved October 13, 2006, from http://www.researchamerica.org/polldata/2004/apha2004.pdf

Yañez, E. (2002). *Clean indoor air and communities of color: Challenges and opportunities*. Washington, DC: Praxis Project.

7

Using Media Advocacy to Influence Policy

Lori Dorfman

LEARNING OBJECTIVES

- Assess how strategic communications can further public health goals.
- Explain the role of mass media in setting the public agenda and framing public health issues, typical news frames for public health issues, and how news might contribute to public health problems.
- Identify the particular perspectives, potential, challenges, and theoretical underpinnings of media advocacy, including strategies to access the media, frame public health problems as social issues, and advance public policy initiatives.

The history of public health is clear: social conditions and the physical environment are important determinants of health. The primary tool available to public health for influencing social conditions and environments is *policy*. Policies define the structures and set the rules by which we live. If public health practitioners are going to improve social conditions and physical environments in lasting and meaningful ways, they must be involved in policy development and policy advocacy. Furthermore, being successful in policy advocacy requires paying attention to the news.

The reach of the news media is intoxicating. In society, the news media largely determine what issues we collectively think about, how we think about them, and what kinds of alternatives are considered viable, which, in turn, influences key policy decisions pertaining to health. The public and policymakers do not consider issues unless they are visible, and they are not visible unless the news has brought them to light. Naturally, public health educators want to take advantage of the vast audience the news media reach. (The examples in this chapter primarily use traditional media—print, television and radio—and all the concepts presented apply equally to social media such as Twitter and Facebook. However, readers should not let the wide reach of social media distract them from keeping a developed strategy and framing approach in place.)

Nonprofit organizations and community activists often are unhappy with the way their issues are presented in the news and typically respond by criticizing the media, ignoring it, or even becoming hostile. These responses are unproductive because they cede power about the public portrayal of their issues to journalists and widen the gulf between journalists and advocates. *Media advocacy* addresses this problem. It is an approach to health communication that differs significantly from traditional mass communication approaches. Media advocacy helps people understand the importance and reach of news coverage, the need to participate actively in shaping such coverage, and the methods to do so effectively. News portrayals of health issues are significant for how they influence policymakers and the public regarding who has responsibility for health. If public health–oriented solutions are to be given full consideration, then advocates talking to journalists (and journalists themselves) must understand how to frame issues from the perspective of *shared accountability* so news coverage is not focused exclusively on individual responsibility. This shared accountability recognizes that health and social problems will only be adequately addressed when all sectors of society (not just the individual) share responsibility for solutions. Media advocacy emphasizes *social accountability*, which typically receives less attention from the news than individually oriented solutions.

Public health practitioners tend to overlook the power of the news media to influence change. Journalists, even when committed to covering social problems, often produce stories that emphasize individual behavior and treatment rather than social factors and prevention.

Reprinted from R. J. Bensley and J. Brookins-Fisher, (Eds.), (2003), *Community Health Education Methods: A Practical Guide* (2nd ed.). Boston: Jones & Bartlett.

Despite the media's enormous reach and potential as a tool for change, public health professionals rarely use mass media to its full advantage. Rather, they tend to use it in its least effective capacity: to convey personal health information to consumers (Wallack & Dorfman, 2001). In contrast, media advocacy harnesses the power of the news to mobilize advocates and apply pressure for policy change.

STEPS FOR DEVELOPING EFFECTIVE MEDIA ADVOCACY CAMPAIGNS

Before public health advocates can harness the power of the news, they have to be clear and precise about why they want to use media advocacy. Four layers of strategy organize the approach to media advocacy campaigns. The first is the *overall strategy*, which defines the ultimate goal of the campaign. Next is the *media strategy*, which is chosen based on appropriateness for the overall strategy. Once advocates have selected a media strategy, they need to determine the specifics of what they want to say and to whom. That is the *message strategy*. Finally, once the other layers of strategy are in place, advocates can figure out how to attract news attention by developing an *access strategy*. Unfortunately, many groups begin by trying to attract journalists' attention without first figuring out why they want that attention and what they will say after they have it. This chapter is designed to prepare readers so they know when to call on journalists and will feel confident about what to say once they have a journalist's attention.

DEVELOP AN OVERALL STRATEGY

The most important part of a media strategy does not concern media at all. Rather, it is the clarification, articulation, and justification of the desired change. The media advocacy prime directive is that "you cannot have a media strategy without an overall strategy." Advocates should begin by asking themselves, "What changes will improve the public's health?" It makes sense for advocates to develop a media strategy only after they know what needs to be accomplished overall and how it will be done. In practical terms, this usually means determining the policy that needs to be enacted, changed, or enforced. The following four questions can help guide the development of an overall strategy:

1. What is the problem or issue?
2. What is a solution or policy (the desired outcome)?
3. Who has the power to make the necessary change?
4. Who must be mobilized to apply the necessary pressure?

The following subsections examine each of these questions in detail.

What Is the Problem or Issue?

Defining the problem is often not as simple as it seems. It is a process rife with social and political tension because different stakeholders will offer competing definitions of the problem. This process is exceptionally important because the ultimate definition of the problem will fundamentally determine the solution. For example, the high school shooting near Littleton, Colorado, in 1999 quickly generated competing definitions of the problem of violence among youth. Problem definitions included the availability of guns, the barrenness of suburban lifestyles, the failure of parents to be involved in their children's lives, the inadequacy of mental health services, and the destructive social cliques of teenagers in high school. News attention to one or the other of such competing issues helps determine the saliency of various policies and, ultimately, which will prevail.

Articulating the problem is important because it will need to be conveyed concisely to a reporter. Public health is often very problem oriented. Thus, those from health departments or social service agencies can endlessly discuss the problem. Indeed, health officials often feel they have a moral and professional obligation to tell journalists everything they know any time they are asked about the problem because they know their issue is of such vital importance. The realities of news today, however, demand that health professionals identify the most critical aspect of the problem and be able to describe it well in just a sentence or two.

Advocates must isolate the piece of the large public health problem that will be addressed specifically. For example, excessive alcohol use is related to more than 75,000 preventable deaths a year in this country (CDC, 2004) and is the number one drug choice for young people (NIAAA, 2004/2005). One way advocates can narrow the problem is by focusing on how alcohol creates problems on college campuses, particularly when it is consumed in large quantities during a short period of time. The problem of binge drinking on college campuses might be narrowed further and defined in terms of price specials at bars nearby that encourage those who are drinking to get drunk. Cheap alcohol is certainly not the only factor leading to alcohol problems on campus, but it is probably an important one. It is also a problem that can be remedied by implementation of a clear policy that would affect the overall alcohol environment.

What Is a Solution or Policy (the Desired Outcome)?

Sometimes advocates are so concerned about focusing attention on the problem they give inadequate attention to the solution. Or, they may not have identified a clear solution. Public health advocates need to identify a solution or policy. The solution need not solve the entire problem, but it should promise to make a difference. Following are some typical inadequate responses:

> "This is a very complex problem with multifaceted solutions."
> "There is no magic bullet."
> "Children are our future and we must do something."
> "The community needs to come together."

Unfortunately, none of these responses provides any concrete direction. Public health advocates need to be clear about what they want to happen: Is a new law necessary? Is more enforcement required? Does the budget need to be changed? Does someone need to take responsibility to do something to protect the community's health? Who? What should they do? When should they do it?

In the example of problems related to alcohol on campus, one solution is to eliminate happy hour price specials that encourage quick consumption of large quantities of alcohol. Advocates might work on only one salient part of the problem or one policy solution at a time (or more), depending on what resources are available.

Who Has the Power to Make the Necessary Change?

The next step is figuring out what person, group, organization, or body has the power to make the desired change. This question identifies the target audience but reflects a fundamental change in what that term means. In this context, there is a difference between traditional use of mass media in public health as a vehicle for public information campaigns to change personal behavior and use of media as an advocacy tool to change policy. In the former, the person with the problem is the one with the power to make the change. For example, the person who drinks too much, smokes, does not exercise, or has a poor diet has the power to change his or her behavior. When using media advocacy to change, implement, or enforce policy, the target is different because the power may reside with a legislator, other elected official, regulatory agency, small business owner, or corporate officer. In addition, the locus of power (or target audience) is likely to change over time. For example, changing a regulation may require focusing on different targets depending on the issue's stage in development.

The primary target for a media advocacy campaign to reduce alcohol problems on and around campus would not be the students who are drinking. Instead, it would be the alcohol vendors and those who regulate them. Eliminating happy hours, to use the policy example mentioned earlier, is not in the power of the students. Once happy hours are gone there will be a beneficial effect regardless of the knowledge and attitude of student drinkers; one avenue for the dangerous behavior would be closed. News coverage generated by media advocacy activities can describe the problem and articulate the demands for solutions so the city government and campus community can more easily move ahead. Advocates must articulate for reporters the reason for the policy and what it will accomplish. Thus, the public learns about the problems alcohol causes on campus via the news, which is perceived as a highly legitimate and credible source.

Who Must Be Mobilized to Apply the Necessary Pressure?

Public health–oriented policies are often hotly contested. Public health goals such as adding fluoride to drinking water, distributing condoms, reducing the speed limit, mandating bicycle or motorcycle helmets, or limiting the availability of alcohol, handguns, or tobacco bring out intense opposition. Many legislators and other policymakers are unlikely to support a controversial change unless constituency groups put pressure on them. The pressure can consist of telephone calls, letters, demonstrations, media coverage, and office visits. The role of news coverage here is twofold. First, media coverage of the issue will let the policymaker know his or her vote or position is being watched and will be part of the public debate. Second, media coverage can help mobilize constituency groups to contact the policymaker or get involved in other ways, thus applying pressure.

Paying attention to these four questions is a good start to creating an overall strategy: What is the problem or issue? What is the desired outcome? Who has the power to make the necessary change? Who must be mobilized to apply the necessary pressure? Once advocates have defined the problem, selected and developed a realistic and achievable policy objective, conducted an analysis to identify the locus for change, and identified and mobilized groups to apply pressure, they can then determine the media, message, and access strategies.

DEVELOP A MEDIA STRATEGY

Traditional forms of mass media interventions emphasize the *information gap* (or *motivation gap)*, which suggests health problems are caused by individuals with the problem or who are at risk of having the problem; these individuals lack either information or sufficient desire to behave in a more healthful manner. Health educators then attempt to provide information to fill the gap. When people have the information and know the facts, it is assumed they will adopt a positive attitude toward the health behavior and act accordingly so the problem will be solved. The role of the media, in this case, is to deliver the solution (knowledge) to the millions of individuals who need it. Media advocacy, on the other hand, focuses on the *power gap* and views health problems as arising from a lack of power to create change in social and physical environments.

Media advocacy can be defined as the strategic use of mass media to advance public policy by applying pressure to policymakers (Wallack, Dorfman, Jernigan, & Themba, 1993). The use of media advocacy has evolved as the definition of health problems has shifted from the individual level to the policy level. What distinguishes media advocacy from traditional health promotion and educational efforts is the goal of the effort (Riley, 2001; see Table 7.1).

Table 7.1 Traditional health communication versus media advocacy

Traditional Health Communication	Media Advocacy
Problem defined at the individual level	Problem defined at the policy level
Health is a personal issue	Health is a social issue
Mass media is used to change behavior	Mass media is used to influence public policy
Short-term focus	Long-term focus

Media advocacy differs in many ways from traditional public health campaigns. It is most marked by an emphasis on the following (Wallack & Dorfman, 2001):

- Linking public health and social problems to inequities in social arrangements rather than to flaws in the individual
- Changing public policy rather than personal health behavior
- Focusing primarily on reaching opinion leaders and policymakers rather than on those who have the problem (the traditional audience of public health communication campaigns)
- Working with groups to increase participation and amplify their voices rather than providing health behavior change messages
- Having a primary goal of reducing the power gap rather than just filling the information gap

In practice, media advocacy uses some of the same media relations techniques that practitioners of social marketing or public information campaigns might use: sending out news releases, pitching stories to journalists, monitoring the media and keeping a list of media contacts, and paying attention to what is newsworthy. Although these practices are frequently used, they do not alone constitute media advocacy. Because media advocacy's target is the power gap, it attempts to motivate social and political involvement rather than changes in personal health behavior (Wallack, Dorfman, & Woodruff, 1997). It is the best media strategy choice when the overall strategy involves changing policy.

DEVELOP A MESSAGE STRATEGY

The message is what is said to the target audience. The overall strategy determines the target audience, which might consist of a single person or a small group, the CEO of a company, or a legislative committee. The message is delivered through the news media. Other mechanisms for delivering the message are used at the same time, of course, because media advocacy is used in combination with community organizing and policy advocacy. Media advocacy adds power and amplification to those strategies by harnessing the news media's reach. It is a mechanism for thrusting the discussion with the target into the public conversation.

Because media advocacy messages are transmitted through the news media, it is useful to examine how the news media typically interpret and represent issues. This process is called framing. Any media advocates' messages will be filtered through the news frame.

Why Framing Matters
News is organized, or framed, to make sense of infinitely sided and shaded issues. Framing is the process of identifying how the issue will be depicted; it is "the package in which the main point of the story is developed, supported, and understood" (Wallack & Dorfman,

1996, p. 299). Inevitably, some elements of a story are left out while others are included. Similarly, some arguments, metaphors, or story lines may be featured prominently, while others are relegated to the margins of the story. News frames are important because the facts, values, or images included in news coverage are accorded legitimacy, while those not emphasized or excluded are marginalized or left out of public discussion. The coverage will significantly contribute to how the issue is felt and talked about by the public.

Journalism has traditions and routines that result in consistent frames, almost like story lines or scripts that reporters gravitate toward, such as heroes and villains, overcoming adversity, and the unexpected or ironic twist of the protector causing harm. Stories have characters, characters have roles, and characters carry out their actions on location in recognizable circumstances within a range of predictable outcomes. Television, in particular, with its two-minute storytelling, uses compact symbols to tell a familiar story. By studying the patterns of news storytelling, advocates can determine the implications for public health.

The Challenge of Framing Public Health Issues in Typical News Frames

Most news, especially television news, tries to *put a face on the issue*. The impact of an issue on an individual's life is often of more interest to news reporters than the policy implications of an issue, in part because reporters believe readers and viewers are more likely to identify emotionally with a particular person's plight. News stories tend to focus on specific, concrete events and use pictures that appeal to and resonate with audiences to tell a short, simple story. Unfortunately, research on television's effects has shown that when viewers see individually focused, event-oriented stories and then are asked what should be done about the problem depicted, the viewers will respond in ways that tend to blame the victim (Iyengar, 1991). Stories about isolated episodes do not help audiences understand how to deliberate about and solve social problems beyond demanding that individuals take more responsibility for themselves. "Following exposure to episodic framing," notes researcher Shanto Iyengar, "Americans describe chronic problems such as poverty and crime not in terms of deep-seated social or economic conditions, but as mere idiosyncratic outcomes" (1991, p. 137). Alternatively, when stories are more issue-oriented, audiences respond differently and include government and social institutions as part of the solution. The latter is the type of response public health advocates usually seek.

A simple way to distinguish between the two story types is to think of the difference between a *portrait* and a *landscape*. In a news story framed as a portrait, one may learn a great deal about an individual or an event, with great drama and detail. But it is hard to see what surrounds that individual or what brought him or her to that moment in time. A landscape pulls back the lens to take a broader view. It may include people and events, but must connect them to the larger social and economic forces. The challenge for media advocates is to make stories about the public health landscape as compelling and interesting as the portrait.

To focus attention on the landscape, media advocates try to frame the content of a news story or the message in that story. Framing for content shifts the individual problem to a social issue. For example, there is a current trend in many state legislatures to introduce youth tobacco access laws that heavily penalize young people who are attempting to purchase tobacco and the clerks who sell tobacco products, but not the storeowners. A way to frame this issue for content is to focus on the responsibility for marketing and promotion that the storeowners and the tobacco companies control. Highlighting the fact that tobacco companies market tobacco products to youth using images that are appealing to this age group (such as cartoon characters, men who are ruggedly independent and rebellious, and thin, independent females) can help shift the focus to the landscape in which the individual young person in that store exists. The primary responsibility for the social issue of youth sales can be shifted from the individual to tobacco industry marketing tactics (Riley, 2001). The industry role in causing the problem is then better understood, and advocates can articulate why it is reasonable to assign responsibility for changing practices to the industry.

Components of a Message

The message is what is to be said to those who have the power to make the change being sought (the target audience). But the message will be delivered in the context of a news story, so it must conform to the needs of journalists for clear, concise statements. Therefore, it is important to keep it simple.

Journalists are not likely to think of the public health aspects of the stories they write, but they are always eager for a new and interesting angle. Public health practitioners can offer ideas to journalists by suggesting stories directly related to the topics on which they work and by thinking about how the public health angle fits in to the news of the day.

To improve reporting from a public health perspective, advocates need to be well versed in social factors and other contextual variables so they can inform journalists of those links. They should be able to fill in the blanks in the following statement.

Every time there is a story on_____, it should include information about _____.

Similarly, advocates should understand how typical news stories might connect to particular health issues and be able to complete the reverse of the same statement. For example, asthma rates began rising in the late 1980s, and studies began to define risk factors such as outdoor pollutants and secondhand smoke (California Center for Health Improvement, 2000). Advocates working to prevent asthma need to determine whether news stories reflect this understanding. If they do not, advocates will know how to focus their discussions with journalists.

Given what is now known from epidemiologists, it is reasonable to expect that whenever there is a story on children's health, it should mention rising asthma rates. Similarly, whenever there is a story on asthma, it should mention children's rates going up, prevention measures for parents, potential environmental policy protections, and the health department as a community resource. It would also be appropriate to include an angle on asthma in stories on environmental tobacco smoke or air quality. Think of it this way:

> Every time there is a story on asthma, it should include information about secondhand smoke.
> Every time there is a story on secondhand smoke, it should include information about asthma.

Advocates can use the same formula to think through other public health issues, their risk factors, and important aspects of prevention that should be included regularly in news stories. They can collect the materials that clearly and simply make their point and have them on hand to send to reporters on short notice when an article on the topic appears. Data and examples should be ready to explain why reporters should include this information in their story.

The message an advocate delivers is usually in the context of an answer to a journalist's question. Journalists will usually ask at least two questions: "What is the problem?" and "What is the solution?" (Dorfman, 1994). It is common for public health professionals and their community allies to spend about 80 percent of their time talking about the problem and 20 percent talking about the solution. Strategically, it is important to reverse the ratio. Advocates should identify the problem briefly but emphasize what needs to be done to solve it.

A practical rule of thumb is that a good message uses concise, direct language to convey at least three elements (Wallack, Woodruff, Dorfman, & Diaz, 1999). One component is the *clear statement of concern*. For example, it is cause for concern there are too many alcohol-related problems on campus. The second component represents the *value dimension*, such as the threat alcohol poses to healthy student life and a nurturing learning environment. The third component elucidates the *policy objective*, for example, the elimination of happy hours in bars near campuses. The components need not always fall in that order, but they are usually all present.

When the latest study was released on drinking on college campuses, reporters sought comments from those who were directly concerned with or affected by the problem. At the University of Iowa, a coalition had formed to try to reduce alcohol problems on and around campus. The coalition had several specific policy goals as its prime directive and had been trained in media advocacy. When the time came to respond to the study, Mary Sue Coleman, then president of the university, told reporters, "Of course, students who drink too much must be responsible for the problems that they cause. But students are not responsible for manufacturing and marketing alcoholic beverages. Students are not responsible for the excessive number of bars within walking distance of our campuses. Students are not responsible for the price specials that encourage drinking to get drunk" (Wilgoren, 2000). In that statement, Dr. Coleman was able to acknowledge the personal responsibility of students but also paint a picture of the landscape surrounding those students that helped illustrate why the policies she sought were both necessary and reasonable. She cannot say everything in one small media bite, but her example goes a long way to define the problem and effectively point to the solution.

Media advocates can develop all the story elements reporters need to tell the public health side of the story. Media bites, like Dr. Coleman's, are essential. In addition, media advocates can prepare compelling visuals to help illustrate their point of view, calculate *social math* so large numbers can be made meaningful, identify *authentic voices* (those advocates who can effectively "put a face on the issue," as reporters might put it) and identify and use evocative symbols in their descriptions of the problem and solution. Having story elements ready that portray the public health frame will make it easier for journalists to cover the story.

DEVELOP AN ACCESS STRATEGY

After advocates have determined an overall strategy, selected a media strategy, and crafted the message, they are ready to attract journalists' attention. At this point, they must think of what parts of the issue will make a good story. By emphasizing those elements, advocates will be framing the issue for access.

Monitoring the News and Building Relationships with Journalists

To work well with journalists, advocates need to understand how they define and report news. Advocates can do this by carefully watching television news, reading newspapers, and listening to the radio. Advocates should regularly scan all sections of the local newspaper for articles that directly or indirectly relate to the advocacy issue. For instance, the sports page may cover an automobile race that is tobacco-sponsored. This may provide an opportunity for a group working on a policy to ban tobacco-sponsored sporting events. Members of the group could respond to the article with a letter to the editor or with an invitation to the reporter who covered the event to learn more about sponsorship. Copies of the article can be sent to other community activists and appropriate legislators (Riley, 2001).

Monitoring means listing and paying attention to the local and relevant national media outlets. For each of the outlets, advocates will have to determine how often it covers the issues that are of concern. Monitoring means noticing what the coverage says about the issue. Does it tell the whole story? Advocates need not conduct a detailed study of the media, but they need enough information to inform their media advocacy efforts. Advocates should read and watch the news critically from a public health perspective. When reading the newspaper, they can ask themselves: Does the article include everything it should given the topic it covers? Are there important aspects missing? Is there a public health aspect to this story that should have been included? These questions can help advocates evaluate the comprehensiveness of a news story and determine the specifics to bring to the attention of the journalist who may do similar stories in the future.

By carefully paying attention to news stories about an issue, advocates can identify which journalists are most interested in a specific topic and what aspect of the topic interests journalists the most. Advocates will also start to see how different symbols and journalistic conventions are used to tell the story. This is the foundation from which they can approach journalists about the aspects of the story not receiving attention (Wallack et al., 1997).

Advocates will have greater success attracting journalists to the story if they have built a relationship with them. The first step to building a relationship is to compile a list of local media contacts. Each entry on the list should include (1) the name of the reporter; (2) telephone and fax numbers; (3) e-mail and mailing addresses; (4) the name of the newspaper, magazine, or television or radio station; (5) the best time to reach the reporter; (6) sections, or beats, the reporter writes about or reports on (for example, sports, columnist, lifestyle, health); and (7) any notes pertaining to interactions to date. Advocates should meet with the reporters who might have an interest in their issue or with those whose beats intersect with the issue. The advocate should introduce herself or himself, explain why she or he has an interest in meeting, and get to know reporters. Advocates need to update the media list regularly because there is a high rate of turnover in the news business. It is therefore important to keep track of contacts as they move on to other news outlets. A relationship at a local television station today may be a relationship at a national news program tomorrow.

Newsworthiness

Framing the issue for access involves making the issue newsworthy. The following questions can help determine newsworthiness (Riley, 2001):

- Is the issue controversial (for example, freedom of speech versus encouraging the sale of illegal products to minors)?
- Is there a milestone event (for example, the introduction of FDA regulations)?
- Is there an anniversary (for example, release of the Surgeon General's report on health consequences of tobacco use)?
- Can irony be used (for example, the contrast between outrage about President Clinton's testimony to special prosecutors and the lack of interest in tobacco company executives who lied to Congress)?
- Can a local issue be connected with a larger or national event (for example, local night spots go smoke-free for the Great American Smokeout)?

Identifying newsworthy components can help turn an issue into a story. Stories have action, plot, and characters. What are they in relation to the topic of interest? Why is it a story now? Why will it matter to the people who read that newspaper or watch that television station?

General Strategies

Four general strategies for getting in the news include: creating news, piggybacking on breaking news, paying for advertisements, and using editorial strategies.

Creating News

Tobacco control advocate Russell Sciandra said, "To gain the media's attention, you can't just say something; you have to do something" (Wallack et al., 1999, p. 39). That *something* need not be elaborate, but it must be newsworthy. Creating news can be as simple as releasing new data or announcing a specific demand. The important part is that it be done publicly and that someone alerts the news media, emphasizing why the story is newsworthy. For example, if advocates know an important document will be released, they could plan a briefing for journalists so they will be prepared or hold a news conference with the group's reaction to it.

Piggybacking on Breaking News

When advocates identify a connection between an issue and news of the day, they should make the story known to journalists. Tobacco control advocates used the occasion of President Clinton's perjury hearings to highlight the fact that tobacco company executives had lied under oath to Congress. Family planning advocates used news hype about Viagra to point out health insurance plans were not covering contraceptives for women, although they were covering Viagra. Piggybacking on breaking news can be achieved in a letter to the editor, with a news conference, or by other actions.

Paid Advertising

Buying space is sometimes the only way to be sure a message gets out unadulterated. In San Francisco, children's advocates used paid advertising to highlight a positive policy change the news media were ignoring. The job market was tight in San Francisco in 2000, and that meant a crisis for child care. Childcare teachers, who were typically paid less than $7 an hour, which was less than parking attendants made, were leaving the field for more lucrative jobs. Families that qualified for subsidized care could not get care because childcare centers did not have the requisite staff. Working with Coleman Advocates for Children and Youth, among others, Mayor Willie Brown took unprecedented action. He allocated $4.1 million to increase the wages of 1,000 childcare workers who were serving low-income families. Never before had the city subsidized the salaries of non-city employees. The advocates were thrilled and immediately alerted the local news media. The reporters, however, refused to cover the story. They did not want to "toot the mayor's horn."

The advocates thought it was a legitimate story and were frustrated by the unresponsive reporters. They decided to tell the story themselves in a full-page ad in the West Coast edition of the *New York Times*. The ad ran on August 7, 2000, during the Democratic national convention, which was being held in San Diego that year. The ad proclaimed "Childcare History in the Making—San Francisco Mayor Willie Brown Sets National Standard for

Quality, Affordable Childcare!" It suggested readers challenge their own mayors to take the same action in their hometowns. Mayor Willie Brown was still talking about the ad six months later when he signed the next budget allocations for childcare.

Editorial Strategies

Letters to the editor, editorials, and op-eds (opinion editorials or opinion pieces found opposite the editorial page) provide other opportunities for bringing attention to a policy solution. Letters are usually 200 words or less and can be written, faxed, or e-mailed to the editor of the newspaper. They are usually in response to a specific article or editorial the paper has published and offer a concise statement of support or objection.

Editorials are unsigned and written by the editorial board of the newspaper. Advocates can make an appointment to talk with the editorial board to ask them to take a position and make a statement about an issue or a pending policy. The meeting is usually attended by the newspaper staff responsible for writing the editorial and those who will make the decision about whether the newspaper will take a position on the issue. Two or three advocates may also be present to speak to various aspects of the issue or represent different perspectives.

If the newspaper decides not to do an editorial, the advocates can ask if the paper would publish an op-ed. Op-eds are usually 600 to 800 words and written from a personal point of view. They describe the problem, solution, and its relevance to the readers. Monitoring should include reviewing op-eds, both to keep tabs on how an issue is being argued and to identify the style the news outlet prefers.

Newspapers often publish on the editorial pages the contact information and instructions for submitting letters and op-eds. Some radio stations and television news programs allow audience members to record commentaries that function like op-eds, although they are usually no more than a few minutes long.

TIPS AND TECHNIQUES FOR SUCCESSFUL MEDIA ADVOCACY

Techniques that can enhance media advocacy's effectiveness include calculating social math, localizing stories, cultivating authentic voices, and reusing the news.

CALCULATE SOCIAL MATH

Social math is the art of making large numbers meaningful, usually by breaking them down and making a relevant, vivid comparison. Calculating social math can illustrate a message. Raw numbers assume the audience already knows something about the issue and why the numbers are important or revealing. Comparisons, on the other hand, can highlight a specific point of view at the same time they deliver basic information.

To calculate social math, restate large numbers in terms of time or place, personalize numbers, or make comparisons that help bring a picture to mind. Consider the following simple facts, which are stated with effective comparisons.

- About 950 packs of cigarettes are being sold in the United States every second of every day (Gloede, 1989).
- A children and youth advocacy group wanted to increase county spending on prevention of violence. To make their point they said, "In San Francisco, there is one police officer for every 18 young people and only one school counselor for every 500 kids" (Coleman Advocates, n.d.).
- Other violence prevention advocates wanted to make clear to the public and their policymakers that availability of firearms was a problem. They said, "Contra Costa County has 700 federally licensed firearms dealers—more than the number of schools, grocery stores and gas stations combined" ("Contra Costa County," 1995).
- Newspaper columnist Ellen Goodman (1998) noted that a worker who helps bury people makes more than one who helps them learn and that the median wage for a funeral attendant is $7.16 an hour, whereas the median wage for a childcare worker is $6.17 an hour. Goodman feels childcare workers are being paid based on what mothers are paid (nothing) and not on what professional teachers earn.
- Public health education professor Meredith Minkler (1999, p. 127) noted, "In a single year one company spent more than $30 million advertising a single sugar-coated cereal. During the same year, the amount spent by the U.S. government on nutrition education for school children was just $50,000 per state."
- A reporter in the *Wall Street Journal* illustrated the amount of chewing tobacco being consumed by writing, "Cigarette sales are down; dip sales are up. Laid out tin-to-tin, the dip sold last year would stretch between New York and Los Angeles 11 times. So there is quite a bit of furtive spitting going on" (Morse, 2000).
- A victim's rights advocate used irony to point out society's skewed priorities and illustrate the need for more resources when he said, "We have more shelters for animals than we have for human victims of abuse" (Stein, 1997).

LOCALIZE STORIES

Every day there is a multitude of news from which to choose. News outlets are tuned in to satellite broadcasts from around the world that operate twenty-four hours daily. Assignment editors, city desk editors, reporters, and producers read several newspapers every day, listen to news radio and police scanners, and monitor wire services. One way advocates can break through that clutter is to alert their news contacts about the local relevance of a story. Questions they can address include the following: "Why does this story matter to people who live here?" and "Why would this story matter to the listeners at this radio station, the viewers of this local television news, or the readers of this newspaper?" When advocates know the answers to those questions, they will know what to tell the reporter. Every reporter has to convince his or her boss why to select one story rather than another. If the story has local relevance, it is much more likely to be pursued.

CULTIVATE AUTHENTIC VOICES

Reporters populate their stories with characters. A common character in health stories is the *victim*, that is, someone who has suffered from or has direct experience with the problem, whatever it might be. If the story is about binge drinking on college campuses, reporters will want to talk to students. If the story is about gun safety in the home, they will want to talk to a parent whose child was killed by a gun in the home. If the story is about immunizations for children, they will want to show a toddler getting a shot.

Reporters focus on characters for two reasons. First, the reporter needs to present evidence in the story that what happened was real and that it happened to a real person. Showing someone with direct experience in the story makes that clear. Second, reporters feel their audience will connect more with the emotion than the facts of a story. People who actually endured a trauma or other experience can be more compelling because they are speaking from experience. They qualify as a "real person," in journalists' parlance.

Besides the usual questions such as "What is the problem?" and "What is the solution?" reporters will ask victims another question: "How do you feel about the tragedy?" The problem, of course, is that if the story does not move much beyond the victim (because it is a portrait rather than a landscape) when audiences see the story they are likely to distance themselves from the individual and say, "That won't happen to me." In some cases they might even blame the victim. Journalists cannot tell stories without characters, and victims can be powerful spokespeople for public health. However, the preferred approach is to change the dynamic and present victims as survivors or *authentic voices*. Authentic voices are survivors who have become advocates. They bring personal experience to the story, just like a victim, but they understand their role as advocates. When an authentic voice gets the question, "How do you feel about this tragedy?" he or she responds, "I feel angry because this tragedy could have been prevented." Then he or she explains how.

Victims become authentic voices with training and experience as they move through their grief and put it to work for prevention. There are many authentic voices in public health to thank for opening up their lives to the public and becoming leaders for change regarding issues such as breast cancer, HIV/AIDS, and tobacco control. For example, in 2000 Mary Leigh Blek became the first chair of the board for the Million Mom March; she had lost her son Matthew to a *Saturday night special* handgun and had been advocating for reasonable gun laws ever since. In 1980, Mothers Against Drunk Driving was created by a small group of women in California after a drunk driver killed Candy Lightner's thirteen-year-old daughter. Survivors have joined with public health advocates to advocate for safer baby cribs, drowning prevention, pedestrian safety, motorcycle helmets, mandatory CPR training, and auto safety, including interior trunk release latches (McLoughlin & Fennell, n.d.). All of these authentic voices have selflessly shared their stories and been willing characters in news stories to help further policies that can save lives.

REUSE THE NEWS

Media advocacy uses mass communication to reach a very small target, which can sometimes consist of only one person. The power comes from the fact that a vast audience has been privy to this conversation between the advocates and the target. It is a public conversation, not a private conversation. To ensure the target understands this, advocates can reuse the news. If their op-ed is published, advocates can clip it, copy it, and send it to the target. They can have the target's constituents copy and send news stories and letters to the editor that have been published. They can also reuse the news to educate reporters who are just coming to the issue or to educate new advocates. They can share clippings and discuss them to become better at framing issues and anticipating the opposition's questions and challenges. News, simply by virtue of having been published, confers legitimacy and credibility on issues. Media advocates reuse the news to remind the target the public is paying attention and knows what it wants done.

OVERCOMING CHALLENGES IN MEDIA ADVOCACY

The biggest barrier to successful media advocacy is in the development of a clear overall strategy, even before getting access to reporters is considered. Other barriers include institutional constraints, not staying *on message*, and being distracted by the opposition. This section discusses strategies for overcoming these barriers.

AVOID HAVING A MURKY STRATEGY

The most important part of media advocacy is developing strategy. If the strategy is not clear and the target has not been well-defined, the media advocacy effort will be diffused and ineffective. Public health advocates sometimes resist simplifying the problem. This simplification is necessary to carve out a viable strategy. Public health problems are complex, and that complexity needs to be addressed. However, not everything can be done at once. Public health problems need to be prioritized into manageable chunks that can be addressed in specific time periods. The alternative, which is to rely upon strategies that remain too large or overly vague, will be ineffective. Goals such as *raising awareness* are not specific enough for media advocacy campaigns. Instead, clear objectives must be stated that identify who must do what to create or change the rules that will ensure healthier social and physical environments.

Advocates must translate general principles into substantive demands. For example, in San Francisco, a campaign to seek justice for a man who unnecessarily died in police custody was transformed into a campaign to change police practices. Demanding justice was too vague and left the action up to others. So the advocates asked themselves: What would justice look like? They decided the offending police officer should be fired and safeguards were put in place to avoid future hires of officers with similar records. Advocates had then defined justice in tangible terms that could be put into practice and used media advocacy to put pressure on the mayor and the police commission to enact the policy changes they desired.

Media advocacy strategies and targets can change over time. In fact, they should change. Targets and strategies will shift in response to circumstances and after the advocates achieve their objectives. Advocates can use the strategy development questions discussed earlier to refocus their efforts and evaluate their strategies. With every new activity, they should ask themselves: How will this help us achieve our objectives? Will this make a clear, positive change in the environment surrounding the people whose health we are concerned about? The answers to those questions can guide strategy and decisions throughout the media advocacy effort.

ALTER PERCEIVED INSTITUTIONAL CONSTRAINTS

Media advocacy is about raising community voices to demand change. In most cases, policy change is the desired outcome. Sometimes policy change will require lobbying, which public agencies and some nonprofit organizations are prohibited from conducting. In most cases, however, public and nonprofit agencies can do a lot that is not considered lobbying. Unfortunately, advocates often stop short of what is allowed and limit their effectiveness needlessly. Organizations such as the Alliance for Justice provide training and consultation to nonprofits to help them maximize their ability to participate legally in the policy process. Constraints are often not as prohibitive as some in the agency might perceive.

Still, media advocacy can be confrontational. Thus, public health practitioners in health departments or other institutions may not be comfortable being *out front* on media advocacy campaigns. Some have a preference for consensus when conflict is what is needed. In these cases, individuals can find roles for themselves in the media advocacy effort that place them more in the background than the foreground. For example, health departments can provide data, resources, meeting space, technical assistance, and other support without compromise.

AVOID BEING DISTRACTED BY THE OPPOSITION

Although media advocates need to construct thoughtful, succinct answers to the questions their opponents will raise, their goal is not to convince the opposition. Media advocates can be distracted by the arguments their opposition puts forward and might be tempted to answer those arguments point by point. Sometimes that is necessary, but often it is a ploy by opponents to frame the issue on their own terms. Instead, media advocates' goal is to motivate and mobilize their supporters to make their voices count with policymakers. Everyone does not have to be convinced the proposal is worth supporting; only those who have decision-making power must be convinced. Media advocacy employs the mass media to make private conversations public so decision makers can be held accountable for their decisions and the impact of those decisions on the public's health. Media advocates need to be vigilant when defining the problem and the solution and focus their attention on the clear and consistent articulation of what they want. Thus, articulating a clear message and staying on message are extremely important.

STAY ON MESSAGE

Staying on message means that whatever advocates may be asked, they do not stray from the key message they are trying to deliver. Staying on message is a skill that can be honed with practice. It is especially helpful to practice aloud, with colleagues. That way, advocates can anticipate what questions they might receive from reporters, decision makers, or the opposition and can craft answers that lead logically from the question to the outcome they seek. Practicing aloud is important because speaking is different from writing or thinking. The right words will flow more easily if they have been said before. At the same time, advocates should not memorize a script because scripts can sound stiff and forced. Instead, frequent practice and feedback sessions will help advocates prepare for staying on message.

INTERVIEW GONE WRONG

Once we have figured out what has to be done, who has to do it, and how to frame the issue, then we have to talk about it, in public and on the record. Talking with journalists is especially important since policy makers pay close attention to the news. Whenever we talk with reporters we have the opportunity to educate them about the problems we see and what to do about them. But talking with reporters can be intimidating. Sometimes it's hard to stay focused on our message, including on the policy goal. Let's use the example of a moratorium on fast food outlets and see what can happen under the pressure of an interview.

Reporter: What should we do about childhood obesity?

Answer: We need to make healthier food more widely available in our communities. One way to do this is to stop building fast-food outlets, so neighborhoods can attract a bigger variety of food options.

So far so good. Let's keep going . . .

Reporter: But no one forces people to go into a McDonald's. What does the number of fast food restaurants have to do with obesity?

Answer: Of course we can't guarantee people will buy fruit instead of french fries or chips, but at least if people have healthy food available instead of junk food, we are headed in the right direction. For example, making produce available in corner stores would make it easier for families to buy healthy food.

Reporter: If people in the neighborhood wanted to purchase that sort of food, wouldn't it already be in the stores? And why should small businesses take the risk of putting expensive, perishable produce on their shelves? Their concern is business, not health.

Answer: People in this neighborhood already purchase that sort of food, but not as often as they want to because they have to travel so far to do it. We want to encourage business owners here to promote health. They should be held accountable for the unhealthy food they carry in their stores and restaurants. Corner stores can start by carrying small quantities of healthy food. They can increase the supply once demand increases.

Now you are off track. These are good points, but you wanted to focus on the specific policy goal of supporting the fast food moratorium in your city. Instead, you find yourself talking about the importance of convenience stores carrying produce. Although this is not a bad idea, you have let your focus stray from your policy goal. Let's try the interview again.

Reporter: What should we do about childhood obesity?

Answer: We need to make healthier food more widely available in our communities. One way to do this is to stop building fast-food outlets so neighborhoods can attract a bigger variety of food options.

Reporter: But no one forces people to go into a McDonald's. What does the number of fast food restaurants have to do with obesity?

Answer: Policymakers can help ensure communities are given a fair chance for health if they pay attention to the environment that affects health. Right now we have plenty of fast food outlets in our neighborhood. What is lacking are places that offer healthier menus with fresh food.

Reporter: Why should government interfere with where businesses locate? Isn't this a free market issue? If there were a demand for other sorts of restaurants, wouldn't businesses like that locate here?

Answer: We have a responsibility, and our policy makers have a responsibility, to be sure neighborhoods don't stack the deck against their residents' health. That's why the moratorium makes sense. We need a breather from fast food to attract other healthier businesses into the neighborhood.

Now you're on the right track. The reporter may follow up with questions about how the fast food moratorium will work, what you hope the outcome will be, or next steps. Or the reporter may ask another distracting question. But by staying on track, you will have the discussion you want to have and stay focused on your priority policy goal.

Source: Berkeley Media Studies Group.

EXPECTED OUTCOMES

When media advocacy is done well, healthy public policy is enacted and implemented. Enacting policies that benefit the public's health is a long-term process, however, with many contributing factors. Media advocacy cannot achieve that end alone but can certainly amplify advocates' voices and accelerate the process. Properly applied, media advocacy can punctuate the advocacy process, add urgency to a campaign, and create visibility. Media advocacy does this by increasing the salience of issues for the public and policymakers through agenda setting and framing. Practicing media advocacy will also increase the capacity of local groups to influence the rules that govern their environments.

INCREASED SKILLS AND POWER

Because policy advocacy is usually a long-term endeavor, it is useful to identify some interim effects and outcomes of media advocacy. The most immediate interim effects of media advocacy are the increases in skills and power of the groups using it. By developing and adapting strategy, advocates can gain skills in critical thinking. By talking with journalists and others about the solutions they seek, advocates develop the confidence necessary to speak effectively in public. They become skillful at framing for content and understanding newsworthiness so they can frame for access. By participating in the policy process, either by meeting with decision makers or mobilizing supporters, advocates exercise their democratic power. These skills build on one another and transfer as advocates work together in a community setting to demand change.

BETTER RELATIONSHIPS WITH JOURNALISTS

An important outcome advocates can expect from media advocacy campaigns is better relationships with journalists. This tangible benefit develops during the course of a media advocacy campaign (and from one campaign to another) because advocates bring good information and interesting stories to reporters. The mutually beneficial relationship helps reporters get what they need to do their job, increases advocates' access to journalists, and, ultimately, makes journalists more responsive. Stated simply, an expected outcome of media advocacy is that certain reporters and advocates end up in each other's Rolodex. For example, after their concerted media advocacy effort to generate news that reframed alcohol as a policy issue, staff at the Marin Institute for the Prevention of Alcohol and Other Drug Problems, located in California, were frequent sources for journalists. Eventually, reporters would call the Marin Institute for comments on stories that had been generated elsewhere. The Marin Institute was now a required source on alcohol policy issues.

INCREASED VISIBILITY AND INFLUENCE

Advocates' increased skills and power, along with their better relationships and influence with reporters, lead to increased visibility for the issue. If successful, advocates will have generated news that put their issue and solution on the policymakers' agenda. Advocates can expect to see their examples used in debate by themselves and eventually by others, shifting the debate toward the advocates' desired outcomes. Advocates' influence will increase with the increased visibility because news coverage confers legitimacy and credibility.

CONCLUSION

Public health educators can harness the power of the news media to advance healthy public policy. They can increase their effectiveness by developing an overall strategy, learning about how the news media operate, developing a specific media strategy, developing a message that frames the issue from a public health perspective, and understanding how to attract journalists' attention. The news media are too important a resource to ignore. If health educators are serious about serving the public and improving its health, they need to be serious about the news and about learning how to better integrate it into prevention efforts.

Media advocacy, however, is not appropriate in every instance. The strategy requires a clear and precise plan for policy change and a constituency that can carry it out. It is a public strategy that is on the record. Media advocates bring public attention to specific individuals. At times they may need to be confrontational and adversarial, depending on the situation. The policies being advocated for are usually controversial. If they were not, there would be no need for a pressure tool and publicity via media advocacy. Advocates should be clear with themselves and their colleagues about what is at stake when choosing to use media advocacy.

Media advocacy is the right choice when public demands must be made and when decision makers must be pressured to protect and promote the public's health.

DISCUSSION QUESTIONS

1. Why is communications important for public health? How is media advocacy different from other communications approaches? When would you use media advocacy?
2. What are the basic elements of media advocacy? What is the relationship between strategy and framing? What would you do to attract news attention? What would you do to be sure you framed the issue to emphasize prevention?
3. How could social media be incorporated into media advocacy efforts to influence policy debate?

REFERENCES

California Center for Health Improvement. (2000, December). Joining forces to fight childhood asthma: A Prop 10 opportunity. *Field Lessons*, pp. 1–8.

Centers for Disease Control and Prevention (CDC). (2004). Alcohol-attributable deaths and years of potential life lost: United States, 2001. *MMWR, 53*, 866–870.

Coleman Advocates for Children and Youth. (2000, August 7). Childcare history in the making— San Francisco Mayor Willie Brown sets national standard for quality, affordable childcare! [Advertisement]. *The New York Times*, West Coast ed., p. A19.

Coleman Advocates for Children and Youth. (n.d.). *Youth time* [Brochure]. San Francisco: Author.

Contra Costa County offers advice on reducing gun use. (1995, July). *The Nation's Health*, p. 11.

Dorfman, L. (1994). *News operations: How television reports on health*. Unpublished doctoral dissertation, University of California, Berkeley.

Gloede, W. F. (1989). Agency execs feel at home in Marlboro country. In E. Thorson (Ed.), *Advertising age: The principles of advertising at work* (pp. 103–105). Lincolnwood, IL: NTC Business Books.

Goodman, E. (1998, January 15). No easy fix for child care. *San Francisco Chronicle*, p. A23.

Iyengar, S. (1991). *Is anyone responsible?* Chicago: University of Chicago Press.

McLoughlin, E., & Fennell, J. (n.d.). Channeling grief into policy change: Survivor advocacy for injury prevention. *Injury Prevention Newsletter*, Vol. 13. San Francisco: The Trauma Foundation. Retrieved October 14, 2006, from http://www.traumaf.org/images/IPNweb.pdf

Minkler, M. (1999). Personal responsibility for health? A review of the arguments and the evidence at century's end. *Health Education and Behavior, 26,* 121–140.

Morse, D. (2000, February 11). If you can't smoke in the office, snuff can be a secret vice. *The Wall Street Journal*, p. A1.

National Institute on Alcohol Abuse and Alcoholism (NIAAA). (2004/2005). Alcohol and development in youth: A multidisciplinary overview. *Alcohol Research & Health, 28*(3), 111–120. Retrieved April 30, 2010, from http://pubs.niaaa.nih.gov/publications/arh283/toc28-3.htm

Riley, B. A. (2001). Media advocacy. In R. J. Bensley & J. Brookins-Fisher (Eds.), *Community health education methods: A practitioner's guide* (pp. 383–409). Sudbury, MA: Jones & Bartlett.

Stein, J., deputy director of the National Organization for Victim Assistance, quoted in J. Shiver Jr. (1997, August 25). Home violence underreported, U.S. study says. *Los Angeles Times*, p. A1.

Wallack, L., & Dorfman, L. (1996). Media advocacy: A strategy for advancing policy and promoting health. *Health Education Quarterly, 23,* 293–317.

Wallack, L., & Dorfman, L. (2001). Putting policy into health communication: The role of media advocacy. In R. E. Rice & C. K. Atkin (Eds.), *Public communication campaigns* (3rd ed., pp. 389–401). Thousand Oaks, CA: Sage.

Wallack, L., Dorfman, L., Jernigan, D., & Themba, M. (1993). *Media advocacy and public health: Power for prevention.* Thousand Oaks, CA: Sage.

Wallack, L., Dorfman, L., & Woodruff, K. (1997). Communications and public health. In F. D. Scutchfield & C. W. Keck (Eds.), *Principles of public health practice* (pp. 183–194). Albany, NY: Delmar.

Wallack, L., Woodruff, K., Dorfman, L., & Diaz, I. (1999). *News for a change: An advocate's guide to working with the media.* Thousand Oaks, CA: Sage.

Wilgoren, J. (2000, March 15). Effort to curb binge drinking in college falls short. *The New York Times*, p. A16.

8

The Impact of Corporate Practices on Health and Health Policy

Nicholas Freudenberg
Sandro Galea

LEARNING OBJECTIVES

- Learn how the business and political activities of corporations influence population health
- Identify the strengths and limitations of campaigns that change corporate practices that are detrimental to population health
- Discuss why government has a right to intervene in markets and regulate corporate practices
- Articulate new directions for research and policymaking that supports corporate practices that promote health and primary prevention

Recently, policymakers, the media, health care advocates, and the public have called attention to the impact of corporate activities on health and disease in the United States. High-profile cases that have galvanized public discourse include: the tobacco settlement that was designed to provide compensation to states for tobacco-related illness, widespread debate over the responsibility of the food and beverage industry for the current epidemic of obesity, and discussions about drug company profits and harmful product side effects. Criminal prosecutions of corporate executives have posed new questions about corporate responsibility. Controversy about corporations and corporate practices has reignited a perennial American conflict regarding appropriate roles for government and markets in political life and in public health.

Within public health, some have urged health professionals to engage corporations to improve health (Wiist, 2006). Few public health commentators, however, have systematically examined corporate practices as social determinants of health or assessed their implications for health policy. While researchers have examined the occupational and environmental health consequences of corporate policies (Geiser & Rosenberg, 2006), very little work has focused on the cumulative impact of consumer exposures to corporate policies. Current interest in the role of social determinants in shaping illness and health has focused on structural characteristics, such as poverty, inequality, and racism (Mechanic, 2002; Wyatt et al., 2003; McGinnis, Williams-Russo, & Knickman, 2002). The research that has considered the impact of corporate activity on health has usually examined the health consequences of a single product or a corporate practice rather than the patterns of behavior by corporations and governments across a variety of industries.

In our view, a systematic investigation of the impact of corporate decisions on health may yield insights that can guide prevention policy. In this review, we consider how fundamental factors, such as the current relationship between markets and government, influence corporate policies and, in turn, how these policies influence health and health behavior. Our primary interest is in *corporate practices*, defined as the business and political activities of corporations. These practices result from companies' decisions about the production, pricing, distribution, and promotion of their products and from their political efforts to create an environment favorable for their businesses. Our goals are to assess the role of corporate practices in determining health, examine their implications for health policy, and suggest directions for policy and research. More broadly, we hope to widen the discussion on social determinants to include corporate practices as a modifiable influence on population health.

Reproduced with permission of Palgrave Macmillan. N. Freudenberg and S. Galea, (2008). *The Impact of Corporate Practices on Health: Implications for Health Policy.* Basingstoke, UK: Palgrave Macmillan.

The authors acknowledge the contributions of Marianne Fahs, Sarah Bradley, Zoe Meleo Erwin, and Erica Sullivan.

Recent literature on social and policy determinants of health (McGinnis et al., 2002; Adler & Newman, 2002; Marmot, 2005; Wilkinson & Pickett, 2006; McKeown, 1980; Link & Phelan, 2005) and the authors' ongoing research (Freudenberg, 2005) informs this inquiry. Corporate practices can both benefit and harm health. Changes in food production and marketing in the first part of the 20th century eliminated most malnutrition in the United States and products developed by the pharmaceutical industry have saved millions of lives are two examples. A better understanding of what leads a company or an industry to choose health-promoting versus health-damaging practices may help to identify new opportunities for policies that encourage primary prevention.

FOUR CORPORATE PRACTICES THAT INFLUENCE HEALTH

Marketing describes corporate strategies and activities to encourage consumption and increase market share and demand. It includes advertising, sales promotions, sponsorship of sports and music events—often particularly targeting those music events which appeal to many youth of color—product placement, viral market-ing, and Web and Internet campaigns (Ewen, 1977; Hawkes, 2006). For example, Merck's heavy marketing of the painkiller Vioxx through direct-to-consumer and physician advertising, its deployment of an army of detail men to encourage physi-cians to prescribe Vioxx (Topol, 2004; Hawthorne, 2003; Brown, 2004; Berenson, 2005), and its advertising campaigns that implied that Vioxx was superior to safer over-the-counter medications (despite the lack of evidence for such a claim) helped to persuade an estimated 20 million consumers to use Vioxx before it was with-drawn, thus magnifying the product's adverse effects on population health (Avorn, 2006).

Retail distribution refers to industry practices that affect product availability at the consumer level. Placement of fast food outlets, supermarkets, or liquor stores; legal or voluntary industry restrictions on who can purchase tobacco or firearms; industry oversight of retail distribution of prescription drugs, firearms, or tobacco; and the allocation of shelf space in supermarkets are all examples of retail decisions that affect product availability and therefore the impact on health. Retail distribu-tion also includes targeting certain communities (for example those that are black, Latino, or lower income) with disproportionate levels of advertising for unhealthy products (Hackbarth et al., 2001; Grier & Kumanyika, 2008).

Pricing practices determine who pays how much for a product and therefore influence access to harmful products. Companies and their retail affiliates decide how much to charge various subgroups of customers, whether or not to engage in legal or illegal price-fixing, whether to oppose or support excise taxes, and how to relate to illicit markets (for example, untaxed tobacco products). Successful efforts by the alcohol and tobacco industries to limit excise taxes contribute to heavier use of these products by low-income and young people, again escalating the adverse health impact of these products (Chaloupka, Cummings, Morley & Horan, 2002; Chaloupka, Grossman & Saffer, 2002).

Courtesy of Corporations and Health Watch, http://www.corporationsandhealth.org/chron.php

TRANS FATS, VIOXX, AND SPORT UTILITY VEHICLES

To understand how corporate practices influence population health, we consider three products that have attracted recent media attention.

TRANS FATS

In 1994, the Center for Science in the Public Interest, a national advocacy organization, petitioned the Food and Drug Administration (FDA) to require that food manufacturers label the trans fatty acid (trans fat) content of their food products. The petition was based on research showing that replacing trans fat with healthier oils could prevent 30,000 to 100,000 premature cardiovascular deaths in the United States each year (Willett et al., 1993; Ascherio et al., 1994). Some researchers have suggested that replacing trans fats with healthier alternatives could reduce the incidence of Type 2 diabetes in the United States by as much as 40 percent (Clandinin & Wilke, 2001; Salmerón et al., 2001). Artificial trans fats are used to enhance the crispness, stability, and flavor of many processed foods (Ascherio et al., 1999). By the late 1990s, 40 percent of U.S. supermarket products contained trans fats. When evidence of harmful effects began to emerge in the early 1990s, sectors of the food industry chose different responses. Some producers rejected the claim that trans fats were harmful and sought to delay any regulatory action by calling for further research (Allison et al., 1995). Throughout the 1990s, food industry groups opposed new FDA regulations on trans fats (Weinraub, 2003). Other companies, however, accepted the call for labeling and looked for ways to reduce the amount of trans fats so that their labels might show lower levels. Yet others, European food companies, moved to substitute safer ingredients for trans fats, demonstrating that companies might opt for health-enhancing practices (Weinraub, 2003).

In 1999, despite the opposition of the food industry, the FDA proposed to require trans fatty acid content on the standard food label. The agency claimed that strengthening food labeling was likely to yield significant health and economic benefits, saving as many as 5,600 lives and $8 billion a year (FDA, 1999). Six years later, the U.S. Institute of Medicine (2005) could not determine a healthful limit of trans fat and urged action to reduce its presence in the American diet. In January 2006, the FDA rule requiring trans fats content on food labels went into effect, but the FDA turned down requests to ban the additive altogether. More recently, several cities and states—including, Boston, New York City, Philadelphia, Montgomery County, Maryland, and the state of California—have banned trans fats in restaurant food. In part as a result of these bans, many food companies have removed trans fat from products sold nationwide, showing that even local regulations can lead to changes in national corporate practices.

VIOXX

Merck Pharmaceuticals obtained FDA approval to market the painkiller Vioxx (generic name, rofecoxib) in 1999. Merck marketing promised that Vioxx would bring pain relief to people with arthritis without the gastrointestinal side effects associated with other medications. Five years later, after more than $10 billion in sales, Merck withdrew Vioxx from the market because a study showed that it doubled the risk of heart attacks and strokes in long-term users (Simons & Stipp, 2004). By then, more than twenty million people had taken the drug and thousands might have experienced adverse events, including death, attributable to Vioxx (Topol, 2004).

Why did so many people take a drug that turned out to be unsafe? First, Merck benefited from a drug-testing system that relied heavily on industry studies rather than on independent review. Their testing regime was developed at the behest of a politically powerful industry (Simons & Stipp, 2004; Topol, 2004). Second, Merck invested hundreds of millions of dollars in promoting Vioxx. In 1997, after a decade of pressure by the drug industry, the FDA issued guidelines that relaxed restrictions on advertising prescription drugs directly to consumers (Hawthorne, 2003), making the United States one of the few countries in the world that allowed this practice. By 2001, spending by pharmaceuticals on direct-to-consumer advertising had more than doubled (Hawthorne, 2003). In six years, Merck spent more than $500 million advertising Vioxx to consumers (Hawthorne, 2003) and in 2003 alone, more than $500 million on Vioxx ads for physicians (Brown, 2004).

The company also developed an aggressive training program for its sales force. A training video told its sales representatives that the drug did not cause heart attacks and encouraged them to avoid questions on that topic (Berenson, 2005). Merck's promotional campaigns and advertisements led many consumers and physicians to believe that Vioxx and other COX-2 inhibitors (the class of drugs that includes Vioxx) were superior painkillers to much less expensive but equally effective over-the-counter alternatives (Brown, 2004). Faced with mounting evidence about the dangers of Vioxx, the FDA adopted a policy of watchful waiting (Topol, 2004), despite the fact that one FDA scientist estimated Vioxx was associated with more than 27,000 heart attacks or deaths linked to cardiac problems (Berenson, 2005).

Finally, Merck ignored warning signs about cardiovascular side effects. Prior to FDA approval, for example, researchers discovered that COX-2 inhibitors interfere with enzymes that prevent cardiovascular disease (Simons, 2004). Another study in 2000 found that people taking Vioxx had three times as many cardiovascular events as those taking naproxen, another pain reliever. Merck attributed these results to the heart-protective effects of naproxen rather than the harmful effects of Vioxx (Simons, 2004). Finally, after another study showed serious cardiovascular problems in those who had taken Vioxx for more than eighteen months (Berenson, 2005), Merck pulled the drug from the market. More recently, some researchers have accused Merck of misrepresenting earlier safety trials that revealed harmful side effects associated with Vioxx use of less than eighteen months (Associated Press, 2006).

SPORT UTILITY VEHICLES

From the early 1990s to 2005, sport utility vehicles (SUVs) were the best-selling and most profitable vehicles made by the U.S. auto industry. SUVs are characterized by a pickup truck underbody, high ground clearance, enclosed rear cargo area, and availability of four-wheel drive (Bradsher, 2002). SUVs, together with pickup trucks and minivans, are considered *light trucks*, a category that has separate safety and fuel efficiency standards than passenger cars. By 2000, light trucks accounted for 40 percent of U.S. motor vehicles, double the 1980 rate (Coate & VanderHoff, 2001).

SUVs pose several health and environmental problems. First, because of their high center of gravity, they are three times more likely to roll over and the rate of occupant fatalities in these rollovers is almost three times higher than for passenger cars (National Highway Traffic Safety Administration, 2005). Second, because of their weight and design, SUVs are more likely than sedans to kill the occupants of cars and pedestrians they hit. An analysis of U.S. traffic fatalities from 1995 to 2001 found that each SUV occupant fatality averted because of the greater weight comes at a cost of 4.3 additional crashes that involve deaths of car occupants, pedestrians, bicyclists, or motorcyclists (White, 2004). Third, SUVs are harder to steer, take longer to stop, and give their drivers a false sense of security that leads to riskier driving (Bradsher, 2002). Fourth, because of high fuel needs, SUVs produce more pollution than passenger cars, contributing to respiratory disease, cancer, and other conditions. SUVs also release up to 47 percent more carbon dioxide than sedans (Environmental Protection Agency, 2004), thus contributing to global warming (Haines & Patz, 2004).

Based on a review of scientific and government reports, Bradsher (2002) estimated that SUVs account for roughly 3,000 annual deaths in the United States. Recent improvements in SUVs have reduced some hazards, although as older vehicles move into the second-hand market, the SUV death toll may increase (Hakim, 2005).

SUVs came to the U.S. auto market through an opportunity created by an exemption from fuel efficiency standards won by automakers in 1975. Since then, the auto industry has used its influence in Washington to oppose changes in fuel standards for SUVs and light trucks, despite the existence of technologies that could improve their efficiency (Doyle, 2000). From 1996 to 2000, Congress passed budgets that prohibited spending any money on fuel-economy research (Bradsher, 2002), ensuring that no new evidence would be available to set new fuel standards. SUVs and pickups were the most profitable auto industry products because of trade protection against imported SUVs. Their simple design led to unit profits ten to twelve times higher than for conventional cars. The auto industry, the nation's largest advertiser, also promoted SUVs heavily, spending more than $9 billion on SUV ads between 1990 and 2001, ads inaccurately suggesting that SUVs were safer than passenger cars (Claybrook, 2006). Once again, profitability trumped health, although in this case some analysts argue that U.S. automakers' short-term focus on profits actually harmed long-term profitability and contributed to the demise of the auto industry, as changing economic conditions reduced the demand for SUVs (Claybrook, 2003).

HOW CORPORATE PRACTICES INFLUENCE HEALTH

The stories that follow illustrate the ways in which specific corporate practices intended to achieve industry goals can result in actions that affect population health. Corporate managers have made decisions that have contributed to tens of thousands of preventable deaths, injuries, and illnesses. But in each case, advocacy, government regulation, and market forces have ultimately reduced the threat to population health. We suggest that the systematic investigation of how companies make decisions that affect health can help identify earlier opportunities for primary prevention.

For all three products, in the absence of safety evidence, corporate practices tried to maximize financial return. Adding trans fats to thousands of processed foods gave the food industry more flexibility in retail markets (for example, longer shelf lives) while magnifying cardiovascular risk for consumers. For Vioxx and SUVs, aggressive advertising of unsafe products increased the population exposed, amplifying negative impacts on health.

In each case, industries conducted extensive public relations and lobbying campaigns and went to court to defeat or delay government regulation, extending both the period of profitability and adverse health impacts. Finally, Ford, General Motors, Merck, and major food companies paid scientists to conduct research to support their positions, contributing to doubt about the evidence that many public health experts believed justified regulation to protect health.

If trans fat, Vioxx, and SUVs were aberrations, they would be alarming but less worthy of analysis. Recent scientific and popular work suggests, however, that corporations regularly make decisions that adversely affect health and that their practices have a substantial impact on U.S. mortality and morbidity (Institute of Medicine, 2005; Bradsher, 2002; Nestle, 2002; Nestle, 2006; Hemenway, 2004; Angell, 2004; Schroeder, 2004). For example, the tobacco and alcohol industries target advertising at young people and heavy users, increasing the harm to health (Chung et al., 2002; Mosher & Johnsson, 2005). The food industry modifies its products by increasing portion size (Young & Nestle, 2003) and adding sweeteners and fats (Bray, Nielsen, & Popkin, 2004; Bray, Paeratakul, & Popkin, 2004), contributing to obesity and diabetes. The tobacco, automobile, and firearm industries make campaign contributions, lobby, and go to court to prevent the government from passing stricter safety standards for their products (Doyle, 2000; Kluger, 1996; Siebel, 2000).

The role of corporations in our daily lives and in the governance of the United States has increased. Between the 1992 and 2004 elections, campaign contributions from the pharmaceutical and the food and beverage industries doubled (Center for Responsive Politics, n.d.). Between 1998 and 2005, food stores' spending on lobbying increased five-fold and pharmaceutical manufacturers tripled their spending (Center for Responsive Politics, n.d.). Since 2000, the number of registered lobbyists in Washington has doubled (Birnbaum, 2005), providing corporations with increased contact with policy makers and greater opportunity to influence legislation. Between 1975 and 2001, total US spending on advertising as a percentage of gross domestic product more than doubled (Galbi, 2001). Corporations have also penetrated more sectors of public life (for example, schools), and other public places have become important sites for advertising (United States General Accounting Office, 2000). As their influence becomes more pervasive, corporations are more able to promote health-damaging behavior.

In the political sphere, as a result of increased lobbying and campaign contributions, many areas of public health oversight have been deregulated and the staff available to monitor industry practices has been reduced (Barstow, Gerstein, & Stein, 2003; Labaton, 2006; Shull & Smith, 2004). At the behest of lobbyists, twenty-two states have banned obesity-related liability lawsuits against fast food restaurants (National Restaurant Association, 2006), and, in its first term, the Bush Administration dropped thirty-one of eighty-five proposed auto safety rules from the National Highway and Auto Safety Administration's agenda (Shull & Smith, 2004).

In the personal sphere, increased advertising has doubled the number of television commercials viewed each year by the average American child, from about 20,000 in 1970 to 40,000 in 2000 (Story & French, 2004). Advertisements for obesogenic processed foods are the most common television ads aimed at children (Walker, 2006). Increasingly, major corporations like McDonald's and Starbucks provide a place away from home and work where people can socialize and consume high-fat products (McGinnis & Foege, 1993).

CORPORATE PRACTICES AND THE SOCIAL PRODUCTION OF POPULATION HEALTH

In past decades, health researchers have disagreed about the most important causes of morbidity and mortality and, therefore, about prevention priorities. The dominant view in the United States is that individual behavior and lifestyle are the primary malleable determinants of health (Mokdad, Marks, Stroup, & Gerberding, 2000; Wilkinson, 1999), suggesting that the goal of policy is to change harmful behaviors. Some United States and European researchers, however, argue that social structures and the distribution of wealth and power are the fundamental causes of disease, and that changes in these factors are needed to achieve improvement in population health (McKeown, 1980; Link & Phelan, 2005; Marmot, 2006; Stampfer, Hu, Manson, Rimm & Willett, 2000).

In our view, a focus on corporate behavior provides common ground for these two approaches. It suggests a policy paradigm that aims to encourage corporate practices that promote healthy behavior. As corporate practices result from specific decisions, they may be more readily changed than underlying social and economic structures in which they are embedded. They offer more immediate opportunities for health promotion than those available to change more entrenched structures. While it is true that corporations, like individuals, make decisions constrained by their social and economic context, identifying policies that make it easier for corporations to choose health should be a public health priority. Strong national standards on pollution control, for example, would make it easier for automakers to produce for the national market than to separately meet California's more stringent requirements (Doyle, 2000), a position recently endorsed by the Obama administration.

To shift the focus of public health policy from individual behavior to corporate practices will require an elucidation of the pathways by which corporate decisions structure the context in which individuals choose behaviors and products. To illustrate, few individuals decide, "Today, I am going to consume an extra-large portion of high fructose corn syrup" (a sweetener linked to obesity and diabetes) or "I'm going to buy a polluting vehicle more likely to kill or injure my neighbors." Rather, these choices are made in a marketplace that produces and advertises certain options and suppresses others—and within a political system that gives certain stakeholders more power and influence than others.

In order to increase opportunities for primary prevention, two changes are needed: a reconceptualization of *lifestyle* and a focused policy agenda that makes it easier for corporate managers to choose health-promoting practices.

BEYOND LIFESTYLE

Historically, health researchers have regarded lifestyle as the sum of behavioral choices in multiple arenas (for example, diet, tobacco, and physical activity), influenced by underlying personal characteristics (for example, orientation to risk and self-efficacy) (Hu, 2001;

Weber, 1946). However, sociologists from Weber on have seen lifestyle as a socially determined pattern of consumption or marker of status (Cockerham, 2005; Williams, 1995). By regarding lifestyle as the consequence of socially constructed choices, it is possible to identify policies that will facilitate healthier lifestyle options.

Free market proponents argue that individuals should have the right to choose what they consume without interference from a *nanny state* (Sullum, 1998), suggesting that lifestyle choices are made in a vacuum. In fact, lifestyle choices are often the direct result of corporate decisions. No consumer ever entered a restaurant demanding a portion of trans fats. Rather, food companies constrain consumer options through decisions made primarily to increase profits. By exposing corporations as the real "nannies" who persuade children to eat to obesity, push drivers to find their inner identity behind the wheel, or encourage patients to solve their social problems with a new drug, health professionals can reframe the discussion about who can be trusted to look after the public's health.

Traditional market proponents have accepted that government has some right to intervene in markets: for example, to ensure that consumers have information to make informed choices, to protect vulnerable groups such as children, or to return unintended costs of a product (*externalities*) from tax payers to producers. Recently, however, more ardent free market advocates have challenged even these roles, a position some label *market fundamentalism* (Stiglitz, 2003). By encouraging more discussion on these issues, health professionals may be able to reframe policy debates to lead to decisions that better protect health. The collapse of financial markets in 2008 after a long period of lax regulation shows the high price of government neglect of its responsibility to safeguard public well-being and provides a window of opportunity for broader public dialogue.

A POLICY AGENDA FOR HEALTH-PROMOTING CORPORATE PRACTICES

Public health advocates have, for the most part, sought reforms governing corporate practices one product, company, or industry at a time. They have advocated strategies, including public education, to enable individual consumers to make more informed choices (Balko, 2005); and legal mandates to label products truthfully (Variyam & Cawley, 2006; Avorn & Shrank, 2006), on the premise that consumers have a right to know (Stiglitz, 1999); and taxation of tobacco, alcohol, and high-calorie, low-nutrient foods (Chaloupka, Wakefield & Czart, 2001; Chaloupka, Grossman & Saffer, 2002; Cook & Moore, 2002; Jacobson & Brownell, 2000) in order to make them less available. Others have suggested banning products like flavored cigarettes designed to appeal to young people (Lewis & Wackowski, 2006), or food advertisements for children ("Marketing food to children," 2005), or requiring higher fuel and safety standards for SUVs to reduce their harmful impact (Union of Concerned Scientists, 2005).

Some advocates have switched from legislative to litigation strategies. Consumer lawsuits have targeted many corporations. Many believe that litigation is particularly effective in getting corporate attention. Beginning with the lawsuits against Big Tobacco in the 1970s, a cadre of lawyers has emerged and shared lessons from their battles against the alcohol, automobile, food, gun, pharmaceutical, and tobacco industries (Mello, Studdert, & Brennan, 2006; Parmet & Daynard, 2000; Lytton, 2004). Public health litigators assert that courts are an important arena in which to seek justice, educate the public, win resources for health promotion, and force companies to change corporate practices by returning externalized costs to their balance sheets.

CAMPAIGNS TO CHANGE CORPORATE PRACTICES

A campaign is a time-limited and place-specific advocacy initiative in which one or more organizations mount coordinated activities to achieve explicit changes in corporate practices perceived to harm health. While these campaigns are often supported by social movements, that is, broader and more ongoing popular mobilizations, the definition used here distinguishes between the more time and objective limited campaigns and the broader social movements.

Campaigns can target individual corporations or an entire industry, or they can seek government action to protect public health. Campaigns can operate at the local, regional, national, or global levels. Most campaigns include coalitions of different constituencies concerned about the health damage caused by a particular corporate practice.

Why Campaigning Is a Smart Strategy for Improving Public Health

Campaigns allow organizations to focus their resources and public attention on a specific problem to bring about changes in corporate practices and policies.

While many public health advocates and researchers point to the deeper social causes of ill health, changing socioeconomic structures, eliminating poverty, and ending discrimination are long-term and worthwhile goals.

Working to change specific corporate practices that harm health provides an opportunity to bring about shorter-term benefits while still addressing deeper causes of health problems. In addition, campaigns offer public health advocates tactical and strategic flexibility. Campaigners can move from the legislature to the courtroom, from local to national forums, or from public health to consumer rights frameworks, as new windows of opportunity open or obstacles block their paths. This flexibility can provide campaigns with an advantage over their often better-financed but less agile opponents.

Finally, at a time when government often abdicates its responsibility from protecting public health from corporate practices, campaigns provide citizens, activists, and professionals an opportunity to take the initiative in promoting health.

Characteristics of a Successful Campaign to Change Health-Damaging Corporate Practices

Successful campaigns can force corporations to modify health-damaging practices, mobilize new constituencies to take action, or encourage public discussion of corporate policies.

While there is no magic formula for success, effective campaigns share some common qualities. First, successful campaigns set specific goals (for example, withdraw a harmful product from the market, change how products are advertised, or pass legislation that sets stricter safety standards). Second, successful campaigns build strong coalitions with others that support their cause, including with community or nonprofit organizations, health professionals, or government officials. A few groups have created innovative relationships with the corporations or the industry they are campaigning against to reach a mutually acceptable compromise. Third, effective campaigns use the media to reach new people, frame the issues, and keep pressure on corporate or government decision makers.

Finally, successful campaigns recognize the significance of intermediate goals, such as raising public awareness about the health impact of industry practices or learning what *not* to do to reach new groups.

Examples of Campaigns to Change Health-Damaging Corporate Practices
Stop Uptown Cigarettes

In 1990, a coalition led by African Americans in Philadelphia mobilized local and national organizations to force the R.J. Reynolds Company to withdraw a planned test marketing of Uptown cigarettes, designed to appeal to African Americans. The campaign included church groups, local and national health leaders, elected officials, and others. The Uptown cigarette campaign was uniquely successful in that it used primarily local grassroots strategies to stop the marketing of Uptown cigarettes before the cigarettes and accompanying promotional products could be distributed to retailers.

Fight KOOL: Stop KOOL Cigarettes Target Marketing

Fight KOOL was a seven-month national campaign launched by the National African American Tobacco Prevention Network. The campaign began in April 2003, and responded specifically to Brown & Williamson (B & W) Tobacco Company, makers of KOOL cigarettes, who were specifically targeting marketing efforts toward African American and Latino youth. Fight KOOL argued such marketing could contribute to widening disparities in health. B & W's marketing campaign, known as KOOL MIXX, was forced to shut down in October 2003 as a result of the grassroots advocacy efforts of Fight KOOL and the simultaneous litigation by several state Attorneys General based on the 1998 *Tobacco Master Settlement Agreement (MSA)* between forty-six states and the five largest tobacco companies.

National Campaign to Close the Newspaper Loophole

In November 2001, Iowans for the Prevention of Gun Violence launched the National Campaign to Close the Newspaper Loophole, a coalition that works to remove classified ads for firearms sold by unlicensed dealers from the nation's newspapers. The campaign's premise was that such advertising made illegal guns more accessible. As a result of this ongoing initiative's primary activity—writing letters to newspaper editors—by August 2005, thirty-three newspapers from across the country had changed their policies to prohibit the advertising of firearms from unlicensed dealers.

Get Alcohol Ads off Public Transit: Marin Institute

In January 2007, the Bay Area Rapid Transit (BART) System voted to end all alcohol advertising on its trains, buses, and shelters. The successful campaign was organized by the Marin Institute, a watchdog group that has been advocating for the reduction of alcohol-related problems since 1987. The group uses grassroots organizing, policy advocacy, and media strategies to reduce environmental influences that encourage alcohol use. By pressuring San Francisco city transportation officials to sign and enforce strict advertising contracts that limit where ads are placed, the campaign has led to a Bay Area public transportation system that disallows all alcohol advertising in buses, on trains, or in transit shelters in school zones. Marin's BART campaign may serve as a model for other municipalities around the nation.

Limitations of Campaigns as a Strategy to Modify Health-Damaging Corporate Practices

While campaigns are an effective way to bring pressure on a company, industry, or government to make changes in health-damaging practices, they have their limitations. These campaigns are generally time limited and focused on challenging a specific corporate practice or policy. While this concentrated and energetic level of activity can help campaigns gain public recognition, it also means that campaigners can run out of funding or lose public support before achieving their goals.

From a public health perspective, campaigns need to achieve persistent and sustained change in order to improve population health, which is sometimes a difficult challenge. It may not be reasonable to expect groups to mobilize against all the many corporate practices that harm health; thus, campaigns should not become a substitute for government responsibility for actively protecting public health. In addition, prolonged campaigning may result in *issue fatigue* among allies, the media, and the public. Moreover, some campaigns encounter well-funded and persistent opposition, which makes victories difficult to achieve. The success of the gun industry and the National Rifle Association in defeating most efforts to reduce gun violence by regulating the gun industry provide an example of this. On the other hand, the success of tobacco control campaigns in reducing public support for the tobacco industry over the last three decades shows that public opinion can change over time.

Courtesy of Corporations and Health Watch: http://www.corporationsandhealth.org/profiles.php

For more information on these and other campaigns, see N. Freudenberg, S. P. Bradley, and M. Serrano (2009). Public health campaigns to change industry practices that damage health: An analysis of 12 case studies. *Health Education and Behavior, 36*(2), 230–249.

While each of these strategies has produced some significant public health advances, in the long run this piecemeal approach seems inadequate to the task of promoting population health and realizing opportunities for primary prevention. Just as researchers and advocates in the occupational and environmental health fields have called for moving beyond regulation of a single substance at a time, often only after a body count has demonstrated damage (Cranor, 2004; Richter & Laster, 2004), public health policy makers concerned about corporate practices need to consider a more comprehensive approach.

A broader agenda could serve to unify many disparate strands of current advocacy, bring together a more cohesive and powerful coalition to advocate in the political arena, and help reframe public debate in more favorable terms. Such an agenda would use language and concepts that appeal to many Americans (Dorfman, Wallack, & Woodruff, 2005; Wallack & Lawrence, 2005) and provide links to other major public issues, such as campaign finance and electoral reform, reduction of corporate crime, health care coverage, and consumer protection.

While the specifics of such a policy agenda can only be forged by key stakeholders—by policymakers, public health professionals, advocacy organizations, and citizens—we suggest the following approaches to stimulate discussion:

• Provide consumers with a right to know the health consequences of legal products and provide companies with a duty to disclose such information. Free market ideology assumes that all parties to commercial transactions have equal information; however, in practice, *buyer beware* is a common experience. Extending the right to know and the duty to disclose beyond the weak protections now offered could provide a legal framework for redefining consumer rights and better balancing the obligations of government and markets. If it were more difficult for producers to externalize the health costs of their products, it might be possible to change the decision-making process by which corporate managers now opt for harmful practices.

• Protect children and other vulnerable populations against targeted advertising that promotes unhealthy behavior. Most Americans oppose such marketing, and many other free market nations restrict such practices. National legislation to protect children could encourage debate on the costs and benefits of recent efforts to extend free speech protection to commercial speech (Gostin & Javitt, 2001; Kunkel, 2001) and unify advocacy across several industries.

• Support measures to level the political playing field. Meaningful campaign finance reform, higher ethical standards for elected officials, more stringent oversight of lobbying, and stronger voter rights will help make it easier for public health advocates to gain electoral, legislative, or litigation support for health-promoting policies and to encourage healthier corporate practices. To date, organized public health has rarely made support of such reforms a priority.

• Increase sanctions for deliberate distortions of science designed to protect corporate interests. Industry campaigns to withhold damaging scientific data and to create scientific uncertainty have hampered efforts to protect public health. By increasing professional, academic, and legal sanctions for such action, it may be possible to make it easier for scientists to resist such pressures.

• A consolidated agenda can significantly strengthen fragmented approaches to encouraging healthier corporate practices, provide a coherent alternative to market advocates who seek to diminish the public role in health, and support the emergence of a social movement that seeks to redefine corporate responsibility. These movements have been the foundation for previous public health advances.

HOW PATTI RUNDALL TOOK ON THE TITANS ONE BABY STEP AT A TIME

What do you do if you see that some of the biggest corporations in the world are putting profits ahead of health and lives? If you're Patti Rundall, you take them on tirelessly, relentlessly, and unflaggingly until they start to make changes, one baby step at a time.

It was 1980 when Patti Rundall—artist and teacher, but not yet a global activist—first heard about the dangerous and misleading marketing tactics of global giant Nestlé. Nestlé was aggressively marketing its baby formula, particularly in developing countries, using promotional tactics that ranged from inaccurate to misleading. Breastfeeding is the most healthy, environmentally friendly, accessible and inexpensive option for infant feeding, providing essential immunity and perfect nutritional balance (World Health Organization, 2008). In developing countries, where clean water can be scarce and money to buy food ever scarcer, breastfeeding is the single most effective preventive intervention for improving the survival and health of children. According to the World Health Organization (WHO), improved breastfeeding practices could save some 1.5 million children's lives per year (WHO, 2008).

To make a profit, Nestlé and other formula corporations had to make a dent in one of the oldest practices in existence. Through their marketing practices they did just that. Mothers in countries around the world, wooed by Nestlé's promises of better infant health, became hooked on free formula samples. Swayed by the implicit endorsement of their medical providers, mothers switched to formula. When they realized formula was not the promised panacea, it was too late. Out of money to buy more formula, without access to clean water to mix formula, and with dwindling supplies of their own breast milk, mothers watched as their infants starved and often died.

Groups including War on Want, Oxfam, and United States-based Infant Formula Action Coalition monitored and catalogued Nestlé's intentional efforts to transition women from breastfeeding to bottle-feeding, captured international attention, and launched a boycott against Nestlé. Rundall joined the fledgling United Kingdom group, Baby Milk Action. Baby Milk Action is a grassroots network that "aims to save lives and to end the avoidable suffering caused by inappropriate infant feeding" by strengthening controls on the marketing of the baby-feeding industry (Brady & Rundall, 2009). At the same time, the International Baby Food Action Network (IBFAN) was formed. IBFAN now has more than two hundred groups in more than one hundred countries.

Baby Milk Action began as a volunteer organization, with virtually no resources, and buoyed the boycott efforts in what was to become the beginning of a thirty-year battle. According to Rundall, "The formula companies have cleverly persuaded women that physiological breast feeding failure is a common . . . occurrence. But the problem lies with lack of support and bad advice . . . that has been influenced by the companies selling formula. With the right support breastfeeding works as it has done for millions of years" (personal communication, January 6, 2010).

IBFAN and Baby Milk Action's roles as brokers of reputable, fact-based information on infant feeding, alongside the action of key figures like Senator Edward Kennedy, helped prompt an unprecedented response from global health governing bodies. In 1981, the World Health Assembly adopted the WHO/UNICEF International Code of Marketing of Breastmilk Substitutes, which provides for "the provision of safe and adequate nutrition for infants, by the protection and promotion of breastfeeding, and by ensuring the proper use of breast-milk substitutes, when these are necessary, on the basis of adequate information and through appropriate marketing and distribution" (WHO, 2008, p. 1). The code restricts baby food companies in the following ways. Baby food companies are not permitted to:

- Promote breast-milk substitutes in hospitals, shops, or among the general public.
- Allow sales personnel to contact mothers.
- Give free samples to mothers, or free or subsidized supplies to hospitals or maternity wards.
- Give gifts to health workers or mothers.
- Promote their products to health workers: any information provided by companies must contain only scientific and factual matters
- Give misleading information
- Allow contact between baby milk company sales personnel and mothers
- Show baby pictures on baby milk labels.

Furthermore, the code specified that baby milk labels must be in a language understood by the mother and must include a clear health warning. Labels are not allowed to contain language that idealizes the use of the product (WHO, 2008).

The code protects the rights of parents who choose to use artificial feeding and of parents who breastfeed to have access to sound, evidence-based, and independent information about infant and young child feeding. Since 1981 more than seventy countries have taken steps to incorporate the code into national legislation.

Although Nestlé was now formally bound to ethical promotional tactics, Rundall's job was not over. In fact, monitoring the nimble efforts of Nestlé (and a growing number of other formula corporations) to exploit loopholes in the new code and to undermine the government's efforts to implement the code correctly requires the continued coordination of multiple organizations. To try to ensure the code is properly implemented in United Kingdom and European legislation, Rundall created the Baby Feeding Law Group, a coalition of health professional and lay organizations that monitors industry actions and works to hold industry accountable. Accountability has proven to be a moving target, and since 1981 there have been more than a dozen World Health Assembly Resolutions that address the new tactics used by Nestlé and other corporations to evade restrictions. These tactics were brought to light through Baby Milk Action dogged attention. Rundall notes, "Regulation of business can't be left to the companies. It's not that companies want to do the wrong thing—it's that they have a fiduciary duty to their shareholders to maximize profits. That's the problem. This pressure and the competition in the world markets means that they will inevitably oppose legislation that protects consumers" ("Patti Rundall," 2003).

The Nestlé boycott continues today, three decades after its launch, as big corporations persist in efforts to edge out breastfeeding, particularly among our most vulnerable populations. Rundall's leadership role has been steady and has earned her an appointment as Officer of the Order of the British Empire in 2000. She has taken a special interest in the issue of sponsorship, corporate partnerships, and public relations and has played a key role in improving transparency in Europe. The corporate influence on health policymaking is often hidden behind the medical profession, and only when governments and professional bodies adopt transparent, independent monitoring and evaluation systems can the thorny issue of conflicts of interest be tackled. Rundall's work resulted in the EU Commission adopting new rules in 2000 that require members of its scientific and food safety bodies to make public declarations of financial links to industry. Rundall continues to pursue this matter as the EU decides whether to approve health claims on children's foods.

Patti represents IBFAN on the European Commission's Platform for Action on Diet and Physical Activity, which challenges Europe's leading food and advertising companies to halt their unethical marketing of foods for children and highlights the risks of commercial involvement in health and education services. Baby Milk Action produced an education pack in 2000 called *Seeing Through the Spin*, which helps students understand how companies use public relations to distort health policies.

Over the years Patti Rundall has consistently shown that grassroots advocacy efforts can thwart big business, particularly when you add a dash of creative, strategic thinking. Rundall owns several shares of Nestlé stock and uses her voice as a stockholder to work from within the corporation's existing systems to drive change (personal communication, June 2009). More recently, Baby Milk Action used social media as a catalyzing force, creating a virtual protest through Facebook and supplying facts to bolster a Twitter-based takeover of Nestlé's Twitter site (#Nestlefamily), originally set up by Nestlé to garner publicity for a corporation-sponsored parenting weekend (Brady & Rundall, 2009). Concessions continue to come from big business. In 2009, after seven years of lobbying following the formula-linked death of a five-day-old baby, formula manufacturers in the United Kingdom were forced to change product labeling to warn parents that formula preparations are not sterile (Brady & Rundall, 2009). Says Rundall, "This type of action is not dependent on money. Many of the best movements in the world are driven by public outrage, not because someone has written a funding proposal" (Maggs, 2003).

Source: Prevention Institute.

CONCLUSION

In summary, we argue that corporate practices are an important determinant of health, and those policies that reduce damaging corporate practices are likely to improve population health. In recent years, public health advocates have developed strategies to bring about policy changes, efforts often opposed by industry and its supporters. A systematic study of both these domains will inform more effective public health policy and practice. In the current political climate, these proposals may seem idealistic, even naïve. In a society that seeks to protect public health, they are common sense.

DISCUSSION QUESTIONS

1. Suppose a conglomerate of beverage manufacturers was lobbying state legislators to oppose an act that would raise the effective price of sugar-sweetened beverages in retail outlets. In what ways would you challenge the beverage industry's efforts? What key components of your advocacy campaign would help ensure its success?
2. If you were planning to investigate the influence of corporate practices on health, what are some research questions you might ask? How might you go about answering them?

REFERENCES

Adler, N., & Newman, K. (2002). Socioeconomic disparities in health: pathways and policies. *Health Affairs, 21*(2), 60–76.

Allison et al. (1995). Trans fatty acids and coronary heart disease risk. Report of the expert panel on trans fatty acids and coronary heart disease. *American Journal of Clinical Nutrition, 62*(3), 655S–708S.

Angell, M. (2004). *The truth about the drug companies: How they deceive us and what to do about it*. New York: Random House.

Ascherio et al. (1994). Trans fatty acids intake and risk of myocardial infarction. *Circulation, 89*(1), 94–101.

Associated Press. (2006, May 19). Vioxx data suggest risk started earlier. *New York Times*.

Avorn, J. (2006). Evaluating drug effects in the post-Vioxx world: There must be a better way. *Circulation, 113*(18), 2173–2176.

Avorn, J., & Shrank, W. (2006). Highlights and a hidden hazard?—The FDA's new labeling regulations. *New England Journal of Medicine, 354*(23), 2409–2411.

Balko, R. (2005). Private matters and "public health." Cato Institute. Retrieved June 26, 2006, from http://www.cato.org/research/articles/balko-050206.html

Barstow, D., Gerstein, R., & Stein, R. (2003, December 22). U.S. rarely seeks charges for deaths in workplace. *New York Times*, p. A1.

Berenson, A. (2005, July 21). In training video, Merck said Vioxx did not increase risk of heart attack. *New York Times*, p. 4.

Birnbaum, J. (2005, June 22). The road to riches is called K street. *Washington Post*, p. A1.

Bradsher, K. (2002). *High and mighty SUVs: The world's most dangerous vehicles and how they got that way*. New York: Public Affairs.

Brady, M., & Rundall, P. (2009, November). *Baby Milk Action Update*, 42. Retrieved December 21, 2009, from http://www.babymilkaction.org/pdfs/update42.pdf

Bray, G., Nielsen, S. J., & Popkin, B. M. (2004). Consumption of high-fructose corn syrup in beverages may play a role in the epidemic of obesity. *Physiology & Behavior, 83*(4), 549–555.

Bray, G., Paeratakul, S., & Popkin, B. M. (2004). Dietary fat and obesity: A review of animal, clinical and epidemiological studies. *Physiology & Behavior, 83*(4), 549–555.

Brown, D. (2004, October 3). Promise and peril of Vioxx casts harsher light on new drugs. *Washington Post*, p. A14.

Center for Responsive Politics. (n.d.). Retrieved June 3, 2006, from http://www.opensecrets.org

Chaloupka, F. J., Cummings, K. M., Morley, C. P., & Horan, J. K. (2002). Tax, price and cigarette smoking: Evidence from the tobacco documents and implications for tobacco company marketing strategies. *Tobacco Control, 11 Supplement 1*, 162–172.

Chaloupka, F. J., Grossman, M., & Saffer, H. (2002). The effects of price on alcohol consumption and alcohol-related problems. *Alcohol Research & Health, 26*(1), 22–34.

Chaloupka, F. J., Wakefield, M., & Czart, C. (2001). Taxing tobacco: The impact of tobacco taxes on cigarette smoking and other tobacco use. In R. L. Rabin & S. D. Sugarman (Eds.), *Regulating tobacco*. New York: Oxford University Press.

Chung et al. (2002). Youth targeting by tobacco manufacturers since the master settlement agreement. *Health Affairs, 21*, 254–263.

Clandinin, M., & Wilke, M. (2001). Do trans fatty acids increase the incidence of Type 2 diabetes? *American Journal of Clinical Nutrition, 73*(6), 1001–1002.

Claybrook, J. (2003). Profit-driven myths and severe public damage: The terrible truth about SUVs. Testimony before the Senate Committee on Commerce, Science and Transportation. Retrieved June 25, 2006, from http://www.citizen.org/documents/JC_SUV_testimony.pdf

Coate, D., & VanderHoff, J. (2001). The truth about light trucks. *Regulation, 24*(1), 22.

Cockerham, W. C. (2005). Health lifestyle theory and the convergence of agency and structure. *Journal of Health and Social Behavior, 46*(1), 51–67.

Cook, P. J., & Moore, M. J. (2002). The economics of alcohol abuse and alcohol control policies. *Health Affairs, 21*(2), 120–133.

Cranor, C. F. (2004). Some legal implications of the precautionary principle: Improving information-generation and legal protections. *International Journal of Occupational Medicine and Environmental Health, 17*(1), 17–34.

Dorfman, L., Wallack, L., & Woodruff, K. (2005). More than a message: framing public health advocacy to change corporate practices. *Health Education & Behavior, 32*(3), 320–36.

Doyle, J. (2000). *Taken for a ride: Detroit's big three and the politics of air pollution.* New York: Four Walls Eight Windows.

Environmental Protection Agency (EPA). (2004). *Control of emissions from new and in-use highway vehicles and engines.* 40 CFR 86.

Ewen, S. (1977). *Captains of consciousness: Advertising and the social roots of the consumer culture.* New York: Basic Books.

Food and Drug Administration (FDA). (1999). Food labeling: Trans fatty acids in nutrition labeling, nutrient content claims and health claims. *Federal Register, 64* (62746).

Freudenberg, N. (2005). Public health advocacy to change corporate practices: Implications for health education practice and research. *Health Education & Behavior, 32*(3), 298–319.

Galbi, D. (2001). Some economics of personal activity and implications for the digital economy. *First Monday, 6*(7). Retrieved September 11, 2006, from http://firstmonday.org/issues/issue6_7/galbi/index.html

Geiser, K., & Rosenberg, B. (2006). The social context of occupational and environmental health. In B. S. Levy, D. H. Wegman, S. L. Barron, & R. K. Sokas (Eds.), *Occupational and environmental health: Recognizing and preventing disease and injury* (5th ed., pp. 21–38). Philadelphia: Lippincott Williams & Wilkins.

Gostin, L. O., & Javitt, G. H. (2001). Health promotion and the first amendment: Government control of the informational environment. *Milbank Quarterly, 79*(4), 547–578.

Grier, S. A., & Kumanyika, S. K. (2008). The context for choice: Health implications of targeted food and beverage marketing to African Americans. *American Journal of Public Health, 98*(9), 1616–1629.

Hackbarth et al. (2001). Collaborative research and action to control the geographic placement of outdoor advertising of alcohol and tobacco products in Chicago. *Public Health Reports, 116*(6), 558–567.

Haines, A., & Patz, J. (2004). Health effects of climate change. *Journal of the American Medical Association, 291*(1), 99–103.

Hakim, D. (2005, June 26). Used SUVs come loaded, with safety concerns. *New York Times.*

Hawkes, C. (2006). Uneven dietary development: Linking the policies and processes of globalization with the nutrition transition, obesity and diet-related chronic diseases. *Global Health, 28*(2), 4.

Hawthorne, F. (2003). *The Merck druggernaut: The inside story of a pharmaceutical giant.* New York: Wiley.

Hemenway, D. (2004). *Private guns, public health*. Ann Arbor: University of Michigan Press.

Hu, F. (2001). Diet, lifestyle, and the risk of type 2 diabetes mellitus in women. *New England Journal of Medicine, 345*(11), 790–797.

Institute of Medicine. (2005). Committee on Prevention of Obesity in Children and Youth. In J. P. Koplan, C. T. Liverman, & V. I. Kraak (Eds.), *Preventing childhood obesity: Health in the balance*. Washington, DC: National Academies Press.

Jacobson, M. F., & Brownell, K. D. (2000). Small taxes on soft drinks and snack foods to promote health. *American Journal of Public Health, 90*(6), 854–857.

Kluger, R. (1996). *Ashes to ashes: America's hundred-year cigarette war, the public health, and the unabashed triumph of Philip Morris*. New York: Knopf.

Kunkel, D. (2001). Children and television advertising. In D. Singer & J. Singer (Eds.), *Children and the media*. Thousand Oaks, CA: Sage.

Labaton, S. (2006, March 10). "Silent tort reform" is overriding states' powers. *New York Times*, p. C5.

LaVeist, T. (2005). Disentangling race and socioeconomic status: A key to understanding health inequalities. *Journal of Urban Health, 82*(2), 26–34.

Lewis, M. J., & Wackowski, O. (2006). Dealing with an innovative industry: A look at flavored cigarettes promoted by mainstream brands. *American Journal of Public Health, 96*(2), 244–251.

Link, B., & Phelan, J. (2005). Fundamental sources of health inequalities. In D. Mechanic (Ed.), *Policy challenges in modern health care*. New York: Rutgers University Press.

Lytton, T. D. (2004). Using litigation to make public health policy: Theoretical and empirical challenges in assessing product liability, tobacco, and gun litigation. *The Journal of Law, Medicine & Ethics, 32*(4), 556–564.

Maggs, L. (2003). Newsmaker: Baby versus the giant—Patti Rundall, policy director, Baby Milk Action. *Third Sector*. Retrieved September 11, 2006, from http://www.thirdsector.co.uk/Channels/Fundraising/Article/619829/NEWSMAKER-Baby-versus-giant—-Patti-Rundall-Policy-director-Baby-Milk-Action

Marketing food to children [Editorial]. (2005). *Lancet, 366*, 2064.

Marmot, M. (2005). Social determinants of health inequalities. *Lancet, 365*(9464), 1099–1104.

Marmot, M. (2006). Status syndrome: a challenge to medicine. *Journal of the American Medical Association, 295*(11), 1304–1307.

McGinnis, J., & Foege, W. (1993). Actual causes of death in the United States. *Journal of the American Medical Association, 270*(18), 2207–2212.

McGinnis, J. M., Williams-Russo, P., & Knickman, J. R. (2002). The case for more active policy attention to health promotion. *Health Affairs, 21*(2), 78–93.

McKeown, T. (1980). *The role of medicine: Dream, mirage, or nemesis?* Princeton, NJ: Princeton University Press.

Mechanic, D. (2002). Disadvantage, inequality, and social policy. *Health Affairs, 21*(2), 48–59.

Mello, M. M., Studdert, D. M., & Brennan, T. A. (2006). Obesity: The new frontier of public health law. *New England Journal of Medicine, 354*(24), 2601–2610.

Mokdad, A., Marks, J., Stroup, D., & Gerberding, J. (2000). Actual causes of death in the United States. *Journal of the American Medical Association, 291*(10), 1238–1245.

Mosher, J., & Johnsson, D. (2005). Flavored alcoholic beverages: An international marketing campaign that targets youth. *Journal of Public Health Policy, 26*(3), 326–342.

National Highway Traffic Safety Administration. US Department of Transportation. (2005). Federal Motor Vehicle Safety Standards: Roof Crush Resistance, 49 CFR Part 571. Docket No. NHTSA-2005-22143. RIN 2127-AG51.

National Restaurant Association. (n.d.). State frivolous-lawsuit legislation. Retrieved September 11, 2006, from http://www.restaurant.org/government/state/nutrition/bills_lawsuits.cfm

Nestle, M. (2002). *Food politics: How the food industry influences nutrition and health.* Berkeley: University of California Press.

Nestle, M. (2006). *What to eat.* New York: North Point Press.

Parmet, W. E. & Daynard, R. A. (2000). The new public health litigation. *Annual Review of Public Health, 21*, 437–454.

Richter, E. D., & Laster, R. (2004). The precautionary principle, epidemiology and the ethics of delay. *International Journal of Occupational Medicine and Environmental Health, 171*, 9–16.

Rundall, P. (2003, July). *Charity Times.* Retrieved December 21, 2009, from http://www.babymilkaction.org/pdfs/charitytimesjune03.pdf

Salmerón et al. (2001). Dietary fat intake and risk of type 2 diabetes in women. *American Journal of Clinical Nutrition, 73*(6), 1019–26.

Schroeder, S. (2004). Tobacco control in the wake of the 1998 master settlement agreement. *New England Journal of Medicine, 350*, 293–301.

Shull, R., & Smith, G. (2004). *The Bush regulatory record: A pattern of failure.* New York: OMB Watch.

Siebel, B. (2000). The case against the gun industry. *Public Health Reports, 115*, 410–418.

Simons, J., & Stipp, D. (2004, November). Will Merck survive Vioxx? *Fortune, 150*, 90–97.

Stampfer M. J., Hu, F. B., Manson, J. E., Rimm, E. B., Willett, W. C. (2000). Primary prevention of coronary heart disease in women through diet and lifestyle. *New England Journal of Medicine, 343*(1), 16–22.

Stiglitz, J. (1999). *On liberty, the right to know, and public discourse: The role of transparency in public life.* Lecture presented at Oxford Amnesty Lecture January 27, 1999, Oxford, United Kingdom.

Stiglitz, J. E. (2003). *Globalization and its discontents.* New York: W.W. Norton.

Story, M., & French, S. (2004). Food advertising and marketing directed at children and adolescents in the U.S. *International Journal of Behavioral Nutrition and Physical Activity, 1*(1), 3.

Sullum, J. (1998). *For your own good: The anti-smoking crusade and the tyranny of public health.* New York: Free Press.

Topol, E. J. (2004). Failing the public health? Rofecoxib, Merck, and the FDA. *The New England Journal of Medicine, 351*(17), 1707–1709.

Union of Concerned Scientists. (2005, August). Fuel economy fraud: Closing the loopholes that increase U.S. oil dependency. Retrieved September 11, 2006, from http://www.ucsusa.org/assets/documents/clean_vehicles/executive_summary_final.pdf

U.S. Department of Transportation, National Highway Traffic Safety Administration. (2005). *Federal motor vehicle safety standards; Roof crush resistance* 49 CFR, Part 571. Docket No. NHTSA-2005–22143. RIN 2127-AG51.

U.S. General Accounting Office. (2000). *Public education: Commercial activities in Schools.* (GAO/HEHS-00–156).

Variyam, J. N, & Cawley, J. (2006). Nutrition labels and obesity (NBER working paper no. 11956). Cambridge, MA: National Bureau of Economic Research.

Walker, R. (2006, April 30). Fitting in. *New York Times Magazine*, p. 22.

Wallack, L., & Lawrence, R. (2005). Talking about public health: Developing America's 'second language.' *American Journal of Public Health, 95*(4), 567–570.

Weber, M. (1946). *Essays in sociology.* New York: Oxford University Press.

Weinraub, J. (2003, November 12). Getting the fat out. *Washington Post*, p. F1.

White, M. (2004). The "arms race" on American roads: The effect of sport utility vehicles and pickup trucks on traffic safety. *Journal of Law and Economics, 47*, 333–353.

WHO. (2008). The International Code of Marketing of Breast-Milk Substitutes: Frequently asked questions. Retrieved December 21, 2009, from http://whqlibdoc.who.int/publications/2008/9789241594295_eng.pdf

Wiist, W. (2006). Public health and the anticorporate movement: rationale and recommendations. *American Journal of Public Health, 96*, 1370–1375.

Wilkinson, R., & Pickett, K. (2006). Income inequality and population health: A review and explanation of the evidence. *Social Science & Medicine, 62*(7), 1768–1784.

Willett et al. (1993). Intake of trans fatty acids and risk of coronary heart disease among women. *Lancet, 341*(8845), 581–585.

Williams, S. J. (1995). Theorizing class, health and lifestyles: Can Bourdieu help us? *Sociology of Health & Illness, 17*, 577–604.

Wyatt et al. (2003). Racism and cardiovascular disease in African Americans. *American Journal of the Medical Sciences, 325*(6), 315–331.

Young, L., & Nestle, M. (2003). Expanding portion sizes in the US marketplace: Implications for nutrition counseling. *Journal of the American Dietetic Association, 103*(2), 231–234.

9

Primary Prevention and Evaluation

Daniel Perales

LEARNING OBJECTIVES

- Identify ways to evaluate primary prevention programs.
- Describe several evaluation models as tools for a systematic method for gathering information about prevention activities and their effectiveness.
- Identify measures to show increased knowledge and behavior change when evaluating program effectiveness.

E valuation is a necessary element for documenting the success of prevention efforts. This chapter is written to illustrate how primary prevention efforts can be evaluated. In fact, because quality primary prevention aims to have an impact on large populations, its effects can be measured by looking at overall population changes over time. In this chapter, the term *program* is defined broadly as a systematic effort to achieve multiple purposes including changing attitudes, knowledge, behaviors, organizational practices, and policies that can help create healthy environments and healthy people. Programs can occur in differing geographical and political settings and with varying purposes and structures (Fink, 2005). Primary prevention programs are specifically defined to forestall or completely prevent the onset of disease or the occurrence of injuries.

Whether programs are designed for *primary prevention* (for example, child immunization programs), *secondary prevention* (such as breast cancer screening), or *tertiary prevention* (as in drug rehabilitation), the programs and the populations they serve benefit greatly from a well-designed and systematically implemented formal evaluation. Therefore, a critical component of any effort intended to effect individual or community-level change is a systematic method for gathering information about the prevention activities and the effectiveness of those activities with regard to the priority population. *Program evaluation* can be defined succinctly as "the diligent investigation of a program's characteristics and merits" (Fink, 2005, p. 4). A more comprehensive definition is "a systematic process for an organization to obtain information on its activities, its impacts, and the effectiveness of its work, so that it can improve its activities and describe its accomplishments" (Mattessich, 2003, p. 3).

It is not uncommon for critics to state that primary prevention efforts are not cost-effective and that evaluation of lifestyle behavior change, in particular, is difficult at best (Russell, 1986). However, beginning with the 1979 landmark publication *Healthy People* (U.S. Department of Health, Education and Welfare, 1979), the value of implementing population-based prevention programs has been resoundingly endorsed by the Institute of Medicine (2003) of the National Academy of Sciences and more recently by a Health Partners Research Foundation study (Maciosek et al., 2006) sponsored by the Centers for Disease Control and Prevention (CDC). Former director of the CDC's Division of Prevention Research and Analytic Methods Steven Teutsch commented on the study's findings:

> Many of the most effective interventions occur at the population level. These include . . . systems to assure access to healthcare, laws and regulations to limit access to tobacco and assure clean air, programs to reduce toxic exposures, interventions to reduce risky behaviors, health education programs and messages, and creation of healthy environments and the availability of healthy foods [2006].

Evaluation is considered so important to public health that the CDC lists evaluation as one of the ten essential public health services (Harrell et al., 1994). Indeed, both the Institute of Medicine and the CDC recognize evaluation is needed to develop evidenced-based prevention programs. In effect, evaluation makes it possible to understand how and why programs work or do not work. This is especially important for primary prevention efforts because of the potential broadscale social and economic impact of such programs on community health.

Although prevention efforts are commonly perceived as focusing primarily on creating individual or group behavioral change with a small scope, primary prevention efforts typically reach statewide and national audiences, especially through policies that can produce communitywide norm changes. For example, in 1988, California voters passed Proposition 99 (the California Tobacco Health Protection Act), which increased the state cigarette tax by 25 cents per pack. The funds were used for health education, a statewide media campaign, and tobacco-related research. These funds were also used to create the statewide California Tobacco Control Program (CTCP). The CTCP uses a comprehensive approach to create social norms around tobacco use by "indirectly influencing current and potential future tobacco users by creating a social milieu and legal climate in which tobacco becomes less desirable, less acceptable, and less accessible" (California Department of Health Services, 1998, p. 3). In this chapter, I will provide several examples of how primary prevention efforts can be evaluated.

THE BENEFITS OF EVALUATION

There are numerous reasons for evaluating a program, including acquiring answers to questions such as these, posed by Rossi, Lipsey, and Freeman (2004, p. 3):

- Is a particular intervention reaching its target population?
- Is the intervention being implemented well?
- Are the intended services being provided?
- Is the intervention effective in attaining the desired goals or benefits?

In addition, program evaluation can identify a program's strengths and weaknesses; modify a program's goals, objectives, and intervention activities based on quantitative or qualitative evaluation feedback or both; validate the program's worth among constituents and stakeholders; and allow program managers to use evaluation findings to improve chances for the program's future funding and sustainability.

Program managers increasingly identify evaluation as an important part of their management responsibility. In addition, evaluation is rapidly becoming an expectation of program grant funding by foundations, nonprofit organizations, and local, state, and federal government agencies. During the past ten or fifteen years, many private and public funding organizations and agencies have incorporated formal evaluation into their requests for proposals. For example, the United Way of America, which raised more than $3.8 billion for social and prevention programs in 2004 (United Way of America, 2006), has been a leader among organizations that fund such programs in promoting and adopting the use of program evaluation (especially outcome evaluation) among its grant recipients. This evaluation emphasis has received surprisingly appreciative responses from program managers (United Way of America, 2000).

THE EVALUATION PROCESS

Evaluators often use various frameworks to conceptualize and develop their evaluation plans. This section of the chapter highlights a few of those frameworks and illustrates how they are linked to the evaluation of primary prevention. The CDC's evaluation framework (see Figure 9.1), developed in 1999, is an excellent way for evaluators and program managers to conceptualize and plan a primary prevention evaluation.

The framework has six steps: engage stakeholders, describe the program, focus the evaluation design, gather credible evidence, justify conclusions, and ensure use and share lessons learned. Each of these steps is described next.

Figure 9.1   The CDC evaluation framework

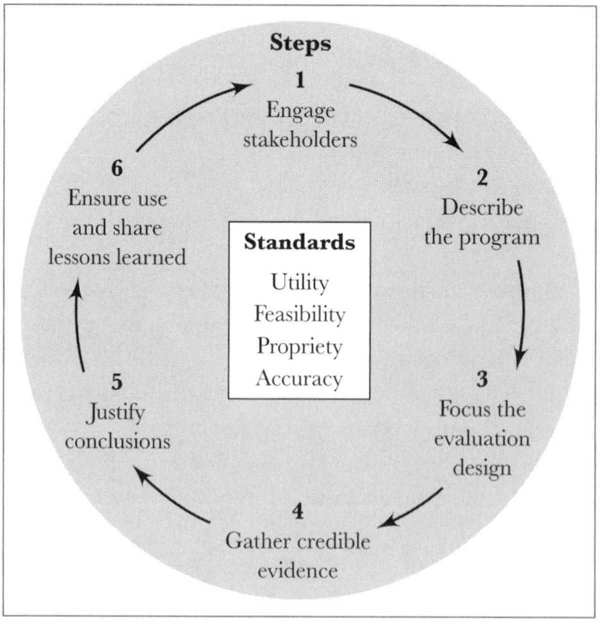

Source: Centers for Disease Control and Prevention (1999).

1. *Engage stakeholders. Stakeholders* are defined as "persons or organizations having an investment in what will be learned from an evaluation and what will be done with the knowledge" (CDC, 1999, p. 5). Stakeholders include those involved in program operations, those served or affected by the program, and primary users of the evaluation. Engaging stakeholders in the evaluation ensures their viewpoints are respected and that the next five steps are more easily implemented.

2. *Describe the program.* A program description is critical to developing the evaluation design and should describe the problem or need, the expected outcomes, the intervention strategies, the resources and community assets that will be used to implement the activities, how the evaluation will assess the program, the social ecological context, and a logic model flowchart that sets forth the key steps that can achieve the desired outcomes.

3. *Focus the evaluation design.* An evaluation must be systematic and focused. Focusing the evaluation design includes establishing a purpose for the evaluation (for example, to assess effects on participants, to assess policy compliance, or to assess program practices), deciding how the evaluation results will be used, and determining a specific evaluation design (experimental, quasi-experimental, or nonexperimental).

4. *Gather credible evidence.* This step begins with gathering information on indicators that can serve as specific measures for program success. Gathering credible evidence requires that multiple information sources, which include people, extant data, and primary data such as surveys, are gathered in sufficient quantity to allow for precise conclusions. Data gathering approaches should also take cultural preferences into account and ensure privacy and confidentiality.

5. *Justify conclusions.* Evaluation conclusions are justified when they are linked to the evidence gathered and judged against agreed values or standards set by the stakeholders. Stakeholders must have confidence the conclusions are justified before they are used for decision making.

6. *Ensure use and share lessons learned.* Deliberate effort is needed to ensure the evaluation processes and findings are used and disseminated appropriately, particularly to the community stakeholders.

INVOLVING STAKEHOLDERS IN ASSET MAPPING AND EVALUATION

The CDC evaluation framework is distinctive because of its emphasis on involving stakeholders. Stakeholder involvement in evaluation is even more critical today as federal, state, and foundation funding increasingly requires community-based coalition involvement in program planning, implementation, and evaluation (Wallerstein, Polascek, & Maltrud, 2002). For example, the W. K. Kellogg Foundation (1998) has an evaluation framework that includes a participatory process that values multiple perspectives and involves people who care about the project. A participatory process also prepares organizations to use evaluation as an ongoing function of management and leadership.

In recent years, participatory evaluation processes such as empowerment evaluation (Fetterman, Kafterian, & Wandersman, 1996) and the more recent emergence of *community-based participatory research* (CBPR, discussed in greater detail in Chapter Ten) have emphasized the importance of collaborative evaluation approaches that incorporate stakeholder participation from beginning to end. Minkler and Wallerstein (2003) define CBPR as a collaborative approach to research that benefits from stakeholder partnerships. They further elaborate:

> [CBPR] equitably involves all partners in the research process and recognizes the unique strengths that each brings. CBPR begins with a research topic of importance to the community with the aim of combining knowledge and action for social change to improve community health and eliminate health disparities [p. 4].

The significance of CBPR in evaluation research was recently emphasized by the Institute of Medicine (2003), which stated public health professionals must understand the major concepts and principles underlying CBPR and achieve competency in this area to engage more effectively in research and practice.

EVALUATING THE NORTH PHILADELPHIA FIREARMS REDUCTION INITIATIVE

Hausman and Becker (2000) used a participatory assessment approach called Rapid Participatory Appraisal (RPA) to address the reduction of youth firearm violence in North Philadelphia and subsequently identify evaluation indicators of success. They developed a key informant questionnaire that incorporated key dimensions of community capacity as previously defined by Kretzmann and McKnight (1993). The questionnaire was reviewed by members of the Community Advisory Board (CAB) of the Firearm Connection: North Philadelphia Firearms Reduction Initiative (NPFRI), a collaboration of health organizations, law enforcement officials, social service agencies, and local residents. Questionnaire wording changes were made on the CAB's recommendations.

Beginning with the CAB and using a snowball technique, the evaluators identified 111 people, 33 of whom were successfully interviewed during a six-month period. After analyzing the results, all interviewees were invited to review the analysis and interpretation, a participatory method that resulted in the interviewees' confirming their comments had been "heard well." The results showed that although firearm violence was a community concern, the most serious problem identified was drugs. Interviewees also cited unemployment, welfare reform, abandoned buildings, trash, and lack of alternative activities for youth as major issues.

The neighborhoods were mapped and resources and activities were identified. However, the data also showed there was a lack of coordination and visibility of those resources. This information resulted in an organizational expansion of the CAB to promote communication and intervention development that resulted in health, law enforcement, and social service partnerships. In addition, the assessment report documenting assets, agencies, and neighborhood information was offered and eagerly accepted by all of the interviewees.

The project funder had specified that reducing firearm violence was to be the purpose for the NPFRI. However, the compelling evidence produced by RPA helped the project and the evaluator convince the funder to support a project and an evaluation that both addressed the funder's primary prevention interest in reducing firearm violence and the community's concern about drugs and opportunities for youth. In effect, the researchers had defined the *real* problem, especially from the community's perspective, and developed capacity-based strategies for overcoming it.

In collaboration with the NPFRI, the evaluator developed indicators of success that were meaningful to the funder and the community stakeholders (see Table 9.1).

Overall, the evaluator felt that by understanding the community through a participatory assessment process, in collaboration with the NPFRI, he was able to develop evaluation indicators that reflected success in ways that were important to the various stakeholders, allowed for the development of strategies for gathering evaluation data from multiple sources with several methods, and used a socioecological perspective to address the identified problems and resources across several levels.

Participatory approaches are not without their difficulties for evaluators. However, evaluators who have learned from their participatory research experiences leave us with sage advice. Wallerstein and Duran (2006) believe that "in CBPR work, we suggest that the most important values are integrity coupled with humility. These values underlie our process with communities, in the science and how we present ourselves, and support our goals in doing this work" (p. 10). Roe and colleagues, in their work with a CDC-funded HIV Planning Council, were even more explicit:

> Empowerment evaluation requires an additional set of professional skills. Evaluators must be flexible, quick-thinking, self-critical, optimistic, and truly interested in the groups they work with and the potential of the community. Collecting this type of data requires the ability to engender trust, coax out stories, process qualitative information, and represent

Table 9.1   Evaluation markers for progress and outcomes in the North Philadelphia Firearms Reduction Initiative

Outcomes	Measures	Evaluation Tools or Methods
Community Capacity Outcomes		
Increased participation of youth and community in specifying key firearm issues and solutions	Participation rates of youth, parents, and community organizations in committee-defined activities	Attendance records; event logs
Increased youth involvement and leadership on gun violence prevention	Youth leadership training participation; youth leadership activities	Attendance records; event logs; youth logs
Increased linkages among community-based organizations and other prevention resources	Number of collaborative efforts; increased use of technical assistance resources	Attendance records; event logs; network maps; committee reports
Increased number of community interventions for safety and control	Number and nature of new intervention activities; new partnerships with police, courts, and health care providers	Event logs; committee reports
Increased intergenerational communication on firearm attitudes, beliefs, and risk behaviors	Number and nature of youth and adult activities	Event logs; satisfaction surveys
Increased awareness and involvement of medical providers	Provider use of monitoring and intervention protocols; number of new links with community organizations	Event logs; health provider survey; committee reports
Community-Indicated Outcomes		
Increased sense of community safety and control	Community residents' sense of safety and control; increased civic involvement	Citywide household survey; repeat interviews; environmental observations
Increased understanding of firearm risks among youth and adults	Changes in community norms	Health provider survey; youth survey; repeat interviews
Health-Related Outcomes		
Reduction of illegal firearm possession among youth	Indications of a downward trend	Data derived from citywide police gun-tracing efforts
Reduction in unintentional and intentional firearm injury among youth	Indications of a downward trend	Data derived from citywide emergency room surveillance

heartfelt experiences. This takes time, energy, and a keen eye for the phrase or the moment that may move a group forward. Evaluators must have an affection for the communities they work with while always maintaining an internal distance from which to observe process and explore empowering strategies [Roe, Berenstein, Goette, & Roe, 1997, p. 321].

Involving stakeholders implies the evaluator knows the community well. Understanding a program and its community setting is critical to evaluation. This process may begin by conducting a needs assessment as part of a formative evaluation. Kretzmann and McKnight (1993) make convincing arguments for conducting assessments that go beyond the traditional focus on needs and problems because such approaches label communities as needy, deficient, and populated by problematic and deficient people whose needs must be met by outsiders. Their asset mapping approach recognizes that all communities have the capacity to address their own problems and that external assistance should be requested by the community itself.

Mapping community capacity through a participatory process can identify key stakeholders and resources that can be used for program development, implementation, and evaluation. The preceding boxed case example of a primary prevention program ("Evaluating the North Philadelphia Firearms Reduction Initiative") describes a participatory asset mapping process and its implications for evaluation.

LOGIC MODELS

Logic models can also be considered planning and evaluation frameworks, since they describe a process from beginning to end. Rossi et al. (2004) note that "simply laying out the logic of the program in this form makes it relatively easy to identify questions the evaluation might appropriately address" (p. 94).

Goldman and Schmalz (2006) believe logic models can help the evaluation do all of the following:

- Identify differences between the ideal program and its real operation
- Frame questions about attribution and contribution
- Specify the nature of questions being asked
- Determine which indicators will (and will not) be measured
- Document accomplishments
- Organize evidence about the program
- Prepare reports and other media
- Tell the program's story

A good primary prevention example of a logic model is the one used by the CDC's VERB Youth Media Campaign (CDC, 2006b). Directed at *tweens* (youth aged nine to twelve), VERB is designed to promote physical activity among young people and prevent

Table 9.2   Elements of the CDC's VERB campaign logic model

Inputs
  Consultants
  Staff
  Research and evaluation
  Contractors
  Community infrastructure
  Partnerships

Activities
  Advertising
  Promotions
  Web sites
  Public relations
  National and community outreach

Outcomes
  Short-term: awareness of campaign brand messages
  Medium-term: changes in subjective norms, beliefs, self-efficacy, and perceived
    behavioral control
  Long-term: engaging in and maintaining physical activity

overweight. The CDC uses the logic model to identify the outcomes for the campaign and link them to each other and to specific activities. The VERB logic model also demonstrates that prevention outcomes are often long-term and hence take time. Table 9.2 shows the basic elements of the VERB campaign logic model.

THE PRECEDE-PROCEED MODEL OF PREVENTION

The *PRECEDE-PROCEED model* is widely recognized for its program planning uses, but it also provides an excellent framework for evaluating primary prevention programs because of its comprehensiveness. In some respects, the PRECEDE-PROCEED model can also be considered a specialized logic model in that it can be used to visualize the expected sequence of program steps from program development to the evaluation of long-term outcomes.

PRECEDE-PROCEED is probably the most widely used planning model in the field of health promotion and health education and has nearly one thousand published applications (Green, 2005). PRECEDE is an acronym for Predisposing, Reinforcing, and Enabling Causes in Educational Diagnosis and Evaluation, and PROCEED is an acronym for Policy, Regulatory, Organizational Constructs in Educational and Environmental Development.

The PRECEDE portion was developed by Lawrence W. Green during the late 1970s from his research and public health experiences in the areas of cost-benefit evaluation, family planning, social factors in health behavior, diffusion and adoption theory, and other models of change (Green, 2005). In 1992, Marshall Kreuter's participation helped create the full PRECEDE-PROCEED model. Kreuter and colleagues describe the model's evolution as follows:

> From its earliest applications in the late 1970s, the model has evolved from a largely linear, causal-chain planning model to an ecological one accounting for a wide range of factors that include social, economic, and environmental determinants of health (Kreuter, De Rosa, Howze, & Baldwin, 2004, p. 448).

A current version of the model (Green & Kreuter, 2005) is presented in Figure 9.2.

As shown in Table 9.3, the model begins with formative evaluation of the first four PRECEDE phases and uses process, impact, and outcome evaluation components of PROCEED to measure and document change on people and their environments.

Some of the applications of the PRECEDE model in the evaluation of successful primary prevention programs include a one-year smoking prevention, exercise, and nutrition educational program that showed a significant decrease in chronic-disease risk factors among 2,283 fourth-graders in New York (Walter, Hofman, Connelly, Barrett, & Kost, 1985); a six-year study by Walter (1989) that showed a significant decrease in cholesterol levels, dietary fat intake, and initiation of smoking in children; and a major study of primary and secondary prevention services in a large HMO that showed a synthesis of clinical medicine and public health population-based approaches to the development and provision of clinical preventive services resulted in decreases in late-stage breast cancer in adult smokers. These prevention services also resulted in increases in child immunization levels and use of bicycle helmets by children (Thompson, Taplin, McAfee, Mandelson, & Smith, 1995).

DEVELOPING EVALUATION QUESTIONS

Evaluation methods are grounded in efforts to answer evaluation questions. Ideally, the questions are derived from the goals and objectives that were collaboratively developed with stakeholders. Rossi et al. (2004) note that good evaluation questions must be reasonable and appropriate. Appropriate and reasonable questions are founded on detailed descriptions that illustrate program structure and activities, priority population characteristics, and knowledge about the problems, needs, and assets. Since many prevention programs operate from finite funding, appropriateness also means the program should be able to answer the questions within the funding time frame and budget. The evaluation questions should also be answerable through the identification of variables that, ideally, can be measured.

Figure 9.2 The PRECEDE-PROCEED model

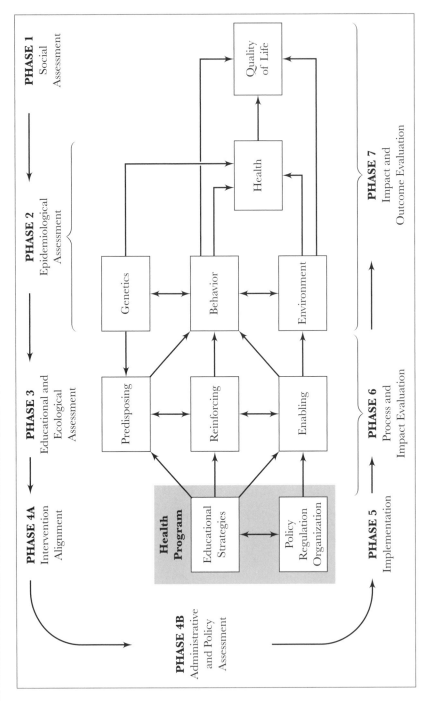

Source: Adapted from Green and Kreuter (2005), fig. 2.1.

Table 9.3 Evaluation Phases of the PRECEDE-PROCEED model

	Phases 1–4: Formative Evaluation	Phases 6 and 7: Process, Impact, and Outcome Evaluation
Phase 1: Social Assessment Quality of life	Assess and document feelings, needs, concerns, assets, and community capacity that describe quality of life.	*Phase 7: Outcome Evaluation* Measure factors that describe overall changes in the quality of life.
Phase 2: Epidemiological Assessment Health conditions	Assess and document health conditions, including morbidity, mortality, disability, and risk factors.	*Phase 7: Outcome Evaluation* Measure and describe the epidemiological indicators that evidence changes in health conditions.

Phase 2: Epidemiological Assessment
  Genetics
  Behavior
  Environment
	Assess and document indicators of health including genetic, behavioral, and environmental factors that affect quality of life.	*Phase 6: Impact Evaluation* Measure and describe the epidemiological and social indicators that document changes in behavior and environments that affect health status.

Phase 3: Educational and Ecological Assessment
  Predisposing
  Reinforcing
  Enabling
	Assess and document the cognitive and social antecedents that influence behaviors that in turn affect health.	*Phase 6: Impact Evaluation* Measure changes in the impact objectives that reflect the predisposing, reinforcing, and enabling factors that promote healthy behaviors and environments.

Phase 4A: Intervention Alignment
  Health Program:
    Educational strategies
    Policy regulation organization
Phase 4B: Administrative and Policy Assessment
	Assess and document administrative resources, regulations, and policies that can affect educational and environmental factors and shape program implementation.	*Phase 6: Process Evaluation* Document and measure process objectives that address program capacity, the activities and strategies that make up the intervention, and the response of practitioners and participants to the intervention's activities.

Phase 5: Implementation	Implement activities that deploy program resources, implement policy and organizational changes, and coordinate the program's interventions.	

Depending on the type of prevention program implemented, the evaluation questions can focus on the program's processes, the intermediate effect of those processes, or the program's final impact or outcomes. Perhaps more important, the evaluation questions can help program managers, stakeholders, and evaluators decide what data should be collected, where data should be collected, and how to collect, analyze, and interpret the data.

EVALUATION DATA

Evaluations are grounded in data. Most adherents of evidence-based designs view collecting quantitative data (*hard data*) as the most appropriate way to measure change. A method of evaluation whereby individual cases, situations, or events are studied to formulate a general principle involves the gathering of qualitative data. This method produces what is often called *soft data*, such as descriptions and opinions.

Prevention researchers (Rimer, Glanz, & Rasband, 2001; Steckler, McLeroy, Goodman, Bird, & McCormick, 1992) recognize there has been an ongoing debate about the role of qualitative versus quantitative prevention research but advocate for the inclusion of both types of data into the definition of evaluation evidence. Indeed, qualitative research is valuable because it can "provide insight not only into what happened but why it happened" (Rimer et al., 2001, p. 234). Table 9.4 describes the advantages and disadvantages of quantitative and qualitative methods.

MEASURING AND EVALUATING PRIMARY PREVENTION PROGRAMS

Primary prevention efforts, especially those requiring significant behavior change (such as smoking cessation), have often been viewed as difficult to measure and evaluate. This is particularly true of efforts that require long-term assessment of effect, such as the reduction in diabetes prevalence rates as a result of primary prevention efforts. The following examples will provide some insight into how primary prevention programs can be measured and evaluated.

When evaluators, stakeholders, and program managers are deciding what type of data they will need to answer their evaluation questions and show the effects of their prevention efforts, they need to consider what they want to measure. This requires an understanding of the program's purpose. Some programs, especially those that are addressing new health issues, will want to know if their intervention activities are affecting the awareness, knowledge, and even attitudes of people. For example, during the early stages of the HIV and AIDS outbreak, it was very important to conduct evaluations that assessed the public's knowledge of how HIV was transmitted to shape prevention strategies (DiClemente, Zorn, & Temoshok, 1986). Nearly two decades later, additional evaluation research proved that

Table 9.4   The pros and cons of quantitative and qualitative approaches to data collection

Quantitative Evaluation	Qualitative Evaluation
Larger numbers (generalizable to a broader population)	Smaller number of people or cases
Deductive generalizations (objectivity; strength of the scientific method; experimental and quasi-experimental designs; statistical analysis)	Inductive process (phenomenological inquiring; naturalistic, holistic; understanding the experience in context; content or case analysis)
Valid, reliable instrument used to gather data; specific administration protocol	Researcher is the instrument; less rigid protocol
Standardized measures used; predetermined response categories;	Able to study selected issues in depth and detail
Rigor	Flexibility
	Understanding of what individual variation means; deepening understanding, insights,
Results easily aggregated for analysis and easily presented	Offers credibility of an outsider making assessment
Can be perceived as biased, predictable, or rigged to obtain certain result	Results are longer, detailed, variable in content, and difficult to analyze
Results easily aggregated for analysis and easily presented	Data include group or individual opinions or perceptions; relationships, anecdotal comments, assessment of quality; descriptions; case studies; unanticipated outcomes.
Data include actual numbers, frequencies or counts of people, events, systems changes, passage of policy and legislation, trends	
Experimental conditions and designs to control or reduce variation in extraneous variables; focus on limited number of predetermined measures	Openness to variation and multiple directions

Source: Adapted from Francisco, Butterfoss, and Capwell (2001).

many of the HIV primary prevention strategies that were developed had been effective in the United States (CDC, 2006a).

As shown in Table 9.5, awareness, knowledge, and attitudes can be measured to only a minimal extent with interviews and surveys. These measures can be indicators that a primary prevention message is at least increasing knowledge. However, much more desirable measures of the effectiveness of prevention program interventions are ones that indicate

Table 9.5   Useful evaluation measures by data collection method

Focus of Measurement	Measures Yielding Quantitative Data	Measures Yielding Qualitative Data
Awareness, knowledge, attitudes	Written instruments (true-or-false items), telephone surveys	Interviews, focus groups
Behavior	Written self-reports with scaled responses	Interviews, focus groups, observations
Skills	Skills tests	Observations
Health status	Medical tests screenings, health risk or hazard appraisals	Interviews, clinical observations
Policy changes	Public records	Observations of compliance
Environmental changes	Written self-reports, public records	Observations, public records
Organizational changes	Public records	Observations, written self-reports
Quality of life	Proxy measures (absenteeism, discrimination, violence rates, clean air, socioeconomic status)	Interviews, focus groups

behavior change. These not only include measures of desired behavior change, such as smoking cessation and increased exercise, but also measures of knowledge-induced behavior change, such as practicing new low-fat food preparation skills or complying with car seat belt laws. Measures of health status change can provide even greater evidence of a primary prevention program's effectiveness. For example, a program designed to reduce risk for diabetes among diagnosed prediabetics will likely incorporate an educational component, a social support component, and a clinical management component. The educational component will include information about diabetes, food preparation, and exercise, all of which can be evaluated with instruments that measure knowledge, food skills, and self-reported changes in attitudes about preventing diabetes. The social support component can be assessed through qualitative and quantitative measures of self-esteem and increased self-efficacy in managing healthier behaviors. However, the clinical component can provide quantitative health status measures such as a decrease in weight loss and normal blood tests that can showcase the biological changes resulting from the knowledge, social support, and behavior change.

Tables 9.6 and 9.7, adapted from materials in the *Local Program Evaluation Planning Guide* issued by the California Department of Health Services' Tobacco Control Section (TCS) in 2004, provide a synopsis of evaluation designs and data collection methods for evaluating TCS-funded prevention programs. Programs funded through the TCS are

Table 9.6   Summary of evaluation designs and measures for behavior change and other interventions

Tobacco Program Plan Type	Individual Behavior Change	Other Change with a Measurable Outcome	Other Change with No Measurable Outcome
Outcome objective	Between July 1, 2005, and June 30, 2008, 100 high-risk smokers will participate in behavior modification-based tobacco cessation services in the community, with at least 50% of the participants who complete the cessation services quitting smoking. Of those, 25 will be smoke-free at one-, three-, and six-month follow-ups.	Between July 1, 2005, and June 30, 2008, the mean number of tobacco advertising signs in the one hundred convenience stores in River City will decrease from 10.6 items per store to no more than 5.0 items per store.	Between July 1, 2005, and June 30, 2006, the California Tobacco-Free Youth project will recruit and form a statewide youth coalition that will develop a statewide youth-focused anti-tobacco social marketing campaign.
Evaluation design	Quasi-experimental: multiple measures of the same participants over time.	Experimental: simple random sample of the 300 tobacco retail stores in River City into 75 intervention group stores and 75 control group stores.	Non-experimental
Process data collection	Focus group of high-risk smokers and other relevant community members to identify barriers and facilitators to recruiting and retaining participants for cessation class. End-of-cessation-class survey of remaining participants to assess satisfaction with content and willingness to quit.	Focus group of tobacco merchants to find out tobacco industry incentives for advertising. Assessment of training provided to the tobacco sign observers. Documentation of the merchant education intervention.	Focus group with selected youth coalition members to identify barriers and facilitators to the development and maintenance of the youth coalition. Review of coalition meeting minutes and other documents that describe development of the social marketing campaign.
Outcome data collection	Telephone interview assessment of smoking status at one-, three-, and six-month follow-ups.	Pre- and post-intervention observations of store signage in the intervention and control groups.	

Table 9.7 Summary of evaluation designs and measures for policy adoption and implementation

Tobacco Program Plan Type	Policy Adoption Only	Implementation Only	Policy Adoption and Implementation	Multiple Policies, Adoption Only
Outcome objective	Between July 1, 2005 and June 30, 2008, at least three low-income housing complexes in San Antonio County will adopt a written cigarette-related fire prevention policy that prohibits smoking in a minimum of 25% of the housing units.	Between July 1, 2005 and June 30, 2008, 100% of all stand-alone bars and bar-restaurants in San Antonio County will maintain compliance with Labor Code 6404.5 prohibiting smoking in bars and restaurants in the incorporated and unincorporated areas of the county.	Between July 1, 2005 and June 30, 2008, a policy will be adopted in San Antonio County that requires all tobacco retailers to obtain a license to sell tobacco products and includes a minimum fee of $100 per year per retailer to conduct compliance checks of retailers at least twice a year.	Between July 1, 2005 and June 30, 2008, San Antonio County will adopt a tobacco retail licensing policy that prohibits tobacco self-service displays and bans the distribution of tobacco gear such as T-shirts and hats with tobacco logos.
Evaluation design	Process	Quasi-experimental; outcome via multiple observations of the same bars and restaurants over time.	Process, quasi-experimental; outcome via multiple observations of the same retailers.	Process
Process data collection	Review of county records related to policy adoption. Key informant interviews with policy county supervisors.		Review of county records related to policy adoption.	Review of county records related to policy adoption. Key informant interviews with policy county supervisors.
Outcome data collection		Semiannual observational surveys of smoking in bars and restaurants.	Semiannual observational surveys of youths' attempts to purchase tobacco.	

required to conduct formal evaluations (California Department of Health Services, 2005). As shown in the tables, the interventions place a strong emphasis on developing policies that can create new social norms (such as smoke-free apartments and parks), complying with existing policies (for example, no smoking in bars and restaurants), and implementing activities that combat the tobacco industry's marketing messages. The evaluation of these interventions uses various evaluation design and data collection methods.

Primary prevention programs often require that evaluators identify measures that are proxy indicators of long-term impact. For example, studies of the laws prohibiting smoking in bars can be used to show the effectiveness of primary prevention public health policies designed to create healthy environments. Such laws are important because they can help prevent the unnecessary workplace deaths of employees, such as bartenders, who not long ago had rates of lung cancer higher than firefighters, miners, duct workers, and dry cleaners (California Department of Health Services, 1981). Weber, Bagwell, Fielding, and Glantz (2003) used observational methods to gather primary data on the long-term compliance with the California Smoke-Free Workplace Law in Los Angeles County in freestanding bars and bar-restaurants. Their observations provided clear evidence the law has been effective at reducing patron and employee smoking in Los Angeles County bars and restaurants. It is therefore likely this compliance will ultimately result in far fewer bar employees developing lung diseases associated with environmental tobacco smoke.

Evaluating policies can also show the primary prevention programs will not harm business. Cowling and Bond (2005) used California state tax revenue data to assess whether the California smoke-free restaurant and bar laws of 1995 and 1998 negatively affected the distribution of revenues between bars and restaurants, since pro-tobacco forces claimed a prohibition on smoking would reduce bar and restaurant revenues. Review of the data revealed that between 1990 and 2002, the effect was just the opposite: passage of both laws was associated with an increase in bar and restaurant revenues. In addition, Eisner, Smith, and Blanc (1998) found the respiratory health of bartenders improved shortly after the law was implemented.

ETHICAL AND LEGAL CONSIDERATIONS

When conducting any kind of evaluation research, evaluators and program managers must be cognizant of several ethical and legal considerations, including the following:

- Anonymity involves protecting the identity of participants. The Health Insurance Portability and Accountability Act (HIPAA) of 1996 provides significant privacy protection for individually acquired health information (U.S. Department of Health and Human Services, 1996).
- Confidentiality is necessary when gathering information on *sensitive issues*, such as substance use. Care should be taken to protect the confidentiality of information gathered from participants.

- Informed consent means advising clients about the nature of the data collection (research) and obtaining their approval to participate.
- Institutional review boards (IRBs) are administrative bodies that review research and evaluation plans to protect the privacy and other rights of participants. Human subject reviews are often required by U.S. government–supported programs, universities, and some state and local agencies. *The Belmont Report* is the "textbook" for ethical standards in research (National Commission, 1979).

MULTICULTURAL AND CULTURALLY COMPETENT EVALUATION

Our increasingly diverse communities require that evaluators develop evaluation plans that acknowledge and respect the differences found in those communities. This is known as *cultural competence*. During a major meeting of evaluators discussing multicultural evaluation, Hanh Cao Yu described the relevance of cultural competence to evaluation as follows:

> [Cultural competence] encompasses the whole evaluation process—from the evaluator's role, to the design and planning, through the reporting and application of findings. Multicultural evaluation also encompasses new approaches to evaluation—approaches that take into account power differentials, culture and systems analyses, and reciprocal relationships between the evaluators and the stakeholders [quoted in Endo & Job, 2003, p. 12].

Multicultural evaluation is essential if the needs of community stakeholders are to be met.

CHOOSING AN EXTERNAL EVALUATOR

Few programs have the internal expertise or time to conduct a formal evaluation and might therefore seek an outside evaluator. However, finding and selecting an evaluator is often difficult. Here are some tips for hiring an evaluator (adapted from Atkinson and Ashton, 2002).

INDICATORS OF A GOOD EVALUATOR

A good evaluator has the following traits:

- Speaks your language and will not talk to you in puzzling *insider's* jargon
- Wants to know your program and will ask questions about your program's history, purpose, and the priority population served by the program

- Has experience evaluating your type of program and will know the terms and acronyms used in such programs. He or she will also know the evaluation designs commonly used for your type of program
- Has experience and knowledge of your program's priority population and will consider the population's characteristics when designing the evaluation
- Has experience using qualitative and quantitative methods (including basic descriptive and inferential statistical methods) and understands how to gather and analyze qualitative information, such as that based on key informant interviews
- Has experience developing data collection instruments for measuring processes and outcomes and will provide you with examples of data collection forms developed for previous program evaluations
- Is willing to evaluate your program's goals and objectives and make recommendations for altering objectives that cannot be properly evaluated within the program's budget. However, a good evaluator recognizes it is the program that guides the evaluation, and not the reverse
- Is willing to develop a flexible evaluation design that can change as the prevention program is implemented
- Is willing to spend time with the program, including observing the program in action, visiting program intervention sites, and scheduling periodic conference calls or face-to-face meetings with program staff to review progress on the program scope of work and evaluation plan
- Is willing to produce periodic evaluation reports necessary for program monitoring and often required by funding agencies
- Is willing to write the final evaluation report that meets the needs of the program manager, the community stakeholders, and the funding agency and that can be used to seek future funding

WORKING WITH YOUR EVALUATOR

A good working relationship with an evaluator is fostered by a clear understanding of roles. However, the program managers also have important evaluation responsibilities, especially to the constituents and funding agencies. Program managers should do all of the following:

- Collaborate with the evaluator to design an evaluation plan that is consistent with the program's objectives and resources
- Ensure the evaluation is conducted within the terms of the evaluation plan, scope of work, and ethical considerations
- Coordinate with the evaluator and supervise the data collection
- Coordinate monthly meetings or conference calls with the evaluator and program staff
- Review and respond to the evaluator's reports

- Ensure information for required progress reports is collected from the evaluator in a timely manner
- Ensure the final evaluation report meets the contracted expectations

CONCLUSION

Despite the complex socioecological environments in which they often operate, primary prevention programs can be evaluated. Indeed, there is increasing recognition that consideration for the social determinants of health (including socioeconomic status, access to services, and public policies) must be incorporated into program evaluation designs for primary prevention programs.

Recognition of the many factors that influence individual and organizational behaviors is a major reason why program evaluation methods have evolved during the past few decades from ones in which researchers controlled the evaluation with minimal involvement of stakeholders, to participatory evaluation methods (such as CBPR and empowerment evaluation) that engage community stakeholders in evaluation decisions.

The complexities of primary prevention efforts should not deter evaluation efforts. Program managers and evaluators should strive to develop interventions that can, within ethical and resource considerations, be evaluated with rigorous evaluation designs to show impact. This rigor is critical, even though prevention scientists recognize that new evaluation designs and statistical techniques are needed to measure the true complexity of primary prevention interventions (Rimer et al., 2001). In addition, such designs can counter the argument that primary prevention programs cannot be evaluated scientifically. Indeed, as illustrated in this chapter, well-designed primary prevention evaluations can show proximate outcomes, such as behavior change, organizational change, and policy compliance, that are likely indicators of long-term impact. In order to move toward more evidence-based primary prevention interventions, program managers and evaluators must take several actions. First, evaluators must continuously increase their prevention program evaluation skills by reading the latest evaluation literature, attending evaluation workshops and conferences, and networking with other prevention evaluators. Second, program managers must recognize that evaluation is not an additional burden but a *necessity* of responsible program management. Third, both evaluators and program managers should join with funding agencies in seeking increases in both the financial and technical assistance resources necessary for rigorous evaluation. I have too often seen funding agencies require evaluation designs that are not supported by the evaluation funds. These resources should extend not just to program managers and evaluators but to community stakeholders. Such support will allow prevention practitioners to unequivocally show the effectiveness of their efforts and continue to add to the growing body of primary prevention knowledge.

DISCUSSION QUESTIONS

1. Which is your favorite evaluation framework or model? Why? If you do not have one, identify a primary prevention issue you are interested in and *walk through* the models listed to identify which one you might prefer.
2. Often prevention programs are evaluated by how many participants attended. Is this an effective way to evaluate behavior change? Why or why not? If no, what might you do differently?
3. Should funding agencies guide program evaluation or should that be left up to the receiving organization? Why or why not?

REFERENCES

Atkinson, A. J., & Ashton, C. (2002). *Planning for results: The safe and drug-free schools and communities program planning and evaluation handbook*. Richmond: Virginia Department of Education.

California Department of Health Services. (1981). *California occupational mortality study, 1979–1981*. Sacramento: Author.

California Department of Health Services, Tobacco Control Section. (1998). *A model for change: The California experience in tobacco control*. Sacramento: Author.

California Department of Health Services, Tobacco Control Section. (2004). *Local program evaluation planning guide*. Sacramento: Author. Retrieved June 6, 2004, from http://www.dhs.ca.gov/ps/cdic/tcs/documents/eval/LPEPlanningGuide.pdf

California Department of Health Services, Tobacco Control Section. (2005). *Local tobacco control interventions*. Sacramento: Author. Retrieved December 30, 2005, from http://www.dhs.ca.gov/tobacco/documents/rfps/RFA05–101.pdf

Centers for Disease Control and Prevention. (1999, September 17). Framework for program evaluation in public health. *Morbidity and Mortality Weekly Report, 48* (RR11), 1–40.

Centers for Disease Control and Prevention. (2006a). Evolution of HIV/AIDS prevention programs, United States, 1981–2006. *Morbidity and Mortality Weekly Report, 55*, 597–603.

Centers for Disease Control and Prevention. (2006b). *Youth media campaign: Logic model*. Atlanta: Author. Retrieved May 28, 2006, from http://www.cdc.gov/youthcampaign/research/logic.htm

Cowling, D. W., & Bond, P. (2005). Smoke-free laws and bar revenues in California: The last call. *Health Economics, 14*, 1273–1281.

DiClemente, R. J., Zorn, J., & Temoshok, L. (1986). Adolescents and AIDS: A survey of knowledge, attitudes, and beliefs about AIDS in San Francisco. *American Journal of Public Health, 76*, 1443–1445.

Eisner, M. D., Smith, A. K., & Blanc, R. D. (1998). Bartenders' respiratory health after establishment of smoke-free bars and taverns. *Journal of the American Medical Association, 280*(22), 1909–1914.

Endo, T., & Job, C. (2003). *Shifting our thinking: Moving from traditional to multicultural evaluation in health: Proceedings from a roundtable discussion*. Woodland Hills: The California Endowment.

Fetterman, D. M., Kafterian, S. J., & Wandersman, A. (1996). *Empowerment evaluation: Knowledge and tools for self-assessment and accountability*. Thousand Oaks, CA: Sage.

Fink, A. (2005). *Evaluation fundamentals: Insights into the outcomes, effectiveness, and quality of health programs* (2nd ed.). Thousand Oaks, CA: Sage.

Francisco, V. T., Butterfoss, F. D., & Capwell, E. M. (2001). Key issues in evaluation: Quantitative and qualitative methods and research design. *Health Promotion Practice, 2*(1), 20–23.

Goldman, K. D., & Schmalz, K. J. (2006). Logic models: The picture worth ten thousand words. *Health Promotion Practice, 7*(1), 8–12.

Green, L. W. (2005). *A resource for instructors, students, health practitioners, and researchers using . . . the PRECEDE-PROCEED model for health program planning and evaluation*. Retrieved January 5, 2006, from http://lgreen.net/index.html

Green, L. W., & Kreuter, M. W. (2005). *Health program planning: An educational and ecological approach* (4th ed.). New York: McGraw-Hill.

Harrell, J. A., et al. (1994). *The essential services of public health*. Washington, DC: American Public Health Association. Retrieved June 5, 2006, from http://www.apha.org/ppp/science/10ES.htm

Hausman, A. J., & Becker, J. (2000). Using participatory research to plan evaluation in violence prevention. *Health Promotion Practice, 1*(4), 331–340.

Institute of Medicine. (2003). *Who will keep the public healthy? Educating public health professionals for the 21st century*. Washington, DC: National Academies Press.

Kretzmann, J. P., & McKnight, J. L. (1993). *Building communities from the inside out: A path toward finding and mobilizing a community's assets*. Evanston, IL: Institute for Policy Research, Northwestern University.

Kreuter, M. W., De Rosa, C., Howze, E. H., & Baldwin, G. T. (2004). Understanding wicked problems: A key to advancing environmental health promotion. *Health Education and Behavior, 31*, 441–454.

Maciosek et al. (2006). Priorities among effective clinical preventive services. Results of a systematic review and analysis. *American Journal of Preventive Medicine, 31*, 90–96.

Mattessich, P. (2003). *Manager's guide to program evaluation: Planning, contracting, and managing for useful results*. Saint Paul, MN: Fieldstone Alliance.

Minkler, M., & Wallerstein, N. (2003). Introduction to community-based participatory research. In M. Minkler & N. Wallerstein (Eds.), *Community-based participatory research for health* (pp. 3–26). San Francisco: Jossey-Bass.

National Commission for the Protection of Human Subjects of Biomedical and Behavioral Research. (1979). *The Belmont Report: Ethical principles and guidelines for the protection of human subjects of research*. Washington, DC: National Institutes of Health. Retrieved July 26, 2006, from http://ohsr.od.nih.gov/guidelines/belmont.html

Rimer, B. K., Glanz, K., & Rasband, G. (2001). Searching for evidence about health education and health behavior interventions. *Health Education and Behavior, 28*, 231–248.

Roe, K. M., Berenstein, C., Goette, C., & Roe, K. (1997). Community building through empowerment: A case study of HIV prevention community planning. In M. Minkler (Ed.), *Community organizing and community building for health* (pp. 308–322). New Brunswick, NJ: Rutgers University Press.

Rossi, P. H., Lipsey, M. W., & Freeman, H. E. (2004). *Evaluation: A systematic approach* (7th ed.). Thousand Oaks, CA: Sage.

Russell, L. B. (1986). *Is prevention better than cure?* Washington, DC: Brookings Institution.

Steckler, A., McLeroy, K. R., Goodman, R. M., Bird, S. T., & McCormick, L. (1992). Toward integrating qualitative and quantitative methods: An introduction. *Health Education Quarterly, 19,* 1–8.

Teutsch, S. (2006). Cost-effectiveness of prevention. *Medscape Today: Perspectives in Prevention from the American College of Preventive Medicine.* Retrieved July 13, 2006, from http://www.medscape.com/viewarticle/540199

Thompson, R. S., Taplin, S. H., McAfee, T. A., Mandelson, M. T., & Smith, A. E. (1995). Primary and secondary prevention services in clinical practice: Twenty years' experience in development, implementation, and evaluation. *Journal of the American Medical Association, 273,* 1130–1135.

U.S. Department of Health, Education and Welfare. (1979). *Healthy people: The surgeon general's report on health promotion and disease prevention.* Washington, DC: Government Printing Office.

U.S. Department of Health and Human Services, Office for Civil Rights. (1996). *Health Insurance Portability and Accountability Act (HIPAA).* Retrieved July 26, 2006, from http://www.hhs.gov/ocr/hipaa

United Way of America. (2000). *Agency experiences with outcome measurement.* Retrieved January 20, 2006, from http://national.unitedway.org/files/pdf/outcomes/AgencyOM.pdf

United Way of America. (2006). *America's number 1 charity: A snapshot of resources raised for 2004–2005.* Retrieved January 20, 2006, from http://national.unitedway.org/files/pdf/200405RDExecutive.pdf.

Wallerstein, N., & Duran, B. (2006). Using community-based participatory research to address health disparities. *Health Promotion Practice, 7*(3), 1–12.

Wallerstein, N., Polascek, M., & Maltrud, K. (2002). Participatory evaluation model for coalitions: The development of systems indicators. *Health Promotion Practice, 3*(3), 361–373.

Walter, H. J. (1989). Primary prevention of chronic disease among children: The school-based Know Your Body intervention trials. *Health Education Quarterly, 16,* 201–214.

Walter, H. J., Hofman, A., Connelly, P. A., Barrett, L. T., & Kost, K. L. (1985). Primary prevention of chronic disease in childhood: Changes in risk factors after one year of intervention. *American Journal of Epidemiology, 122,* 772–781.

Weber, M. D., Bagwell, D. A., Fielding, J. E., & Glantz, S. A. (2003). Long-term compliance with California's Smoke-Free Workplace Law among bars and restaurants in Los Angeles County. *Tobacco Control, 12,* 269–273.

W. K. Kellogg Foundation. (1998). *Evaluation handbook: Philosophy and expectations.* Battle Creek, MI: Author. Retrieved January 17, 2006, from http://www.wkkf.org/pubs/Tools/Evaluation/Pub770.pdf

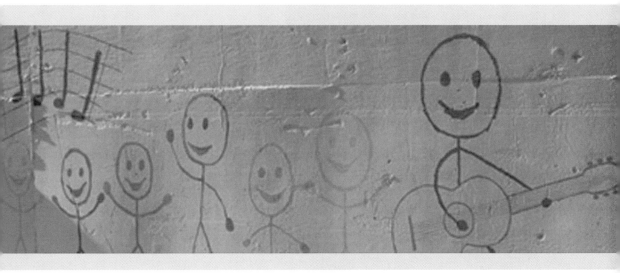

PREVENTION IN CONTEXT

Part Three explores the application of prevention efforts that correspond to a range of contemporary health issues. Each chapter puts the current practice of prevention into context through specific examples and emphasizes the integral role of prevention in improving community environments and changing social norms. In addition, each notes how improving norms and environments will be reflected in improved health.

The links between environmental exposures and health outcomes are well documented among conditions that include cancer, asthma, and developmental disabilities. Environmental exposures are preventable and disproportionately affect disfranchised communities. In Chapter Ten, "Preventing Injustices in Environmental Health and Exposures," Stephanie Farquhar, Neha Patel, and Molly Chidsey first describe environmental health and explain how it can be approached from a prevention perspective and then focus on injustices in environmental exposures and how they can be redressed. Traditional risk assessment for environmental exposure does not focus on prevention but rather responds to crises of illness or injury. The authors propose two prevention approaches critical to achieving environmental justice. The *precautionary principle* borrows from the medical oath to "do no harm" and places the burden of demonstrating safety prior to public exposure on those who produce chemicals and other substances. Community-based *participatory research* is a vital primary prevention strategy that addresses the need for community capacity building and involvement of key stakeholders in decisions that affect community health.

The physical environment in which we live, work, and play has a fundamental impact on health and behaviors that affect health. Health outcomes are affected directly by the environment when, for instance, the siting of a truck depot increases diesel emissions in a neighborhood. Environmental factors also affect health impacts. For example, a community without sidewalks is associated with people who walk less and are therefore at risk of increased rates of chronic disease.

However, the specific decisions about how the environment is built, such as street design, are generally made without considering their impact on health. In Chapter Eleven, "Health and the Built Environment," Howard Frumkin and Andrew Dannenberg describe the developing emphasis on the *built environment* and its emerging links with health. They make a compelling case for the critical role that changes to the physical environment can have in preventing our most serious health problems. The authors explain why health leaders need to work with new partners and new disciplines and influence those who make built environment decisions (including city planners and traffic engineers) to broaden their health and prevention perspective.

Our choices about what and how much to eat are made in the context of our social, physical, and cultural environment. The accessibility and availability of food, coupled with advertising and pricing, form the food environment. Leslie Mikkelsen, Catherine Erickson, Juliet Sims, and Marion Nestle, in Chapter Twelve, "Creating Healthy Food Environments to Prevent Chronic Disease," link the current U.S. food environment to a range of nutrition-related chronic diseases that are resulting in significant increases in illness and death. They describe the need to prevent these diseases by transforming the food environment and discuss several primary prevention strategies that hold great promise for improving nutrition and related health outcomes at the community level. The authors also present new approaches that address policy areas, including access to healthy food, affordability, and advertising.

Violence can affect every family and community, and disfranchised communities are more at risk than any others. The public is generally skeptical about violence, assuming it is natural and that nothing can be done about it. In Chapter Thirteen, "A Public Health Approach to Preventing Violence," Deborah Prothrow-Stith and Rachel Davis describe violence as a learned behavior that is therefore preventable; it can be unlearned or not learned in the first place. Dr. Prothrow-Stith was one of the first prevention advocates in the country to frame violence as a public health issue and to propose the application of public health solutions. In laying out a public health approach to preventing violence, the authors point out that like other health issues, understanding what underlies violence gives one the capacity to prevent it. An accompanying sidebar by Dionne Smith Coker-Appiah, Mysha R. Wynn, and Donald Parker describes Project LOVE, a community-based approach to preventing adolescent dating violence.

For more than a quarter of a century, HIV has been a high-profile public health issue, and prevention efforts have focused primarily on addressing individual behavior change. In Chapter Fourteen, "The Limits of Behavioral Interventions for HIV Prevention," Dan Wohlfeiler and Jonathan Ellen suggest this focus on behavior change is necessary but insufficient to achieve sustainable change. Instead, the authors recommend that HIV advocates take their cues from primary prevention successes and focus on structural-level solutions that address the social, economic, and political systems in which we live and in which sexual decisions are made. They describe the need to target the sexual networks that lead to increased risk-taking behavior and point out the ultimate outcome of HIV prevention efforts is not merely a reduction in risk-taking behavior but also a sustained decrease in the rate of new infections.

Authored by Anita M. Wells, GiShawn A. Mance, and M. Taqi Tirmazi, Chapter Fifteen, "Mental Health in the Realm of Primary Prevention," is a timely addition to the text. The authors argue that poor mental health outcomes are far from inevitable and point out how a primary prevention framework to mental health could be adopted for otherwise often marginalized populations, such as veterans, immigrant youth, and urban youth. By using a social determinants framework that includes "environmental and systemic factors that influence the development of mental illness" the authors lay out specific strategies for primary prevention. A sidebar contribution by Joseph P. Gone addresses the role culture needs to play in primary prevention for Native Americans. Prevention Institute's sidebar contribution describes how the Health System Behavioral Health and Recovery Services in San Mateo County, California, developed an interdisciplinary planning process in 2008 to determine strategies that emphasize primary prevention and complement existing treatment services for mental health.

10

Preventing Injustices in Environmental Health and Exposures

Stephanie Ann Farquhar
Neha Patel
Molly Chidsey
Sidebar contributors:
Nancy M. Goff, Peter Murchie

LEARNING OBJECTIVES

- Describe the concept of *environmental health* and how it can be approached from a *prevention perspective*.
- Begin to learn why low-income communities and communities of color have higher than average levels of toxic exposures (and increases in related disease) and how the environmental justice movement emerged in response to these disparities.
- Describe two preventive approaches to environmental health, the *precautionary principle* and *community-based participatory research*, and learn how each approach can be integrated with traditional risk assessment of community environmental exposures.

Environment matters. The same environmental problems that contribute to poor air and water quality and to blight and neighborhood deterioration also contribute to negative mental and physical health outcomes. Cancer, asthma, birth defects, developmental disabilities, infertility, and Parkinson's disease are on the rise, and they are linked to chemical exposures from air, water, food, and products and practices used in our schools, homes, neighborhoods, and workplaces. These health problems are widespread, affecting nearly one of every two Americans (Pew Environmental Health Commission, 2001).

Health problems related to environmental exposures are also very expensive and cost $325 billion yearly in health care costs, loss of productivity, and special education programs (Pew Environmental Health Commission, 2001). An estimated $54.9 billion is spent annually on pediatric diseases linked to environmental pollutants alone (Landrigan, Schechter, Lipton, Fahs, & Schwartz, 2002).

If environmental health is the assessment and control of the environment and related health outcomes (a more complete definition will be given in the section in this chapter on environmental health), *environmental justice* provides one way to examine and discuss the unequal nature of exposures and health outcomes. Environmental justice as a framework and a practice acknowledges that pollution and related health effects fall disproportionately on residents living in economically and politically disadvantaged communities (Bryant, 1995). And there are clear patterns, in that low-income people and people of color are typically the most affected. Furthermore, the same residents who are already facing a multitude of environmental threats are often excluded from the very decisions and environmental policies that threaten their communities' health.

The traditional environmental risk assessments that are widely used to evaluate exposure and related health outcomes frequently fail to examine exposures among the most vulnerable residents, the synergistic effect of exposure to multiple environmental health problems, or the social or political aspects associated with exposure and risk decisions. Traditional risk assessment evaluates new technologies and products by calculating the mathematical likelihood exposure will threaten our health. This approach requires us to prove a product, practice, or chemical is harmful before discontinuing its manufacture or use.

This chapter presents two approaches that can be used to augment the types of information and solutions obtained using the more traditional risk assessment approach. These two supplemental methods, the *precautionary principle* and *community-based participatory research*, explicitly involve residents and other stakeholders and consider the social and political aspects of environmental exposure. Two case studies from Portland, Oregon, illustrate the potential power of local resident and government involvement and make manifest a preventive framework that seeks equity in environmental health burden and benefit.

ENVIRONMENTAL HEALTH

The *Journal of Environmental Health Perspectives* defines environmental health as "those aspects of human disease and injury that are determined or influenced by factors in the environment," including "direct pathological effects of various chemical, physical, and biological agents, as well as the effects on health of the broad physical and social environment, which includes housing, urban development, land-use and transportation, industry, and agriculture" (Environmental Health Perspectives, n.d.). It should be noted that when using the terms environment and environmental health, we are drawing from this broader definition, which considers the *built* and *social environments* in addition to chemical and other exposures in the physical environment.

The environmental health movement developed in response to an increased awareness of the effects of toxic chemicals on the environment and human health. Significant dates and benchmark achievements associated with the environmental health movement are presented in Exhibit 10.1.

EXHIBIT 10.1 BENCHMARK ACHIEVEMENTS IN ENVIRONMENTAL HEALTH

1960s

Rachel Carson's *Silent Spring* exposes the hazards of the pesticide DDT and brings a new public awareness to the impact of widely released chemicals on health and the environment.

1970s

Twenty million people celebrate the first Earth Day.
President Nixon creates the Environmental Protection Agency (EPA).
Congress amends the Clean Air Act, restricts use of lead-based paint, bans DDT, and phases out PCB production.

1980s

Congress creates the Superfund to clean up hazardous waste sites.
Safer disposal of nuclear waste becomes a priority.

1990s

> The Toxics Release Inventory is created, designed to track emissions from certain industry groups.
>
> The Pollution Prevention Act changes the focus of pollution policies to preventive source reduction.
>
> An executive order protects children from health risks associated with environmental factors, including asthma and lead poisoning.
>
> The United Nations Rio Earth Summit leads to the agreement on the Climate Change Convention and the Kyoto Protocol.

THE IMPACT OF ENVIRONMENTAL EXPOSURE

Despite some limited progress in the past decades, pollution continues to threaten our health, and some communities are more exposed than others. Hundreds of contaminants accumulate in our bodies through exposure to cleaning products, plastics, fuels, pesticides, and cosmetics. A study conducted by researchers at Mount Sinai School of Medicine in New York and the Environmental Working Group found a total of 167 industrial compounds, pollutants, and other chemicals in the blood and urine of nine volunteers, none of whom had worked with or had any significant exposure to chemicals (Thornton, McCally, & Houlihan, 2002). Of the 167 chemicals found, 76 are known to cause cancer in humans or animals, 94 are toxic to the brain and nervous system, and 79 cause birth defects or abnormal development. In 2005, the Centers for Disease Control and Prevention (CDC) issued its third report on *body burden* (chemical load) and measured 148 chemicals or their breakdown products in the blood or urine of approximately 2,400 people who participated in the National Health and Nutrition Examination Survey (NHANES) from 1999 to 2002 (CDC, 2005). Other biomonitoring studies have detected high concentrations of certain classes of flame retardants in wildlife and human blood, milk, and tissues (Hites, 2004). It should also be noted that although exposure regulations are based on the assessment of single products or practices, we are exposed to a multitude of chemicals, and the potential synergistic effect of these exposures is typically not evaluated and can be more damaging to health than any one single exposure.

Many chronic and acute diseases are strongly associated with products and practices used in our schools, homes, parks, and workplaces. The incidence of asthma has nearly doubled in the past twenty-five years, and certain populations are disproportionately affected by this disease, particularly children and the urban poor (Solomon, 2002). Incidences of breast, thyroid, kidney, liver, skin, lung (in females), testicular, brain, esophageal, and bladder cancer and non-Hodgkin's lymphoma have all increased during the past twenty-five years (Houlihan, Wiles, Thayer, & Gray, 2003; Schettler, 2002). Nervous system disorders

TRIPLE INJUSTICE OF CLIMATE CHANGE

Peter Murchie

Climate change is not just a problem for the future; its impacts are currently felt globally. There is an urgency to take action now to help reduce future warming and to adapt to the current level of warming (Intergovernmental Panel on Climate Change, 2007). The body of scientific research related to climate change has grown significantly in the past twenty years. In 2007 the Intergovernmental Panel on Climate Change (IPCC) found that global warming is "unequivocal" and primarily due to human emissions (IPCC, 2007). In addition, the global models scientists use to predict the potential change have underestimated the rapidly increasing emissions of greenhouse gases (Canadell, 2007).

Globally we are witnessing average surface air temperature increases, weather and climate extremes, a reduction in sea ice in the Arctic, in Greenland and in parts of Antarctica, and rising sea levels. In the United States, researchers have observed changed precipitation patterns, impacts on habitat and wildlife, retreating glaciers, early snowmelt, a decline of forest health and catastrophic fires, changes in planting zones and crop ranges, an expansion of ranges of pest- and vector-borne disease species, drought, increased flooding, and the relocation of native Alaskan communities due to erosion and melting permafrost.

Public health impacts such as social disruption, forced migration, and increased rates of asthma are predicted. Threats to well-being will likely disproportionately impact vulnerable populations such as children, the elderly, and the poor (Ebi, Sussman, & Wilbanks, 2008). Poor populations and communities of color might be hit the hardest by climate-related threats to housing, rising energy costs, and threats to culture and social stability. In fact, new research highlights the triple injustice of climate change; that is, people of color and poor communities are less responsible for climate change, have less capacity to adapt to changes, and yet will suffer the most from it. For example, African Americans make up 13 percent of the U.S. population and on average emit nearly 20 percent less greenhouse gases than non-Hispanic whites per capita (Hoerner & Robinson, 2008).

Currently, technologies, policies, and plans are being developed to reduce greenhouse gas emissions. Internationally, countries have negotiated treaties, such as Kyoto, and multi-lateral and bi-lateral agreements to reduce emissions and establish green development funding for the developing world. In the United States, the EPA is pursuing regulation of greenhouse gas emissions under the Clean Air Act, and Congress is debating new legislation that would cap greenhouse gas emissions. Governments at the national, state, and local levels are developing climate action plans and using incentives to encourage investment in clean energy and green development.

Increasingly there has been a call to support the communities hit by the triple injustice of climate change. New policies and programs to support energy efficiency and weatherization efforts will also provide new green job opportunities in the renewable energy, energy efficiency, and weatherization trades. In sum, these efforts may help slow climate change and its public health, social, environmental and economic consequences.

such as autism, learning impairments, and Parkinson's disease are also on the rise (Blaxill, 2004; Houlihan et al., 2003). In a study of twenty autistic children, Edelson and Cantor (1999) found all subjects had liver detoxification profiles outside of normal. Development of Parkinson's disease is strongly associated with exposure to pesticides and other toxic agents (Brown, Rumsby, Capleton, Rushton, & Levy, 2006; Wang, Li, Chou, & Bronstein, 2006).

DISPARITIES IN HEALTH OUTCOMES

Given the high average levels of toxic exposures and increases in related disease, it is especially distressing that exposure-related health outcomes disproportionately burden low-income communities and communities of color. For example, as noted earlier, asthma rates are increasing (Solomon, 2002). This chronic disease alone costs Americans $14 billion annually and accounts for more than 14 million lost school days and 1.8 million emergency room visits each year (Smart, 2004). But the burden of this disease that is linked to indoor and outdoor air quality is not evenly distributed. Disproportionate numbers of people of color and people from low-income households live in *nonattainment areas* (areas that persistently fail to meet the federally established ambient air quality standards) and may be exposed to higher than average levels of indoor and outdoor pollution. Approximately three times as many African Americans as whites die from complications related to asthma, and the hospitalization rate for African Americans and Latinos is three to four times the rate for whites (Grant, Lyttle, & Weiss, 2000). Asthma also affects children disproportionately. Although they make up only 25 percent of the population, children account for 40 percent of all asthma cases (Solomon, 2002), and five times more children than adults die from asthma each year.

Lead poisoning is another environmental health threat that disproportionately affects poor inner-city African American children. Lead poisoning affects an estimated 434,000 American preschoolers, or 2.2 percent of the under-five age group, yet African American children continue to be much more likely to be poisoned by lead than white children (Meyer et al., 2003). More than 22 percent of African American children living in pre-1946 housing have high blood lead levels, compared with 5.6 percent of white children and 13 percent of Mexican American children living in older homes. Effects of exposure on behavior are potentially devastating. Even very low levels of exposure can result in reduced IQ, and an estimated 16 percent of juvenile delinquent behavior in the United States is attributable to high lead exposure (Wakefield, 2002).

There is also a *double injustice* in terms of unequal exposure and unequal access to prevention and treatment. Populations that are at a higher risk of exposure to environmental contaminants are also more likely to have little or no access to adequate health care. This lack of access makes it more difficult for certain groups to seek early detection, preventive care, and care after becoming sick. More than 45 million Americans, including 10 million children, are without health insurance today, and the cumulative effect of increased risk and less care is potentially devastating (Institute of Medicine, 2002). A 2001 Commonwealth Fund survey revealed that Hispanics and African Americans were most likely to be uninsured, as 46 percent of working-age Hispanics and 33 percent of working-age African Americans lacked insurance for all or part of the twelve months prior to the survey. In comparison, only 20 percent of both whites and Asian Americans aged 18 to 64 lacked health coverage for all or part of the previous twelve months (Collins et al., 2002). However, there is hope on the horizon, as the sweeping health reform legislation of 2009 will provide more equitable access to health care. Yet, even though more equitable health coverage will soon exist in the United States, the differential exposure to environmental toxins by race or social class will continue to prevail.

Furthermore, as evidenced by Hurricanes Katrina and Rita in 2005, natural disasters are another aspect of the environment that tends to disproportionately affect poor communities and residents of color. This exposure occurs through both subsequent toxic exposures (such as contaminated floodwater) and a more general inability to flee unsafe conditions. A community's potential for exposure to hazards, which include asbestos, lead and contaminated soil and water, is determined in part by its ability to access resources in the aftermath of a disaster. Furthermore, the conditions of people's lives before the disaster occurs (for example, their employment status, education, social support system, housing situation, and access to health care, financial credit, and legal services) contributes to their level of vulnerability or security in terms of exposure risks and the recovery process (Blaikie, Cannon, Davis, & Wisner, 1994; Bolin & Stanford, 1998; Farquhar & Wing, 2003; Donner & Rodriguez, 2008). Furthermore, people of color experience longer recoveries from natural disasters, have limited access to insurance, and use aid and relief organizations differently than the rest of the population (Natural Hazards Research and Applications Information Center, 2001; Fothergill, Maestas, and Darlington DeRouen, 1999).

ENVIRONMENTAL JUSTICE

The environmental justice movement emerged in response to the recognition that environmental exposure disproportionately affects the economically and politically disadvantaged. The movement also emerged out of frustration with the exclusion of affected populations in environmental health decisions. The EPA defines environmental justice as "the fair treatment and meaningful involvement of all people regardless of race, color, national origin, or income with respect to the development, implementation, and enforcement of environmental laws, regulations, and policies" (1992, p. 2). As mentioned previously, if environmental health is the science and control of environmental threats to health, environmental justice provides us with the tools, language, and framework to examine inequity in environmental exposure and decision making.

DR. ROBERT BULLARD

The year 1978 witnessed the largest polychlorinated biphenyl (PCB) spill ever recorded in the United States. Oil laced with PCB was illegally dumped along 210 miles of roadway in North Carolina (Bullard, Glenn, & Torres, 2004). Four years later, in 1982, Warren County, a poor and mostly African American county, was selected for disposal of the contaminated soil. Protests erupted in response to the decision, and although opponents were not able to block the siting of the PCB landfill, the battle that ensued in Warren County brought environmental justice into public view (Bullard & Johnson, 1997).

Robert Bullard, sociology professor at Clark Atlanta University and director of the Environmental Justice Resource Center, has been instrumental in the quest for environmental justice. When Bullard's wife, Linda McKeever Bullard, filed a lawsuit (*Bean* v. *Southwestern Waste Management*) that opposed the placement of a landfill in the middle of a predominantly black, middle-class, homeowning suburban neighborhood (Dicum, 2006), her husband collected data to support her case.

His research revealed that 100 percent of the city-owned landfills in Houston were in black neighborhoods, even though blacks made up only 25 percent of the population. Similarly, six out of eight of the city-owned incinerators were in predominantly black neighborhoods. Of the privately owned landfills, three out of four were located in predominantly black neighborhoods. Bullard concluded that in the absence of zoning in Houston, these decisions had to have been made by government officials (Dicum, 2006).

The United Church of Christ Commission for Racial Justice (UCCCRJ) responded by publishing a study in 1987, *Toxic Waste and Race* (Bullard & Johnson, 1997). The study documented that three in five African Americans lived in communities with abandoned toxic waste sites, three in five lived in communities with one or more active waste sites, and three of the five largest commercial hazardous waste landfills were located in predominantly African American or Latino communities. In fact, these three large commercial hazardous waste landfills accounted for 40 percent of the nation's total hazardous waste landfill capacity in 1987.

Among other publications documenting environmental injustice, *Dumping in Dixie: Race, Class, and Environmental Quality* (Bullard, 1990) chronicled environmental justice struggles in the South. Grassroots organizations began to spring up in reaction to such findings.

Bullard helped plan the first National People of Color Environmental Leadership Summit in 1991, which generated the organizing principles of the environmental justice movement. He went on to help the Clinton administration write the executive order that required federal agencies to consider environmental justice in their programs (Motavalli, 1998), and he served on the Environmental Protection Agency's National Advisory Council for Environmental Policy and Technology, offering direction in regard to complaints filed under the antidiscriminatory Title VI of the Civil Rights Act of 1964 (Motavalli, 1998).

According to Bullard, "The environmental justice movement has basically redefined what environmentalism is all about. It basically says that the environment is everything: where we live, work, play, go to school, as well as the physical and natural world. And so we can't separate the physical environment from the cultural environment" (Schweizer, 1999, p. 1).

Source: Prevention Institute.

The environmental justice movement is marked by several landmark events, which are presented in Exhibit 10.2. Warren County, North Carolina, is widely recognized as the birthplace of the environmental justice movement. In 1982, this predominantly African American county, with more industry than any other North Carolina county, held demonstrations against the siting of a hazardous waste landfill. The following year, a study of several southern states by the General Accounting Office found that three out of four landfills were sited near communities with a non-white majority. In 1987, the UCCCRJ issued a report that showed race to be the most significant factor nationally in determining the location of hazardous waste facility sites, with three out of every five African Americans and Hispanics living in a community in close proximity to unregulated toxic waste sites (EPA, 2003). Other studies corroborate that a greater number of environmentally hazardous waste sites and polluting industries are located in low-income communities and communities of color (Faber & Krieg, 2002) and that a higher risk of cancer is associated with airborne toxics in socioeconomically disadvantaged communities and African American communities (Apelberg, Buckley, & White, 2005; Lopez, 2002).

The results of these and other studies, paired with effective local organizing efforts that challenged the government to respond to disproportionate exposure, led to the establishment of the EPA's Office of Environmental Justice in 1992 and the 1994 Executive

EXHIBIT 10.2   LANDMARK EVENTS IN ENVIRONMENTAL JUSTICE

1964

> Congress passes the Civil Rights Act, Title VI, which prohibits the use of federal funds to discriminate on the basis of race, color, or national origin.

1971

> The Council on Environmental Quality's annual report acknowledges that racial discrimination adversely affects the urban poor and the quality of their environment.

1979

> Linda McKeever Bullard files a lawsuit, *Bean* v. *Southwestern Waste Management*, on behalf of Houston's Northeast Community Action Group, challenging the siting of a waste facility.

1982

> Warren County residents protest the siting of a PCB landfill in Warren County, North Carolina.

1983

> The General Accounting Office publishes *Siting of Hazardous Landfills and Their Correlation with Racial and Economic Status of Surrounding Communities*, which found that three-quarters of all off-site commercial hazardous waste facilities in EPA Region IV were located in African American communities.

1987

> The United Church of Christ Commission for Racial Justice (UCCCRJ) issues *Toxic Wastes and Race in the United States*, a report that correlated waste facility siting and race.

1991

> The first National People of Color Environmental Leadership Summit is held in Washington, DC, with more than one thousand participants.

1998

The UCCCRJ convenes grassroots environmental justice, civil rights, and academic leaders to challenge the chemical company Shintech's permit application, halting the company's efforts to build a PVC plant in Louisiana.

2001

The National Black Environmental Justice Network coordinates the Congressional Black Caucus Hearing on environmental justice in Washington, DC.

Order No. 12898, whereby President Clinton directed eleven federal agencies to incorporate environmental justice into their policies (EPA, 2003).

One of the common responses to the issue of disproportionate exposure and unhealthy neighborhoods is the suggestion that people simply move from health-threatening neighborhoods. What is frequently underappreciated is that the same residents who bear the burden of environmental exposures are also less likely to have the means to move away from a stressful physical environment (Greenberg, Schneider, & Choi, 1994; Evans & Kratrowitz, 2002). And if residents are able to relocate, others may simply move in and take their place, leaving the new residents vulnerable to the same set of health problems. A population's location might determine its exposure, but a lack of access to resources, including education, employment, and social mobility, can limit health-protective options (Williams, 1990).

HEALTH IMPACT ASSESSMENT

Nancy M. Goff

Health Impact Assessment (HIA) is a combination of methods and tools used to determine the distribution of health effects of a policy, program, or project within a particular population (European Centre for Health Policy, 1999). HIA is not a strict methodology; rather, it includes a series of steps to ensure health is considered in all types of decisions. Its goal is to provide evidenced-based information that will be used to maximize the positive and minimize the negative impacts of social, economic, political, or environmental decisions.

HIA draws from several different methodologies, including risk assessment, precautionary approaches, and community-based participatory research (CBPR). Like CBPR, HIA has an explicit focus on community participation, democracy, and equity. The full participation of communities in issue selection, assessment, and advocacy is ideal in HIA, although this gold standard of participation is sometimes hindered by the immediacy of decision-making timelines. Also embedded in HIA is the precautionary principle, as it aims to predict and mitigate harm. Unlike traditional risk assessment, HIA examines the health effects of projects and policies before rather than after they are implemented.

HIAs have been conducted around the globe for the last decade, but the lack of trained practitioners, available resources, and knowledge has limited the institutionalization of the approach in the United States. In Oregon, a group of public health practitioners has been working to overcome some of these barriers through a collaborative, multi-stakeholder process.

In June 2008, representatives from public, nonprofit, health care and private sectors completed Oregon's first HIA on the Columbia River Crossing (CRC) Project, a proposal to rebuild an existing interstate highway bridge connecting Oregon and Washington. The five CRC design alternatives proposed different combinations of traffic lanes, bike and pedestrian facilities, and public transportation options. An analysis conducted by the Multnomah County Health Department predicted potential health impacts through changes in air pollution and noise, traffic safety conditions, and the availability of opportunities for physical activity. The results of the analysis were presented in a comment letter in response to the project's *Draft Environmental Impact Statement*. Advocacy groups used the results to testify at public hearings and engage potentially affected communities. To date, the project outcome remains unknown, but the HIA was considered successful in that it built capacity and raised awareness about HIA and the consequences of the CRC Project.

Additional Resources

Centers for Disease Control and Prevention, Healthy Places Initiative: http://www.cdc.gov/healthyplaces/hia.htm

Multnomah County Health Department, Columbia River Crossing Health Impact Assessment: http://www.mchealth.org/documents/CRC_%20DEIS_response.pdf

Oregon Public Health Division, Health Impact Assessment Program: http://www.healthoregon.org/hia

UCLA HIA Clearinghouse: http://www.ph.ucla.edu/hs/hiaclic/index.htm

TWO PREVENTIVE APPROACHES TO ENVIRONMENTAL HEALTH

So how do we measure exposure, determine health effects, quantify risk, and inform policy and practice? For the last several decades, environmental public health and the study of exposure and related health outcomes has been guided by the risk analysis model. This model assesses new technologies and products by calculating the mathematical likelihood they will threaten our health. It typically includes four steps: *hazard identification, dose-response evaluation, exposure assessment*, and *risk characterization*. The quantitative risk assessment model allows commercial and industrial interests to require that harm be "scientifically" proven before discontinuing a process or product (Myers & Raffensperger, 2005). The primary deficit of quantitative risk assessment is that it frequently fails to consider most social and cultural factors and the broader costs to the environment or to future generations. Furthermore, assessing risk based on a single exposure to a single chemical does not take into account the combinations of chemicals people are exposed to daily or other individual differences, such as nutrition, immune system health, and age.

We propose two approaches that can be integrated with traditional risk assessment in an effort to obtain more complete information about what types of exposures communities are facing. The *precautionary principle* is based on a preventive approach to local policy and decision making around environmental exposures and health outcomes, whereas *community-based participatory research* is based on the meaningful and significant participation of community residents in assessing environmental health problems and seeking solutions to them. Both offer methodologies for public health practitioners and researchers working with affected communities and are guided by principles of equality, justice, and prevention; both can be used to augment the types and quality of information we obtain using more traditional approaches for assessing risk.

PRECAUTIONARY PRINCIPLE

Today, more than eighty-five thousand industrial chemicals are registered for use in the United States, and an average of twenty-three hundred more are registered each year. Yet toxicological data exist for only 7 percent of the registered chemicals, meaning that tens of thousand of chemicals are not registered (Goldman & Koduru, 2000). This makes it difficult for us to know definitively which products or toxic contaminants threaten our health and environment. In fact, the U.S. Toxic Substance Control Act does not require chemical companies to perform basic health and safety tests on their products (Goldman & Koduru, 2000; Schettler, 2002; Thorton et al., 2002). The responsibility falls to the federal government and the public to demonstrate a chemical poses an *unreasonable risk* to society. In the current regulatory system, a chemical is generally considered safe until proven harmful. In other words, a chemical is innocent until proven guilty. This can mean by the time the evidence of harm is apparent, many people (typically low-income or people of color) have already developed symptoms and health problems.

TOXICS RESOLUTION IN MULTNOMAH COUNTY AND THE CITY OF PORTLAND

In September 2004, the Portland City Council and the Multnomah County Board of Commissioners became the first government bodies in Oregon to unanimously adopt the precautionary principle as the basis for reducing toxics in city and county government operations to protect public health. The resolution is as follows:

> *Every resident* of Portland and Multnomah County has an *equal right* to a healthy and safe environment. In order to achieve this goal locally, our government, residents, and businesses must work together to ensure that our air, water, soil, and food are safe. As a first step in reaching this goal and developing the toxics reduction strategy called for by the resolution, the Sustainable Development Commission and the Oregon Center for Environmental Health recommend the city and county resolve to create a Toxics Reduction Strategy for government operations utilizing the Precautionary Principle [Multnomah County Board of Commissioners, 2004].

Although Portland and Multnomah County are often perceived as having a healthy environment, particular neighborhoods were challenged with toxic threats to human health. For example, fourteen air toxics in the county exceed health-based benchmarks, with six pollutants more than ten times national health standards (Multnomah County Health Department, 2003). Similarly, a section of the lower Willamette River in Portland is listed as a Superfund site, designating it as one of the most polluted rivers in the country. Demographic data from the 2000 census indicate that whereas only 1.7 percent of Oregon residents are African American, they make up 60 to 95 percent of the total population living within a few blocks of the 7-mile stretch of the lower Willamette River designated as the Portland Harbor Superfund site (U.S. Census Bureau, 2000).

Work to develop the resolution began in the spring of 2003 through a collaboration between the Sustainable Development Commission of Portland and Multnomah County (SDC) and the Oregon Center for Environmental Health (OCEH). The SDC is an appointed citizen advisory board charged with making policy recommendations to the city and county to ensure a sustainable future. The OCEH is an environmental and health advocacy organization that works to protect public health and the environment by promoting alternatives to the use, manufacture, release, and disposal of toxic chemicals.

The SDC and the OCEH convened workshops and work groups with area residents and other key stakeholders, including government officials and community members, to develop a dialogue on using precaution as a basis for protective environmental and public health policy. Following the adoption of the resolution, a more formal work group of community members and city and county staff was formed in 2005 to develop a process to reduce the purchase and use of toxics in city and county operations. Although the work group has made significant steps forward, development of the strategy has progressed slowly. However, allowing ample time for stakeholder participation and input and moving through the proper channels of city and county government during the development of the strategy will help ensure the implementation is supported and purchasing practices are amended.

Every phase of this local effort has incorporated the tenets of the precautionary principle, including prevention of new toxic pollution and inclusion of stakeholders. A complete proposed toxics reduction strategy was presented to the county board of commissioners and the city council in May 2006 and was unanimously adopted. The proposed reduction strategy provided specific directives for both agencies to reduce the impact of toxic pollution on all residents.

In an effort to address the limitations of a traditional risk assessment model, an international group that included scientists, government officials, lawyers, and labor and grassroots environmental activists (such as leaders from the Science and Environmental Health Network and the Center for Health, Environment and Justice) convened at the Wingspread Conference Center in Wisconsin in 1998 (Montague, 1998). In the same spirit of medicine's principle of *first do no harm*, this group called for a more preventive and protective approach to environmental assessment through the Wingspread Statement on the Precautionary Principle developed at the conference, as follows:

> When an activity raises threats of harm to human health or the environment, precautionary measures should be taken even if some cause-and-effect relationships are not fully established scientifically. In this context the proponent of an activity, rather than the public, should bear the burden of proof. The process of applying the precautionary principle must be open, informed and democratic and must include potentially affected parties [Myers & Raffensperger, 2005].

During the past decade, especially in European countries, the precautionary principle has emerged as one of the leading environmental health frameworks in shaping new policy that prevents harm and that allows for participation of community residents and leaders.

Although facing constant challenges by industry and manufacturers who would be asked to prove their products are safe, the precautionary principle has produced some victories (Myers & Raffensperger, 2005). The U.S. Toxic Substances Control Act authorizes the EPA to halt marketing and require safety testing or other measures for any substance determined to pose an unreasonable risk (EPA, 1976). Similarly, the CDC has begun monitoring human exposure to chemicals, collecting data that can be used to inform future precautionary policies (CDC, 2003). The White House Policy Declaration on Environment and Trade from 1999 acknowledges a precautionary approach is an essential element of the U.S. regulatory system since regulators often have to make decisions in the absence of full scientific certainty (Wirth, 2002).

This framework provides policymakers and communities with a more comprehensive way to estimate the full costs of a product or practice. The precautionary principle considers both *seen costs* (for example, equipment purchase and hazardous waste disposal costs) and *hidden costs* (such as insurance and hazardous waste liability, employee health benefits, and impact on social and cultural well-being) associated with substance manufacture, use, and disposal. Adoption of the principle has been shown to initiate economic development by creating new opportunities for local businesses to provide safer products, processes, and technologies (Ackerman & Massey, 2002).

Despite a few early successes, including the adoption of a set of purchasing guidelines based on the precautionary principle by the City and County of San Francisco (San Francisco Commission on the Environment, 2003), the approach has been underutilized by local government, businesses, and policymakers in the United States. This approach, which calls for transparency, democracy, and preventive action, requires a systematic change in the way we think as well as in the way we act. Rather than asking how much harm is acceptable, we must determine the least amount of harm that can be achieved. The principle can also be used to protect communities from exposure and related health outcomes as described in the preceding case study.

COMMUNITY-BASED PARTICIPATORY RESEARCH

Community-based participatory research (CBPR) creates an opportunity for the individuals and groups who are most affected by potential environmental health threats to influence policy and practice. Environmental justice advocates demand more than clean air and water and insist on the participation of all people as equal partners in decision making, regardless of class, race, ethnicity, or national origin (EPA, 1998; Kuehn, 1996). Community organizations and federal agencies alike have called for the inclusion of community residents in assessing and characterizing risk assessment and establishing policy (O'Fallon & Dearry,

2002). On November 4, 2005, EPA Administrator Steve Johnson issued a memorandum that identified national environmental justice priorities and called for ensuring greater public participation in the agency's development of and implementation of environmental regulations and policies.

Some environmental health research has united communities and researchers to challenge a few of the basic assumptions of traditional science, such as the supposition that research must maintain objectivity and remain detached from participants (Lynn, 2000; Minkler, 2000; O'Fallon & Dearry, 2002). CBPR, a collaborative approach to research that equitably and meaningfully involves all partners in every step of the research process, encourages equal partnerships between community members and academic investigators (Israel, Schulz, Parker, & Becker, 1998; Keeler et al., 2002). CBPR has its roots in the work of American researchers in the mid-twentieth century, notably the psychologist Kurt Lewin, who were frustrated by the inability of traditional research methods to understand complex phenomena and experiences. Much of the most innovative CBPR work has been conducted in developing countries by researchers, educators, and activists (for example, Paolo Freire in Brazil) who are interested in empowerment and social change. An important step of CBPR is the shared translation and dissemination of research findings with the broader community, including residents, policymakers, and the media, so they can be applied to future policy and practice.

The CBPR approach has been widely used by environmental justice researchers and activists and has the potential to achieve social change and also create a healthier and less polluted environment. For example, the National Institute of Environmental Health Sciences (NIEHS) has promoted and supported the use of CBPR to research environmentally related disease. One of the studies funded by NIEHS, the Southeast Halifax project, was a partnership among the University of North Carolina at Chapel Hill, Concerned Citizens of Tillery, and the North Carolina Student Rural Health Coalition. This community-academic partnership determined that corporate hog operations were more concentrated in poor non-white areas and that there was a marked increase in reported headache, runny nose, sore throat, excessive coughing, diarrhea, and burning eyes in those areas compared to communities not located near intensive livestock operations (Wing & Wolf, 2000).

USING CBPR TO ASSESS COMMUNITY EXCELLENCE IN ENVIRONMENTAL HEALTH

Following a participatory model of environmental health assessment, the Multnomah County Health Department in Portland, Oregon, collaborated with several organizations and dozens of residents to form the Protocol for Assessing Community Excellence (PACE) Coalition between 2002 and 2005. The PACE Coalition was guided by the Protocol for Assessing Community Excellence in Environmental Health, developed in 1995 by the National Association of County and City Health Officials and the CDC as a series of thirteen steps designed to help local health officials work collaboratively with communities to: identify populations at disproportionate risk of environmental exposure; assess and prioritize environmental health concerns; and create an action plan and evaluation. The following discussion highlights the process used to complete one of the most vital preliminaries of the thirteen PACE steps, the process of defining and characterizing the community.

The vision of the PACE Coalition members was to create a network of individuals and local organizations who take an active role in setting an environmental health and environmental justice agenda for their Portland communities. As the initiator of the PACE Coalition, the Multnomah County Health Department (MCHD) sought to establish the department's programmatic priorities based on resident input and participation, rather than on narrowly defined and short-term federal funding opportunities (that some health department representatives referred to as the "environmental health issue du jour").

Although MCHD recognized there was an unequal burden on certain communities in Multnomah County, they did not have the internal capacity or the public's consent to address environmental justice issues. The environmental health services department in the MCHD reflected a more common approach to environmental disease diagnosis and control, such as illnesses and injuries related to swimming pools, vectors, and food safety. This more traditional mandate, paired with a general mistrust by the public of county agencies, made it difficult for the MCHD to begin to conduct a comprehensive and participatory assessment of environmental health needs. To build relationships with the broader community, the MCHD hired two community *connectors* (organizers) to reach out to residents and encourage their participation in the PACE Coalition. Hiring the community connectors demonstrated the MCHD's commitment to a different way of doing business, especially since the hiring happened during state and county budget cuts.

Community Selection

The more than sixty member PACE Coalition structured meetings to develop leadership among community members and ease among agency partners who might not have been used to working with communities. An assessment team, including representatives from the health department, local residents, community-based organizations, and a local university, gathered census data and maps documenting the exposure level of dozens of indicators ranging from potential *brownfields* (contaminated sites) to solid-waste facilities in the county to determine which areas were most heavily affected by environmental health hazards. After a community discussion of the findings, the Inner North/Northeast area of Portland was selected as the community of greatest immediate concern.

Community Outreach

The community connectors and the assessment team began conducting extensive outreach to community leaders and residents in the affordable housing communities of Inner North/Northeast Portland to generate a top-ten list of environmental health concerns: mold and mildew, pesticides, indoor air quality, outdoor air quality, brownfields, lead, trash and garbage, lack of meeting places, water quality, and lack of green spaces. The discussions between community residents and members of the PACE assessment team included both the physical and the social environment and acknowledged their complex interplay. For example, many residents talked about feeling unsafe or the lack of community meeting places as threats to environmental health and well-being.

The coalition members, especially the staff from the MCHD, committed themselves to identifying funding that could support sustained efforts in one or more of these identified priority areas. The partnerships created during the PACE process led to the acquisition of a million dollar Healthy Homes grant designed to create home-based interventions for improvement of asthma control in low-income children. Outcomes of the Healthy Homes grant included improved health for individual families and an increased understanding of the connection between health and housing. Four of the five cities in Multnomah County had no housing code and the City of Portland housing code did not define a relationship between health and housing; subsequently, the cities have revised housing code recommendations so they now reflect the connection between housing and health.

CONCLUSION

To adequately address disproportionate exposure, the discipline and practice of environmental health must identify ways to involve communities, government agencies, and academic partners in eliminating and preventing injustices in environmental health and exposures. Government and local leaders should be invited to play a key role in rehabilitating our communities and in planning for a healthier and safer environment. In both of the Portland case studies, the projects were largely facilitated and supported by innovative thinkers in the city and county governments. In cities and counties that lack a progressive health department or city council, however, community residents can still initiate the assessment and prioritization of environmental health needs by generating awareness and by gathering a critical mass. For example, concerned residents can use community-organizing tactics and hold town meetings, conduct resident surveys, or gather their own data that can then be presented to government and local leaders as evidence of environmental exposure. The citizen-led *bucket brigades* that are cropping up in towns and cities across the United States provide one example. Residents take air samples with a bucket provided by an international environmental group called the Bucket Brigade and analyze the air samples in a lab. Community residents can then present the assessment results to educate public leaders and pressure industries and governments to identify solutions to poor air quality.

Furthermore, with the wider acceptance of CBPR principles and methods, community residents should feel increasingly comfortable approaching academics and researchers to help them investigate environmental toxins and potential health effects. *Science shops* are one model of CBPR whereby residents and community groups work with university-based researchers to examine and address environmental health problems. The term *science* includes the natural and social sciences and humanities; the term *shop* reflects the notion that the university should be used by community members to address research questions posed by the local community. Researchers at science shops can use existing data, collect new data, or help facilitate a new research project created and conducted by community members to answer the research question posed by the community.

Public health practitioners and researchers should consider ways to use the precautionary principle and CBPR in tandem to supplement traditional risk assessment methods. In fact, the two approaches share many qualities and principles that may facilitate their blending. For example, both approaches advocate for an open and democratic process of decision making. Both approaches value laypeople's knowledge, in contrast to experts' knowledge, which is the primary driver of traditional risk assessment methods. In addition, each approach has inherent limitations that might be eliminated when the two approaches are combined. For example, an assessment using the precautionary principle may not clearly acknowledge disproportionate environmental exposure; CBPR tends to explicitly identify and address the causes of injustice and inequality. Conversely, CBPR might not consider the value of *precaution* or seek to prevent exposure before the health problems are manifested, whereas prevention is at the core of the precautionary principle. Implementation of these approaches, alone or together, provides the opportunity to create a dialogue with community stakeholders and local environmental health leaders that can wholly transform the assessment of environmental risks and the creation of preventive solutions.

DISCUSSION QUESTIONS

1. The text highlights Dr. Robert Bullard and the work he did with landfill data. What other types of environmental health issues might affect politically and economically disadvantaged communities? Use the following issues to start your discussion: sanitation, safe walking areas, violence.

2. What kinds of strategies would you use in your community to develop a dialogue to address higher than average levels of exposure to an environmental toxin? How might you find common ground about this issue if you were collaborating with community members of different backgrounds (including different socioeconomic status, race, ethnicity, or national origin).

3. What *seen* and *hidden* costs and benefits might be impacted by an organizational or worksite environmental health change strategy? How would you communicate these differences to the president or leader of your organization?

REFERENCES

Ackerman, F., & Massey, R. (2002, August). *Prospering with precaution: Employment, economics, and the precautionary principle.* Boston: Global Development and Environment Institute, Tufts University. Retrieved October 16, 2006, from http://ase.tufts.edu/gdae/policy_research/PrecautionAHTAug02.pdf

Apelberg, B. J., Buckley, T. J., & White, R. H. (2005). Socioeconomic and racial disparities in cancer risk from air toxics in Maryland. *Environmental Health Perspectives, 113,* 693–699.

Blaikie, P., Cannon, T., Davis, I., & Wisner, B. (1994). *At risk: Natural hazards, people's vulnerability, and disasters.* New York: Routledge.

Blaxill, M. F. (2004). What's going on? The question of time trends in autism. *Public Health Reports, 119,* 536–551.

Bolin, R., & Stanford, L. (1998). The Northridge earthquake: Community-based approaches to unmet recovery needs. *Disasters, 22,* 21–38.

Brown, T. P., Rumsby, P. C., Capleton, A. C., Rushton, L., & Levy, L. S. (2006). Pesticides and Parkinson's disease—Is there a link? *Environmental Health Perspectives, 114*(2), 156–164.

Bryant, B. (1995). *Environmental justice, issues, policies, and solutions.* Washington, DC: Island Press.

Bullard, R. D. (1990). *Dumping in Dixie: Race, class, and environmental quality.* Boulder, CO: Westview Press.

Bullard, R. D., Glenn, S. J., & Torres, A. O. (Eds.). (2004). *Highway robbery: Transportation racism and new routes to equity.* Boston: South End Press.

Bullard, R. D., & Johnson, G. S. (1997). *Just transportation: Dismantling race and class barriers to mobility.* Stony Creek, CT: New Society.

Bullard, R. D., & Wright, B. H. (1993). Environmental justice for all: Community perspectives of health and research needs. *Toxicology and Industrial Health, 9,* 821–841.

Campaign for Safe Cosmetics. (2005, October 8). Governor signs safe cosmetics bill: New law heightens scrutiny of industry safety. Retrieved July 5, 2005, from http://www.safecosmetics.org/newsroom/press.cfm?pressReleaseID=13

Campaign for Safe Cosmetics. (n.d.-a). About us. Retrieved July 5, 2006, from http://www.safecosmetics.org/about

Campaign for Safe Cosmetics. (n.d.-b). Frequently asked questions. Retrieved June 5, 2006, from http://www.safecosmetics.org/faqs

Canadell, J. G., et al. (2007). Contributions to accelerating atmospheric CO_2 growth from economic activity, carbon intensity, and efficiency of natural sinks. *Proceedings of the National Academy of Science, 104*(47), 18866–18870.

Centers for Disease Control and Prevention. (2003). *Second national report on human exposure to environmental chemicals.* National Center for Environmental Health, Division of Laboratory Sciences. (NCEH Publ. No. 02–0716). Atlanta: Author.

Centers for Disease Control and Prevention. (2005). *Third national report on human exposure to environmental chemicals*. National Center for Environmental Health, Division of Laboratory Sciences. (NCEH Publ. No. 05-0570). Atlanta: Author.

Collins et al. (2002). *Diverse communities, common concerns: Assessing health care quality for minority Americans*. New York: Commonwealth Fund.

Dicum, G. (2006, March 14). Justice in time: Meet Robert Bullard, the father of environmental justice. *Grist Magazine*. Retrieved October 16, 2006, from http://www.grist.org/news/maindish/2006/03/14/dicum

Donner, W., & Rodriguez, H. (2008). Population composition, migration, and inequality: The influence of demographic changes on disaster risk and vulnerability. *Social Forces, 87*(2), 1089–1114.

Ebi, K. L., Sussman, F. G., & Wilbanks, T. J. (2008). Analyses of the effects of global change on human health and welfare and human systems. In J. L. Gamble (Ed.), A report by the U.S. Climate Change Science Program and the Subcommittee on Global Change Research. Washington, DC: U.S. Environmental Protection Agency.

Edelson, S. B., & Cantor, D. S. (1999). Autism: Xenobiotic influences. *Journal of Advancement in Medicine, 12*, 35–47.

Environmental Health Perspectives, Science Education. (n.d). Frequently asked questions. Retrieved July 26, 2006, from http://www.ehponline.org/science-ed/faq.html

Environmental Protection Agency. (1976). *Toxic Substances Control Act*. Retrieved January 23, 2006, from http://www.epa.gov/region5/defs/html/tsca.htm

Environmental Protection Agency. (1992). Environmental equity: Reducing risk for all communities. In R. M. Wolcott & W. A. Banks (Eds.), *Workgroup Report to the Administrator*, Vol. 1. Rep. No. EPA 230-R-92–008. Washington, DC: Author.

Environmental Protection Agency. (1998). *Final guidance for incorporating environmental justice concerns in EPA's NEPA compliance analyses*. Washington, DC: Author.

Environmental Protection Agency. (2003, July 25). *History of environmental justice*. Retrieved January 4, 2005, from http://www.epa.gov/envjustice/History

European Centre for Health Policy, WHO Regional Office for Europe. (1999). *Gothenburg Consensus Paper. Health Impact Assessment: Main Concepts and Suggested Approach*. Brussels: WHO.

Evans, G. W., & Kantrowitz, E. (2002). Socioeconomic status and health: The potential role of environmental risk exposure. *Annual Review of Public Health, 23*, 303–331.

Faber, D. R., & Krieg, E. J. (2002). Unequal exposure to ecological hazards: Environmental injustices in the Commonwealth of Massachusetts. *Environmental Health Perspectives, 110*(Suppl. 2), 277–288.

Farquhar, S. A., & Wing, S. (2003). Methodological and ethical considerations of community-driven environmental justice research: Examination of two case studies from rural North Carolina. In M. Minkler & N. Wallerstein (Eds.), *Community-based participatory research for health* (pp. 221–241). San Francisco: Jossey-Bass.

Fothergill, A., Maestas, E., & Darlington DeRouen, J. (1999). Race, ethnicity, and disasters in the United States: A review of the literature. *Disasters, 23*, 156–173.

Goldman, L. R., & Koduru, S. (2000). Environmental chemicals in the environment and developmental toxicity to children: A public health and policy perspective. *Environmental Health Perspectives, 108*, 443–448.

Grant, E. N., Lyttle, C. S., & Weiss, K. B. (2000). The relation of socioeconomic factors and racial/ethnic differences in U.S. asthma mortality. *American Journal of Public Health, 90*, 1923–1925.

Greenberg, M., Schneider, D., & Choi, D. (1994). Neighborhood quality in areas with multiple technological and behavioral hazards. *Geographical Review, 84*, 1–15.

Health Care Without Harm. (2002a). *Aggregate exposures to phthalates in humans*. Washington, DC: Author.

Health Care Without Harm (with Women's Environmental Network, UK, & Swedish Society for Nature Conservation). (2002b). *Pretty nasty: Phthalates in European cosmetic products*. Stockholm, Sweden: Author.

Hites, R. A. (2004). Polybrominated diphenyl ethers in the environment and in people: A meta-analysis of concentrations. *Environmental Science and Technology, 38*, 945–956.

Hoerner, J. A., & Robinson, N. (2008). *A climate of change: African Americans, global warming, and a just climate policy for the U.S.* Retrieved May 5, 2010, from http://www.rprogress.org/publications/2008/climateofchange.pdf

Houlihan, J., Brody, C., & Schwan, B. (2002, July 8). *Not too pretty: Phthalates, beauty products, and the FDA*. Washington, DC: Environmental Working Group, Health Care Without Harm.

Houlihan, J., Wiles, R., Thayer, K., & Gray, S. (2003). *Body burden: The pollution in people*. Washington, DC: Environmental Working Group, Health Care Without Harm.

Institute of Medicine. (2002). *Unequal treatment: Confronting racial and ethnic disparities in health care*. Washington, DC: National Academies Press.

Intergovernmental Panel on Climate Change. (2007). *Climate change 2007: Synthesis report*. Geneva, Switzerland: Author.

Israel, B. A., Schulz, A. J., Parker, E. A., & Becker, A. B. (1998). Review of community-based research: Assessing partnership approaches to improve public health. *Annual Review of Public Health, 19*, 173–202.

Keeler et al. (2002). Assessment of personal and community-level exposures to particulate matter among children with asthma in Detroit, Michigan, as part of Community Action Against Asthma (CAAA). *Environmental Health Perspectives, 110*(Suppl. 2), 173–181.

Kuehn, R. (1996). The environmental justice implications of quantitative risk assessment. *University of Illinois Law Review, 38*, 103–172.

Landrigan, P. J., Schechter, C. B., Lipton, J. M., Fahs, M. C., & Schwartz, J. (2002). Environmental pollutants and disease in American children: Estimates of morbidity, mortality, and costs for lead poisoning, asthma, cancer, and developmental disabilities. *Environmental Health Perspectives, 110*, 721–728.

Lopez, R. (2002). Segregation and black/white differences in exposure to air toxics in 1990. *Environmental Health Perspectives, 110*(Suppl. 2), 289–295.

Lynn, F. M. (2000). Community-scientist collaboration in environmental research. *American Behavioral Scientist, 44*, 649–663.

Meyer et al. (2003, September 12). Surveillance for elevated blood lead levels among children—United States, 1997–2001. *Morbidity and Mortality Weekly Report, 52*(SS10), 1–21.

Minkler, M. (2000). Using participatory action to build healthy communities. *Public Health Reports, 115*, 191–198.

Montague, P. (1998, February 18). The precautionary principle. *Rachel's Environment and Health News*, #586. Retrieved October 16, 2006, from http://www.rachel.org/bulletin/pdf/Rachels_Environment_Health_News_532.pdf

Motavalli, J. (1998, July–August). Dr. Robert Bullard: Some people don't have "the complexion for protection." *E: The Environmental Magazine, 9*(4). Retrieved June 3, 2006, from http://www.emagazine.com/index.php?toc&issue=11

Multnomah County Board of Commissioners. (2004). Precautionary principal resolutions. Portland, OR: Author. Retrieved July 26, 2006, from http://www.besafenet.com/ppc/docs/environmental_precaution/ENV_OR_Rep.pdf

Multnomah County Health Department. (2003). *The environmental health of Multnomah County.* Portland, OR: Author.

Myers, N. J., & Raffensperger, C. (Eds.). (2005). *Precautionary tools for reshaping environmental policy.* Cambridge, MA: MIT Press.

Natural Hazards Research and Applications Information Center. (2001). *Holistic disaster recovery: Ideas for building local sustainability after a natural disaster.* Retrieved July 20, 2002, from http://www.colorado.edu/hazards/holistic_recovery

Not Too Pretty. (2003). *Poisoned cosmetics, not too pretty.* Retrieved October 15, 2006, from http://www.nottoopretty.org

O'Fallon, L., & Dearry, A. (2002). Community-based participatory research as a tool to advance environmental health sciences. *Environmental Health Perspectives, 110*(Suppl. 2), 155–159.

Pew Environmental Health Commission. (2001). *Transition report to the new administration: Strengthening our public health defense against environmental threats.* Baltimore: Pew Environmental Health Commission, Johns Hopkins School of Public Health.

San Francisco Commission on the Environment. (2003). *White paper: The precautionary principle and the City and County of San Francisco.* San Francisco. Retrieved November 15, 2006, from http://www.environmentalcommons.org/precaution-white-paper.pdf

Schettler, T. (2002). Changing patterns of disease: Human health and the environment. *San Francisco Medical Society, 75*(9), 10–13.

Schweizer, E. (1999, July). Environmental justice: An interview with Robert Bullard. *Earth First! Journal*, pp. 1–5. Retrieved October 16, 2006, from http://www.ejrc.cau.edu/earthfirstinterviewrb.htm

Smart, B. A. (2004, Fall). The costs of asthma and allergy. *Allergy and Asthma Advocate.* Retrieved October 16, 2006, from http://www.aaaai.org/patients/advocate/2004/fall/costs.stm

Solomon, G. M. (2002). Rare and common diseases in environmental health. *San Francisco Medical Society, 75*(9).

Thornton, J. W., McCally, M., & Houlihan, J. (2002). Biomonitoring of industrial pollutants: Health and policy implications of the chemical body burden. *Public Health Reports, 117*, 315–323.

U.S. Census Bureau. (2000). *Census data for the state of Oregon.* Retrieved May 11, 2006, from http://www.census.gov/census2000/states/or.html

Wakefield, J. (2002). The lead effect? *Environmental Health Perspectives, 110*, A574–A580.

Wang, X. F., Li, S., Chou, A. P., & Bronstein, J. M. (2006). Inhibitory effects of pesticides on proteasome activity: Implication in Parkinson's disease. *Neurobiology of Disease, 23*, 198–205.

Williams, D. R. (1990). Socioeconomic differentials in health: A review and redirection. *Social Psychology Quarterly, 53*, 81–99.

Wing, S., & Wolf, S. (2000). Intensive livestock operation, health, and quality of life among eastern North Carolina residents. *Environmental Health Perspectives, 108*, 233–238.

Wirth, D. A. (2002). Precaution in international environmental policy and U.S. law and practice. *North American Environmental Law and Policy, 10*, 219–268.

11

Health and the Built Environment

Howard Frumkin
Andrew L. Dannenberg

LEARNING OBJECTIVES

- Begin to learn how features of the built environment (from occupational ergonomics to buildings to neighborhood design and characteristics) affect population health.
- Identify strategies to improve environments so that illness and injury decrease at the same time that health increases.
- Explain reasons why features of suburban community design may undermine social capital and sense of community.
- Understand the rationale behind identifying and paying attention to several at-risk populations when planning improvements for the built environment.

The *built environment* refers to the many components of our surroundings formed by human acts of creation or modification. Almost all the settings in which we live, work, study, and play are parts of the built environment.

Many features of the built environment affect health. These range in scale from the design of furniture in a room to the layout of a home or office building to the infrastructure of the neighborhood and metropolitan area in which one lives. The built environment concept includes fixed objects, such as sidewalks. It also includes activities that give rise to the built environment, such as architecture and urban planning, and functions that are embedded in and directly dependent on physical infrastructure, such as transportation and energy production. The concept of the built environment includes contact with nature, since most urban and suburban dwellers encounter nature primarily in backyards, parks, and other places that are designed and built by people.

This chapter focuses on the links between health and the built environment on various scales and on strategies to help create health-promoting environments (such as parks to promote physical activity) and to reduce health-damaging environments (such as automobile-dependent communities with increased air pollution).

THE SMALL SCALE

The built environment on a small scale refers to tools and other implements people use, wear, or occupy. Examples include computer keyboards and office furniture. The scientific study of these small-scale environments draws on both ergonomics and biomechanics. Details of the health issues related to small-scale environments are beyond the scope of this chapter.

THE INTERMEDIATE SCALE

People spend much of their time in buildings (for example, in homes, schools, workplaces, stores, and places of worship), which represent perhaps the most familiar examples of the built environment. Physical conditions of buildings such as noise levels, temperature, humidity, and lighting may have a major effect on comfort, productivity, and health. In addition, the design of built environments can affect injury risk. The following discussion focuses on a few of these issues.

LIGHTING

The level and quality of indoor lighting affects several aspects of health and well-being (Smith, 2000). Good lighting supports and restores normal circadian rhythms (Duffy &

Wright, 2005). In schools and workplaces, adequate natural lighting (or *daylighting*) is associated with improved subjective well-being, academic performance and behavior, and task performance, whereas glare is associated with diminished performance (Heschong, 2003a, 2003b; Kuller & Lindsten, 1992). Bright nighttime lighting may help shift workers adjust to schedule changes, although data are not definitive (Knauth & Hornberger, 2003). Well-designed lighting might help alleviate seasonal depression (Lewy, Kern, Rosenthal, & Wehr, 1982), speed recovery from severe depression (Beauchemin & Hays, 1996), and improve sleep patterns in people with insomnia (Lack & Wright, 1993) and with dementia (Van Someren, Kessler, Mirmirann, & Swaab, 1997).

CROWDING

Crowding is both an objectively measurable condition in terms of the number of people per unit area (density) and a subjective experience reflecting loss of privacy, loss of control, or overstimulation (Maxwell, 2006). Crowding may occur in many indoor settings, including primary environments (such as the home, school, and workplace) and more transient secondary environments (such as a train or a department store).

Crowding has negative effects on health and well-being. Children from crowded homes demonstrate diminished motivation and aggressive or withdrawn behavior (Aiello, Nicosia, & Thompson, 1979; Saegert, 1982). Crowding is associated with less cooperative behavior among young children (Aiello et al., 1979) and with more disruptive, aggressive, and hostile behavior (Maxwell, 2003; Saegert, 1982), inattentiveness (Evans, Saegert, & Harris, 2001), or withdrawal from classroom participation among older children (Loo & Smetana, 1978). Crowding at home and in classrooms is associated with lower academic achievement (Evans, Lepore, Shejwal, & Palsane, 1998; Maxwell, 2003; Saegert, 1982). Similar effects, such as stress, psychological dysfunction, and impaired interpersonal relations, have been associated with crowding among adults in community and institutional settings (Evans, 2003). Crowded indoor environments may also increase the risk of infectious disease transmission (Lienhardt, 2001). It appears important for built environments to offer adequate space and privacy to avoid some of the adverse aspects of crowding.

INJURY RISK

Substantial numbers of unintentional injuries occur in and around buildings. The home environment is the setting for more than thirty thousand fatal injuries and thirteen million nonfatal injuries per year in the United States (National Safety Council [NSC], 2004). The majority of these injuries occur among young children, the elderly, and the poor (NSC, 2004). Two categories of injury, falls and burns, illustrate the magnitude of the problem and the potential for environmental design to reduce risk.

Falls are the leading single cause of fatal and nonfatal unintentional injuries in homes (Runyan & Casteel, 2004). Children are at risk of falls through open windows or railings, off rooftops and other elevations, and down stairs (Staunton, Frumkin, & Dannenberg, 2006). Design features that can reduce risk include window guards and window stops, limited access to rooftops and other elevations, and closely spaced posts on guard rails (American Academy of Pediatrics, 2001; Bergner, Mayer, & Harris, 1971; Istre et al., 2003). The elderly are also at risk of home falls (Cayless, 2001; Gill, Williams, Robison, & Tinetti, 1999; Sattin, Rodriguez, DeVito, & Wingo, 1998). Environmental interventions that might reduce the risk of falls in the elderly include removing throw rugs and other tripping hazards, using non slip mats in tubs and showers, installing grab bars in bathrooms, installing handrails on both sides of stairways, and improving lighting throughout the home (Centers for Disease Control and Prevention [CDC], 2005).

Residential burns are also a leading cause of injury, accounting for about 2,200 deaths and more than 250,000 injuries in the United States each year (NSC, 2004). Most fatal burns result from home fires, whereas most nonfatal burns result from scalds, thermal burns, and electrical burns. Environmental interventions that reduce the risk of burns include smoke detectors (Runyan et al., 2005), indoor sprinkler systems (Cote, 1984), and reduced hot water heater temperature settings (Erdmann, Feldman, Rivara, Heimbach, & Wall, 1991; Feldman, Schaller, Feldman, & McMillon, 1978). Other strategies for reducing burn injuries include using child-resistant lighters, roll-up cords for electric coffeepots, kitchens with shorter distances between the stove and the sink, and cooking pans and kettles designed to reduce the probability of tipping (Staunton et al., 2006).

FROM NEIGHBORHOOD TO METROPOLIS

At a larger scale, the built environment consists of neighborhoods, towns, and cities. For many centuries, towns and cities were relatively dense, walkable places where people lived and worked in close quarters (Hall, 1998; Mumford, 1961). Over the course of time, however, a combination of technical advances, cultural values, commercial opportunities, and policy initiatives led to the geographical expansion of cities in a pattern commonly known as *sprawl* (Bullard, 1990; Cervero, 1989; Fishman, 1987; Garreau, 1991; Gillham, 2002; Jackson, 1985; Whyte, 1958). As automobiles became the predominant form of transportation, transit use, walking, and bicycling declined. Automobiles enabled people to live farther from their workplaces, schools, and other destinations and to travel these distances regularly.

These developments led directly to land use changes. Land development since World War II has occurred at much lower density than prevailed in traditional cities and towns. Accordingly, the distances people routinely travel are greater. Different land uses, including residential, commercial, educational, recreational, and others, are separated, a phenomenon known by planners as *low land use mix*. Suburban street networks feature low *connectivity*. The prototypical neighborhood is no longer a walkable grid in a small town or city where homes are located near stores, workplaces, and schools and where bus or trolley service is available for longer journeys. Instead, the prototypical neighborhood is characterized by a low-density suburban subdivision with poorly connected serpentine roads that require an automobile trip for nearly every errand. There is a well-established link between land use and travel behavior: cities with low residential density, low connectivity, and related indicators are associated with less walking and bicycling and more automobile travel (Cervero & Gorham, 1995; Cervero & Kockelman, 1997; Frank & Pivo, 1995; Newman & Kenworthy, 1999; Transportation Research Board, 2005).

Features of the built environment combine with cultural preferences, public policy, and other factors to determine travel behavior. In the Netherlands, 28 percent of all trips in urban areas are on bicycles and 18 percent are on foot; in England, these figures are 4 percent and 12 percent, and in the United States, 1 percent and 6 percent, respectively (Pucher & Dijkstra, 2003). Approximately 25 percent of all trips in the United States are less than one mile, and of these, 75 percent are by car (Koplan & Dietz, 1999).

Transportation and land use patterns, which are key aspects of the built environment, can affect health and well-being. For example, the heavy reliance on automobiles for transportation has implications for air quality and safety. Similarly, low-density land development with separation of different land uses has implications for physical activity and for water quantity and quality. These transportation and land use patterns may also affect mental health and social capital.

PHYSICAL ACTIVITY

Sedentary lifestyles have become the norm in the United States. More than half of American adults are physically inactive on a regular basis, and just over one in four Americans reports no leisure-time physical activity at all (Macera et al., 2003). In 2000, only 26.2 percent of adults were classified as meeting recommended levels of physical activity (defined as any physical activity for at least thirty minutes a day at least five days a week or vigorous physical activity for at least twenty minutes at least three days a week). This pattern is similar among children aged nine to thirteen, 61.5 percent of whom participate in no organized physical activity outside of school (Duke, Huhman, & Heitzler, 2003).

A sedentary lifestyle, in turn, increases the risk of cardiovascular disease, stroke, and all-cause mortality, whereas physical activity prolongs life (Lee & Paffenbarger, 2000; U.S. Department of Health and Human Services, 1996; Wannamethee, Shaper, & Walker, 1998; Wannamethee, Shaper, Walker, & Ebrahim, 1998). Low physical fitness produces cardiovascular risk comparable to, and in some studies greater than, the risk of hypertension, high cholesterol, diabetes, and even smoking (Blair et al., 1996; Wei et al., 1999). Physical activity also appears to be protective against cancer (Bauman, 2004; Kampert, Blair, Barlow, & Kohl, 1996; Lee, 2003).

Beyond the direct effects on health, physical inactivity is also a risk factor for weight gain. Overweight and obesity are on the rise. (Overweight is defined as a *body mass index* [BMI] of at least 25 kg/m^2, and obesity as a BMI of at least 30 kg/m^2.) In 1960, only 24 percent of Americans were overweight, but by 1990, that proportion had increased to 33 percent (Kuczmarski, Flegal, Campbell, & Johnson, 1994). During the same interval, the prevalence of obesity nearly doubled (Flegal, Carroll, Kuczmarski, & Johnson, 1998). According to data from the CDC's Behavioral Risk Factor Surveillance System, this trend continued during the 1990s, with the prevalence of obesity increasing from 12.0 percent in 1991 to 20.9 percent in 2001 (Mokdad et al., 1999, 2001, 2003).

Being overweight or obese, in turn, is a well-established risk factor for a number of diseases, including the following: ischemic heart disease, hypertension, stroke, dyslipidemia, osteoarthritis, gallbladder disease, and some cancers. Obese people die at as much as 2.5 times the rate of nonobese people (Must et al., 1999; Sesso, Paffenbarger, & Lee, 1998; Shaper, Wannamethee, & Walker, 1997; Wannamethee, Shaper, & Walker, 1998; Willett, Dietz, & Colditz, 1999). Overweight people face as much as an eighteenfold increase in the risk of type 2 diabetes, and the current epidemic of type 2 diabetes tracks closely with the increase in overweight (Mokdad et al., 2001; Must et al., 1999). Obese people have increased risks of some cancers, such as colorectal, prostate, and breast (Calle, Rodriguez, Walker-Thurmond, & Thun, 2003). Obesity is also associated with depression (Stunkard, Faith, & Allison, 2003).

The built environment plays a role in sedentary lifestyles, overweight, and obesity. As noted earlier, people in suburbs and exurbs drive more and walk less than people in cities and towns. Transportation research has also focused on neighborhood *walkability* with respect to travel behavior. *Highly walkable* neighborhoods are characterized by high density, high land use mix, high connectivity, good walking infrastructure, pleasing aesthetics, and safety. In general, people in highly walkable neighborhoods record more walking trips per week, especially for errands and going to work (Craig, Brownson, Cragg, & Dunn, 2002; Frank & Pivo, 1995; Kockelman, 1997; Powell, Martin, & Chowdhury, 2003; Saelens, Sallis, Black, & Chen, 2003). This finding translates into a higher total amount of physical activity with its associated health benefits.

Research has started to examine the entire hypothesized causal chain, from environmental features to physical activity to health risk factors to health outcomes. Although this is a complex set of relationships, with many variables operating on many different spatial scales, emerging evidence supports the notion that certain built environments, known by some as *active living environments*, promote physical activity and good health (Frank, Andresen, & Schmid, 2004; French, Story, & Jeffery, 2001; Handy, Boarnet, Ewing, & Killingsworth, 2002; Humpel, Owen, & Leslie, 2002; Kahn & Kellert, 2002; Saelens, Sallis, & Frank, 2003; Sallis, Bauman, & Pratt, 1998; Transportation Research Board, 2005; Trost, Owen, Bauman, Sallis, & Brown, 2002).

AIR POLLUTION AND RESPIRATORY DISEASES

Motor vehicles are a leading source of air pollution, especially carbon monoxide, carbon dioxide, particulate matter, oxides of nitrogen (NOx), and hydrocarbons (Environmental Protection Agency [EPA], 2006). In the presence of sunlight, NOx and hydrocarbons form ozone. In the United States, cars and trucks account for approximately 33 percent of NOx and 30 percent of human hydrocarbon emissions (EPA, 2006). In automobile-dependent metropolitan areas, the relative contribution of mobile sources might increase substantially. These pollutants, especially NOx, hydrocarbons, ozone, and particulate matter, account for a substantial part of the air pollution burden of U.S. cities. Certain pollutants, such as carbon monoxide, reach their highest concentrations alongside roadways, which increases the exposure risk for homes, schools, and other places near heavy traffic routes. Other pollutants, most notably ozone, are formed from precursors over time. As the precursors move downwind from their sources, the highest ozone levels might occur miles away. Thus vehicle-related air pollution might be a problem throughout entire regions.

The health hazards of air pollution are well established. Ozone is an airway irritant, and higher ozone levels are associated with more respiratory symptoms, worse lung function, more frequent emergency room visits and hospitalizations, more medication use, and more absenteeism from school and work (Bell & Samet, 2005). People with asthma and other respiratory diseases are especially susceptible to such adverse effects. Particulate matter is associated with many of the same respiratory effects and also with cardiovascular disease, lung cancer, and increased mortality (Brook et al., 2004; Dockery et al., 1993; Pope et al., 1995).

Motor vehicle emissions are a source of carbon dioxide and other greenhouse gases, including methane, NOx, and volatile organic compounds (VOCs). As a result, automobile traffic is a major contributor to global climate change, accounting for approximately 29 percent of U.S. greenhouse gas emissions (U.S. Department of Transportation, 2010). During the 1990s, greenhouse gases from mobile sources increased 18 percent, primarily a reflection of an increase in vehicle-miles traveled (EPA, 2001). Global climate change, in turn, is expected to threaten human health in several ways, including through the direct effects of heat, aggravation of some air pollutants, and increased prevalence of some infectious diseases (Epstein, 2000; Haines & Patz, 2004; National Assessment Synthesis Team, 2000).

A built environment that reinforces automobile dependence contributes to air pollution, which threatens health. This effect is mitigated by cleaner-burning, more fuel-efficient vehicles, but technical improvements are counteracted by increased vehicle-miles traveled. Conversely, a built environment that reduces travel demand by placing trip origins and destinations close together or that promotes alternatives to automobile travel might reduce air emissions.

MOTOR VEHICLE CRASHES

In the United States, automobiles claim more than forty thousand lives every year (National Highway Traffic Safety Administration [NHTSA], 2004). Automobile crashes are the leading cause of death among persons between one and twenty-four years old (CDC, 1999). They account for 3.4 million nonfatal injuries each year and cost an estimated $200 billion (CDC, 1999). Thanks to safer cars and roads, laws that discourage drunk driving, and other measures, rates of automobile fatalities and injuries per driver and per mile driven have decreased substantially. Still, the absolute toll of automobile crashes remains high.

The automobile is a relatively dangerous mode of travel. Depending on the assumptions used, a mile of automobile travel is between thirty and several hundred times more likely to result in the traveler's death than a mile of bus, train, or airplane travel (Halperin, 1993). Built environments that entail more time in an automobile would be expected to increase an individual's probability of a motor vehicle crash (Lourens, Vissers, & Jessurum, 1999).

In automobile-oriented environments such as suburban and exurban communities, several additional aspects of driving add to the risk of crashes. First, suburban roads may pose a special hazard, especially major commercial thoroughfares and *feeder* roads that combine high speed, high traffic volume, and frequent *curb cuts* where drivers enter and exit stores and other destinations (Ossenbruggen, Pendharkar, & Ivan, 2001). In addition, suburban drivers often travel longer distances to commute, transport their children, and run errands, which results in tired, busy people. Fatigue is an important risk factor for traffic crashes (Horne & Reyner, 1995; Pack, Cucchiara, Schwab, Rodgman, & Pack, 1994). The increasing use of cellular phones while driving further amplifies the risk of crashes (Laberge-Nadeau et al., 2003; Redelmeier & Tibshirani, 1997).

Denser metropolitan areas that require shorter trip distances and rely more on walking and public transportation have lower automobile fatality rates for both drivers and passengers than more sprawling cities (NHTSA, 2004). In a recent study of 448 counties in the largest 101 metropolitan areas in the United States, for every 1 percent decrease in the level of sprawl (as measured by density and other factors), the traffic fatality rate fell by 1.49 percent and pedestrian fatality rates fell by 1.47 to 3.56 percent. This suggests "urban sprawl was directly related to traffic fatalities and pedestrian fatalities" (Ewing, Schieber, & Zegeer, 2003). Reducing time spent in automobiles can therefore be considered a form of primary prevention. As noted by injury expert Ian Roberts (1993, p. 437), "Strategies which reduce the need for car travel or substitute car travel with safer forms of transport would substantially reduce population death rates."

PEDESTRIAN INJURIES AND FATALITIES

The implications of the built environment for pedestrian safety are more complex. Annually, automobiles cause about 5,000 fatalities and 110,000 injuries among pedestrians nationwide. In a built environment oriented more toward motorized than nonmotorized travel, a mile of walking or biking is more likely to be fatal than a mile of driving. In 2001, a mile of walking was twenty-three times more likely to kill a pedestrian, and a mile of biking was twelve times more likely to kill a bicyclist than a mile of driving was likely to kill a car occupant (Ernst & McCann, 2002).

Fortunately, pedestrian and bicyclist injury and fatality rates are decreasing in most industrialized nations, including the United States (Pucher & Dijkstra, 2003). In terms of public health, this is a Pyrrhic victory, since it reflects reduced walking and bicycling.

For example, data from the National Personal Transportation Survey show half of U.S. children are driven to school in a private vehicle and approximately one-third travel by school bus, whereas fewer than one in seven trips to school is made on foot or bicycle, a substantial decline from a generation ago (Dellinger & Staunton, 2002). In the 1999 nationwide HealthStyles survey, the two leading reported barriers to walking or biking to school were distance and traffic. Although safety was not offered as a perceived barrier, the concern with traffic is presumably a safety concern (Dellinger & Staunton, 2002). Parental concerns about the dangers of heavy traffic are well-founded. For example, a New Zealand policy that temporarily restricted automobile use resulted in a 46.4 percent decline in child pedestrian mortality (Roberts, Marshall, & Norton, 1992).

Design of the built environment helps determine traffic volume and defines another factor that affects pedestrian and bicyclist safety: physical infrastructure. Environmental modifications that help protect pedestrians and bicyclists include separating pedestrians from vehicles, making pedestrians more visible and conspicuous to drivers, and reducing vehicle speeds (Retting, Ferguson, & McCartt, 2003). Pedestrian-activated crossing signals, favorable traffic signal timing, and no-right-on-red laws can all help separate pedestrians from vehicles in time. They can be spatially separated with pedestrian overpasses, wide sidewalks on both sides of the street, and pedestrian refuge islands in the middle of wide streets. One strategy used in some European cities is to ban motor vehicles from designated streets or entire zones. Furthermore, separate paths and other infrastructure for pedestrians and bicyclists help prevent injuries from motor vehicles (Pucher & Dijkstra, 2003). Methods to make pedestrians more conspicuous to drivers include increased roadway lighting, raised intersections and crosswalks, and *bulb-outs* that extend the sidewalk corners into the street. Vehicle speeds can be reduced with traffic circles, narrowed traffic lanes, curving or zigzag roadways, raised intersections, and speed bumps. These techniques are collectively known as *traffic calming* (Elvik, 2001; Sarkar, Nederveen, & Pols, 1997; Shaw, 1994), and there is good evidence these measures help prevent pedestrian injuries and fatalities (Bunn et al., 2003; Retting et al., 2003).

The apparent trade-off between pedestrian travel and pedestrian safety is not inevitable. Under the right circumstances, higher levels of walking and bicycling are associated with lower rates of injuries and fatalities to pedestrians and cyclists. In the Netherlands and Germany, countries where walking and bicycling are far more common than in the United States, pedestrians and cyclists are killed at far lower rates than in the United States (Pucher & Dijkstra, 2000). In observational studies of intersections in both Sweden and Ontario, heavier pedestrian and bicycle traffic predicted lower rates of collisions with automobiles (Ekman, 1996; Leden, 2002). This relationship was confirmed in studies of California cities, Danish towns, and European countries (Jacobsen, 2003). A paradox exists, therefore, and it contains an important public health opportunity: whereas lower pedestrian and bicyclist injury rates might result from built environments that decrease walking and bicycling, a marked increase in foot and bicycle trips brings associated benefits (such as greater awareness among drivers and better roads and paths) and also decreases the number of pedestrian and bicyclist injuries.

WATER QUANTITY AND QUALITY

Features of the built environment might threaten the quantity and quality of the water supply. Land converted from forest and grassland to residential and commercial buildings yields extensive impervious surfaces such as rooftops, driveways, roads, and parking lots that do not effectively absorb rainwater and replenish groundwater aquifers (Noble, 1999; Zielinski, 2000). In suburban Indianapolis during a period of nearly twenty years, an 18 percent increase in impervious areas resulted in an estimated 80 percent increase in annual average rainwater runoff (Bhaduri, Harbor, Engel, & Grove, 2000). About half of U.S. communities depend on groundwater for their drinking water; such communities are at risk of water shortages if increased impervious surfaces prevent adequate groundwater recharge. High-density development confined to limited areas and balanced by preserved greenspace (especially along waterways) may limit the impact of impervious surfaces on a watershed. The amount of impervious surface has been identified as a key environmental indicator, much like air pollutant levels (Arnold & Gibbons, 1996).

Features of the built environment may affect water quality by increasing water pollution that occurs when rainfall or snowmelt deposits contaminants into surface water such as lakes, rivers, wetlands, and coastal waters. Such contaminants include oil, grease, and toxic chemicals from roads, parking lots, and other surfaces, as well as sediment from improperly managed construction sites. Suburban development increases surface-water levels of contaminants such as polycyclic aromatic hydrocarbons, zinc, and organic waste (Callender & Rice, 2000; Dierberg, 1991; Van Metre, Mahler, & Furlong, 2000). Surface runoff may also carry microbial contaminants from feces of pets and wildlife (Bannerman, Owens, Dodds, & Hornewer, 1993) or in sediment. The result is that waterways downstream from developed areas might be contaminated after significant rainfalls, increasing the risk of waterborne diseases (Curriero, Patz, Rose, & Lele, 2001; Gannon & Musse, 1989). In addition, in suburban developments that rely on wells and septic tanks, well water might be contaminated if the density of septic systems overwhelms the soil's ability to accommodate the wastes.

Water quantity and quality may be threatened by land use and development patterns. Source water protection, both upstream and in residential areas, is an important aspect of health protection often overlooked in decisions about the built environment.

NATURE CONTACT

An atrium with trees and plants, an urban park, and a grassy backyard are examples of built environments that offer opportunities for nature contact. People might find tranquility in certain natural environments, a soothing, restorative, even healing sense. Nature contact may help through mechanisms such as attention restoration and reduced stress (Ulrich, Simons, Losito, & Fiorito, 1991).

Some built environments offer visual access to nature, such as nature views through windows. Studies suggest improved attention and decreased distractibility in apartment dwellers and in college students in dormitories who have views of nature from their windows (R. Kaplan, 2001; Tennessen & Cimprich, 1995). Other studies have found that views of nature were associated with reduced sick call visits in prisoners (E. O. Moore, 1981), fewer headaches in employees (R. Kaplan, 1992; S. Kaplan, Talbot, & Kaplan, 1988), shorter postoperative hospital stays, and less need for pain medication in cholecystectomy patients (Ulrich, 1984).

A series of studies among residents of inner-city housing projects in Chicago compared two configurations of otherwise identical buildings, some with barren surroundings and others surrounded by trees. Living in a building with nearby trees was associated with higher levels of attention and greater effectiveness in managing major life issues, lower levels of aggression and violence among women, and lower levels of reported crime (Kuo, 2001; Kuo & Sullivan, 2001a, 2001b).

Some built environments go beyond visual access and offer people the chance to work or play in natural settings. Residents of retirement communities report that living within pleasant landscaped grounds is important (Browne, 1992), and office employees report plants make them feel calmer and more relaxed (Larsen, Adams, Deal, Kweon, & Tyler, 1998; Randall, Shoemaker, Relf, & Geller, 1992). In urban settings, gardens and gardening have been linked to a range of social benefits, ranging from improved property values to greater conviviality (see, for example, Patel, 1992). A study of children with attention deficit hyperactivity disorder found that playing in natural settings reduced ADHD symptoms more than playing in built settings (Kuo & Taylor, 2004). It has been suggested that regular opportunities for nature contact provide an essential (and diminishing) aspect of wholesome child development (Louv, 2005).

Contact with nature increasingly seems to offer health benefits, a principle that can be applied in many ways to building and community design.

MENTAL HEALTH

The built environment might have an effect on mental health if people find some places soothing and restorative and other places irritating and depressing. Tradition and research in architecture, geography, landscape architecture, urban planning, and environmental psychology support this concept (Alexander et al., 1997; Frumkin, 2003; Gallagher, 1993; R. Kaplan, 2001; Kaplan, & Ryan, 1998; Tuan, 1977; Whyte, 1980). Some observers think living in ugly or unpleasant places may adversely affect mental health. James Howard Kunstler (1993, 2005) suggests that sprawling suburban developments are isolating, disaggregated, and neurologically punishing and may contribute to obesity and depression.

Another set of links between the built environment and mental health pertains to the stressful effects of driving. Markers of this stress include increased heart rate and blood pressure and increased levels of stress hormones measured in urine. Driving-related stress is aggravated by certain personality traits, high levels of life stress in general, and situations such as crowded roads, unpredictability, and rude behavior by other drivers. It is therefore no surprise that automobile commuting that involves unavoidable, time-pressured driving performed ten times a week at crowded times of day has long been recognized as a stressor (Frumkin, 2004). Various studies have linked automobile commuting in congestion with increased blood pressure, back pain, cardiovascular disease, and self-reported stress (Belkic et al., 1994; Koslowsky, Kluger, & Reich, 1995; Magnusson, Pope, Wilder, & Areskoug, 1996; Novaco, Stokols, Campbell, & Stokols, 1979; Pietri et al., 1992; Stokols, Novaco, Stokols, & Campbell, 1978). As people spend more time on more crowded roads, an increase in these health outcomes might be expected.

One possible indicator of such problems is aggressive driving. Substantial proportions of drivers report aggressive feelings while driving and confess to such behaviors as swearing out loud at other drivers, making threatening or hostile gestures, and even feeling they "could gladly kill" other drivers (Hauber, 1980; Parry, 1968; Snow, 2000; Turner, Layton, & Simons, 1975). These aggressive thoughts can escalate into episodes that have come to be called *road rage*, such as when "an angry or impatient driver tries to kill or injure another driver after a traffic dispute" (Rathbone & Huckabee, 1999). According to the American Automobile Association's Foundation for Traffic Safety, the interval from 1990 to 1996 saw a 51 percent increase in reported incidents of road rage. The foundation documented ten thousand reports of such incidents, resulting in 12,610 injuries and 218 deaths (Mizell, 1997). A variety of weapons were used, including guns, knives, clubs, fists, feet, and, in some cases, the vehicle itself.

Road rage is not well understood. Risk factors include male sex and psychological predispositions (Dahlen & Ragan, 2004; Smart, Stoduto, Mann, & Adlaf, 2004). Stress at home or work may combine with stress while driving to elicit anger (Hartley & el Hassani, 1994; Novaco, 1991). Data from Australia, Canada, and Europe suggest traffic volume, travel distance, and the amount of time spent driving are risk factors (Harding, Morgan, Indermaur, Ferrante, & Blagg, 1998; Parker, Lajunen, & Summala, 2002; Smart et al., 2004). Long delays on crowded roads are likely to be a contributing factor.

It seems reasonable to hypothesize that anger and frustration among drivers are not restricted to their cars. When angry people arrive at work or at home, what are the implications for work and family relations? If the phenomenon known as *commuting stress* affects well-being and social relationships both on the roads and off, and if this set of problems is aggravated by increasingly long and difficult commutes on crowded roads, then the built environment may in this manner threaten mental health.

SOCIAL CAPITAL

Social capital refers to the attitudes (such as trust and reciprocity) and behaviors (such as civic engagement and participation) that bind a community or a society together (Portes, 1998). A closely related concept is *sense of community*. Social capital, especially more and better social relationships, is associated with health benefits (House, Landis, & Umberson, 1988; Kawachi, 1999). Conversely, conditions corresponding to low social capital, which include social isolation, social stratification, and income inequality, are, independent of income and poverty, associated with higher all-cause mortality, infant mortality, and mortality from a variety of specific causes. (G. A. Kaplan, Pamuk, Lynch, Cohen, & Balfour, 1996; Kawachi & Kennedy, 1999; Kawachi, Kennedy, Lochner, & Prothrow-Stith, 1997; Kennedy, Kawachi, & Prothrow-Stith, 1996; Lynch, Smith, Kaplan, & House, 2000; Lynch et al., 1998; Stanistreet, Scott-Samuel, & Bellis, 1999; Wilkinson, 1996).

Many factors, ranging from television and computer use to employment patterns, affect levels of social capital. The built environment may play a role (Calthorpe, 1993; Mo & Wilkie, 1997; Putnam, 2000). After the Second World War, many Americans flocked to newly developing suburbs, drawn in part by the promised sense of community. In Park Forest, Illinois, in the 1950s, William Whyte (1956) observed an almost frantic pace of socializing, a "hotbed of participation." Investigators in Levittown, on New York's Long Island, described many social organizations that formed during the 1950s, such as babysitting co-ops, Tupperware parties, Little League, and service on the school board and PTA (Baxandall & Ewen, 2000).

But other observers have noted adverse consequences of suburban design on social capital. For example, Ewing believes "strong communities of place, where neighbors interact, have a sense of belonging, and have a feeling of responsibility for one another are harder to find" in suburbs than in traditional small towns or cities (1997, p. 117).

Several features of suburban community design may undermine social capital. First, urban sprawl and associated long commutes restrict the time and energy people have available for civic involvement. Putnam (2000) reports commute time is one of the most important demographic variables in predicting civic involvement. He writes "each ten additional minutes in daily commuting time cuts involvement in community affairs by 10 percent— fewer public meetings attended, fewer committees chaired, fewer petitions signed, fewer church services attended, and so on" (p. 213).

Second, the built environment can foster or prevent opportunities for spontaneous, informal social interaction. Traditional towns and cities typically include *great good places*, such as the "cafés, coffee shops, bookstores, bars, hair salons, and other hangouts at the heart of a community" where people may gather to socialize (Oldenburg, 1989). In contrast, recently developed suburbs tend to lack such places.

Third, the built environment could affect social capital by either promoting or devaluing the public realm. People who use exercise machines at home or relax in their backyards rather than jog or picnic in parks may have little feeling for parks and other public assets. Recent voting trends suggest suburban voters prefer limited government programs and place little emphasis on such social goals as eliminating discrimination and reducing poverty. They also tend to reject initiatives such as park acquisition and mass transit (Oliver, 2001; Putnam, 2000; Teaford & Kilpinen, 1997).

Fourth, relatively homogeneous communities segregated by social class and race may obviate the political discourse that is important to social capital. Oliver (2001) suggests that in homogeneous suburban communities, social conflicts between citizens are transformed into conflicts between political institutions. This removes incentives for people to become personally involved in the political process, reducing levels of civic participation.

Finally, many homogeneous suburban neighborhoods offer housing appropriate to only one stage in the life cycle, so that couples who wanted large houses and lots while raising children will need to leave the neighborhood when they are ready to downsize to smaller lodging. The use of property taxes to fund schools may be a further incentive for empty nesters to move away from communities with young families. The systematic departure of families after living in a neighborhood for twenty years reduces social capital.

Such evidence suggests that features of the built environment may either promote or diminish social capital (Burchell et al., 1998; Frumkin, Frank, & Jackson, 2004). In general, evidence suggests that walkability, public spaces, and mixed uses are associated with improvements in social capital, whereas automobile dependence, absence of public spaces, and low density have a negative impact. In these ways, the built environment may indirectly but significantly affect health.

POPULATIONS AT SPECIAL RISK

As with many environmental exposures, features of the built environment are likely to affect some groups more than others. Groups that deserve special attention in this regard include women, children, the elderly, poor people, people of color, and people with disabilities.

WOMEN

In automobile-dependent areas, women play a disproportionate role as chauffeurs who are often tasked with driving children to school, play dates, or soccer games; taking elderly parents to the doctor; and running errands to the grocery store, post office, or bank. One study found that two-thirds of all chauffeur trips are made by women and that married women with school-aged children were averaging more than five automobile trips a day, 21 percent more than the average for men (Surface Transportation Policy Project, 2002). Among women, 50.4 percent of trips were made for chauffeuring, compared with 41.1 percent among men. Time spent in the car per day averaged sixty-six minutes for married women with school-aged children and seventy-five minutes for single mothers. The image of the suburban *soccer mom* in a minivan turned out to reflect long hours at the wheel providing transportation and delivery services. For women in suburban and exurban areas faced with a large burden of driving, the built environment must seem very much a women's health issue.

CHILDREN

Children are also a vulnerable population in several ways. First, the burdens of air pollution fall heavily on children, since they breathe disproportionately more air than adults, have more outdoor exposure time, and have developing respiratory systems (Etzel & Balk, 2003). Asthma prevalence is high in children, and asthmatic children are especially susceptible to exposure to ozone and other respiratory irritants. Ozone increases acute respiratory symptoms in children in the short term and may impair lung growth (Künzli et al., 1997) and increase the probability of developing asthma following long-term exposure (McConnell et al., 2002). This is an issue in densely trafficked areas, such as alongside busy roadways, and it is an issue on a regional scale when high levels of driving increase the air pollution burden.

Second, children have been hard hit by the physical inactivity associated with shifting travel patterns. The disappearance of walking and bicycling to school, discussed earlier, together with other changes in activity patterns and diet, have contributed to a rapid increase in childhood overweight and obesity (Hedley et al., 2004; Ogden, Flegal, Carroll, & Johnson, 2002). The consequences include low self-esteem; increased risk of diabetes, hyperlipidemia, and other diseases; and an increased risk of being overweight in adulthood (Dietz, 1998; Serdula et al., 1993). Third, children are especially susceptible to automobile-related injuries and fatalities, particularly when they are pedestrians or bicyclists (Schieber & Thompson, 1996). Fourth, children need certain cues and stimuli from their environment for normal development; these may include contact with nature and opportunities to navigate and learn wayfinding (Bronfenbrenner, 1979; Louv, 2005; R. C. Moore, 1997; Spencer & Woolley, 2000). Children in built environments that feature little nature contact or that require being driven everywhere instead of walking or bicycling (and exploring) might suffer as a result. Finally, the decline of social capital may be especially worrisome for children. The adage "it takes a village to raise a child" reflects a traditional understanding, supported by both theory and empirical research, that children benefit from cohesive communities (Earls & Carlson, 2001; Morrow, 2002).

THE ELDERLY

The elderly represent the fastest-growing age segment of the U.S. population. Aging inevitably includes declines in function such as impaired vision and mobility. Many elderly people become unable to drive. Accordingly, elderly persons are disfranchised in communities in which driving is the only practical means of transportation and in which walkable destinations are scarce. In contrast, walkable communities, where destinations such as stores, libraries, and churches are in close proximity to people's homes, offer ideal opportunities for elders to maintain their mobility and independence. Physical activity is a powerful protector of health in the elderly (Mazzeo, Cavanagh, & Evans, 1998).

POOR PEOPLE AND PEOPLE OF COLOR

Poor people and people of color are affected in many ways by the design of the built environment. John Kain (1968) identified a systematic spatial mismatch in which blacks were trapped in the inner city by housing discrimination, while the job base was increasingly moving outward. "Sprawl is related to poverty and inequality," Paul Jargowsky (2002, p. 51) observes, "mainly because sprawl creates a greater degree of separation between the income classes." For city dwellers without automobiles, public transit rarely provides affordable, efficient access to suburban jobs (Bullard & Johnson, 1997; Bullard, Johnson, & Torres, 2000). The health consequences of poverty, especially in urban centers, are widely recognized (Berkman & Kawachi, 2000; Marmot & Wilkinson, 1999).

Some specific health effects of the built environment fall disproportionately on poor people and people of color. For example, home injury risks are more common among disadvantaged populations, who frequently rent housing in poorly maintained buildings (Cubbin, LeClere, & Smith, 2000; Shenassa, Stubbendick, & Brown, 2004). Pedestrian fatalities follow a similar pattern. In suburban Orange County, California, Latinos make up 28 percent of the population but account for 43 percent of pedestrian fatalities (Marosi, 1999). In the Virginia suburbs of Washington, DC, Hispanics make up 8 percent of the population but account for 21 percent of pedestrian fatalities (Moreno & Sipress, 1999). The reasons for this disproportionate impact are complex and may involve the probability of being a pedestrian (perhaps related to low access to automobiles and public transportation), road design in areas where members of minority groups walk, and behavioral and cultural factors. Built environment interventions to reduce injuries should target such disadvantaged populations.

PEOPLE WITH DISABILITIES

Finally, aspects of the built environment have a major impact on the health and well-being of people with disabilities. Transportation systems designed for cars rather than pedestrians are especially unfriendly to those with special transportation needs. People in wheelchairs need sidewalks and paths that are sufficiently wide and level to allow safe and convenient passage, with curb cuts at appropriate locations. People with visual impairments need audible pedestrian signals at intersections to facilitate safe crossings (Barlow et al., 2003). Crossing signals need to be timed to allow people with disabilities enough time to reach the other side. In some cases, traffic-calming measures designed to protect most pedestrians, such as roundabouts, pose special challenges for those who are blind. Careful planning is needed to provide safe and convenient mobility for all, and design guidelines are available (American Association of State Highway and Transportation Officials, 2001; Institute of Transportation Engineers, 1998). Undertaking such changes requires an awareness of the needs of people with disabilities, as well as a broader orientation to safe, nonmotorized travel.

CONCLUSION

The built environment may affect health and well-being on many spatial scales, from a piece of furniture to an entire metropolitan area. The built environment also affects cardiovascular, respiratory, and mental health and influences sense of community. Recognizing these links, the health sciences have identified many opportunities to create built environments that prevent injury and illness and promote health. Ergonomists help design safe, comfortable furniture; industrial hygienists help assess and control indoor air problems; and sanitarians help control rodent infestations in buildings. Equally important, professionals in other fields also shape the health and safety of built environments. Architects design buildings, planners lay out neighborhoods, landscape architects create parks, and traffic engineers design roadways. All these professionals play a major, if sometimes unrecognized, role in public health.

A health impact assessment (HIA) is a new tool that offers promise for bringing attention to the prospective health consequences of decisions in the design of the built environment (Dannenberg et al., 2006; Kemm, Parry, & Palmer, 2004). An HIA is defined as "a combination of procedures, methods, and tools by which a policy, program, or project may be judged as to its potential effects on the health of a population and the distribution of those effects within the population" (European Centre for Health Policy, 1999). An HIA can be used to improve communication between local health departments and community decision makers, enabling the latter to consider improved designs that favor health promotion or minimize adverse effects on health.

One example of a comprehensive approach to the built environment is known as *smart growth*, a set of land use and transportation principles that include mixed land uses, higher density balanced by the preservation of green spaces, transportation alternatives (including pedestrian infrastructure and transit), attractive communities with a strong sense of place, and effective, coordinated regional planning based on community and stakeholder participation (Bollier, 1998; Calthorpe, 1993; Calthorpe & Fulton, 2001; Congress for the New Urbanism, 2000; Langdon, 1994; Local Government Commission, 1991; Newman & Kenworthy, 1999). Smart growth has been recognized as offering a range of health benefits (Frumkin et al., 2004), and planners and health professionals are increasingly cooperating to implement and evaluate smart growth principles.

Most aspects of the built environment are designed and constructed to achieve many goals, of which health is only one; others include efficiency, profitability, environmental performance, and aesthetics. However, the health implications of the built environment are increasingly being recognized and documented with rigorous evidence.

Health professionals and other community leaders need to act on this evidence, contributing their perspective to the planning and design of the built environment. Activities that can be used by local citizens to enhance community well-being include participating in public hearings with zoning and planning boards, writing letters to newspapers, and joining local groups that advocate for public health and environmental improvements. All citizens can benefit when places are designed to optimize community well-being.

DISCUSSION QUESTIONS

1. Think about your work or living conditions. Which of the built environment issues mentioned in the chapter are both feasible and important to address to promote health in your community? Describe why in detail.
2. What types of strategies would you use to try to improve your physical environment? How would you begin to make the change? Think about the role of health impact assessment (HIA).
3. Although a smart growth environment with sidewalks, green spaces, and mixed land uses provides opportunities to increase levels of physical activity in the community, this kind of environment does not guarantee community residents will become physically active. How might health professionals motivate individuals and communities to take advantage of available opportunities for active living?

REFERENCES

Aiello, J. R., Nicosia, G., & Thompson, D. E. (1979). Physiological, social, and behavioral consequences of crowding on children and adolescents. *Child Development, 50*, 195–202.

Alexander, C., Ishikawa, S., Silverstein, M., Jacobson, M., Fiksdahl-King, I., & Angel, S. (1997). *A pattern language: Towns, buildings, construction.* New York: Oxford University Press.

American Academy of Pediatrics. (2001). Falls from heights: Windows, roofs, and balconies. *Pediatrics, 107*, 1188–1191.

American Association of State Highway and Transportation Officials. (2001). *A policy on geometric design of highways and streets* (4th ed.). Publ. No. GDHS-4. Washington, DC: Author.

Arnold, C. L., & Gibbons, C. J. (1996). Impervious surface coverage: The emergence of a key environmental indicator. *Journal of the American Planning Association, 62*, 243–258.

Bannerman, R. T., Owens, D. W., Dodds, R. B., & Hornewer, N. J. (1993). Sources of pollutants in Wisconsin stormwater. *Water Science and Technology, 28*, 241–259.

Barlow, J. M., Bentzen, B. L., Tabor, L. S., & Pedestrian and Bicycle Information Center. (2003, May). *Accessible pedestrian signals: Synthesis and guide to best practice.* Washington, DC: National Research Council. Retrieved October 17, 2006, from http://www.walkinginfo.org/aps/home.cfm

Bauman, A. E. (2004). Updating the evidence that physical activity is good for health: An epidemiological review, 2000–2003. *Journal of Science and Medicine in Sport, 7*(1 Suppl.), 6–19.

Baxandall, R., & Ewen, E. (2000). *Picture windows: How the suburbs happened.* New York: Basic Books.

Beauchemin, K. M., & Hays, P. (1996). Sunny hospital rooms expedite recovery from severe and refractory depression. *Journal of Affective Disorders, 40*, 49–51.

Belkic et al. (1994). Mechanisms of cardiac risk among professional drivers. *Scandinavian Journal of Work and Environmental Health, 20*, 73–86.

Bell, M. L., & Samet, J. M. (2005). Air pollution. In H. Frumkin (Ed.), *Environmental health: From global to local* (pp. 331–361). San Francisco: Jossey-Bass.

Bergner, L., Mayer, S., & Harris, D. (1971). Falls from heights: A childhood epidemic in an urban area. *American Journal of Public Health, 61*, 90–96.

Berkman, L. F., & Kawachi, I. (2000). *Social epidemiology.* New York: Oxford University Press.

Bhaduri, B., Harbor, J., Engel, B., & Grove, M. (2000). Assessing watershed-scale long-term hydrologic impacts of land-use change using a GIS-NPS model. *Environmental Management, 26*, 643–658.

Blair et al. (1996). Influences of cardiorespiratory fitness and other precursors on cardiovascular disease and all-cause mortality in men and women. *Journal of the American Medical Association, 276*, 205–210.

Bollier, D. (1998). *How smart growth can stop sprawl.* Washington, DC: Essential Books.

Bronfenbrenner, U. (1979). *The ecology of human development.* Cambridge, MA: Harvard University Press.

Brook et al. (2004). Air pollution and cardiovascular disease: A statement for healthcare professionals from the Expert Panel on Population and Prevention Science of the American Heart Association. *Circulation, 109*, 2655–2671.

Browne, A. (1992). The role of nature for the promotion of well-being in the elderly. In D. Relf (Ed.), *The role of horticulture in human well-being and social development* (pp. 75–79). Portland, OR: Timber Press.

Bullard, R. D. (1990). *Dumping in Dixie: Race, class, and environmental quality.* Boulder, CO: Westview Press.

Bullard, R. D., & Johnson, G. S. (Eds.). (1997). *Just transportation: Dismantling race and class barriers to mobility.* Stony Creek, CT: New Society.

Bullard, R. D., Johnson, G. S., & Torres, A. O. (2000). *Sprawl city: Race, politics, and planning in Atlanta.* Washington, DC: Island Press.

Bunn et al. (2003). Area-wide traffic calming for preventing traffic related injuries. *Cochrane Database of Systematic Reviews, 1*, art. CD003110.

Burchell et al. (1998). *The costs of sprawl—revisited.* Transportation Research Board Rep. No. 39. Washington, DC: National Academies Press.

Calle, E. E., Rodriguez, C., Walker-Thurmond, K., & Thun, M. J. (2003). Overweight, obesity, and mortality from cancer in a prospectively studied cohort of U.S. adults. *New England Journal of Medicine, 348*, 1625–1638.

Callender, E., & Rice, K. C. (2000). The urban environmental gradient: Anthropogenic influences on the spatial and temporal distributions of lead and zinc in sediments. *Environmental Science and Technology, 34*, 232–238.

Calthorpe, P. (1993). *The next American metropolis: Ecology, community, and the American dream.* Princeton, NJ: Princeton Architectural Press.

Calthorpe, P., & Fulton, W. (2001). *The regional city: Planning for the end of sprawl.* Washington, DC: Island Press.

Cayless, S. M. (2001). Slip, trip and fall accidents: Relationship to building features and use of coroners' reports in ascribing cause. *Applied Ergonomics, 32*, 155–162.

Centers for Disease Control and Prevention. (1999). Motor vehicle safety: A 20th-century public health achievement. *Morbidity and Mortality Weekly Report, 48*, 369–374.

Centers for Disease Control and Prevention, National Center for Injury Prevention and Control. (2005). *Falls and hip fractures among older adults.* Retrieved October 17, 2006, from http://www.cdc.gov/ncipc/factsheets/falls.htm

Cervero, R. (1989). *America's suburban centers: The land use–transportation link.* Boston: Unwin Hyman.

Cervero, R., & Gorham, R. (1995). Commuting in transit versus automobile neighborhoods. *Journal of the American Planning Association, 61*, 210–225.

Cervero, R., & Kockelman, K. (1997). Travel demand and the three Ds: Density, diversity, and design. *Transportation Research Record, 2*, 199–219.

Congress for the New Urbanism. (2000). *Charter for the new urbanism.* New York: McGraw-Hill.

Cote, A. (1984). Field test and evaluation of residential sprinkler system: Part III. *Fire Technology, 20*, 41–46.

Craig, C. L., Brownson, R. C., Cragg, S. E., & Dunn, A. L. (2002). Exploring the effect of the environment on physical activity: A study examining walking to work. *American Journal of Preventive Medicine, 23*(Suppl. 2), 36–43.

Cubbin, C., LeClere, F. B., & Smith, G. S. (2000). Socioeconomic status and injury mortality: Individual and neighbourhood determinants. *Journal of Epidemiology and Community Health, 54*, 517–524.

Curriero, F. C., Patz, J. A., Rose, J. B., & Lele, S. D. (2001). The association between extreme precipitation and waterborne disease outbreaks in the United States, 1948–1994. *American Journal of Public Health, 91*, 1194–1199.

Dahlen, E. R., & Ragan, K. M. (2004). Validation of the propensity for angry driving scale. *Journal of Safety Research, 35*, 557–563.

Dannenberg et al. (2006). Growing the field of health impact assessment in the United States: An agenda for research and practice. *American Journal of Public Health, 96*, 262–270.

Dellinger, A. M., & Staunton, C. E. (2002). Barriers to children walking and biking to school: United States, 1999. *Morbidity and Mortality Weekly Review, 51*, 701–704.

Dierberg, F. E. (1991). Non-point source loadings of nutrients and dissolved organic carbon from an agricultural-suburban watershed in east central Florida. *Water Research, 25*, 363–374.

Dietz, W. H. (1998). Health consequences of obesity in youth: Childhood predictors of adult disease. *Pediatrics, 101*, 518–525.

Dockery et al. (1993). An association between air pollution and mortality in six U.S. cities. *New England Journal of Medicine, 329*, 1753–1759.

Duffy, J. F., & Wright, K. P., Jr. (2005). Entrainment of the human circadian system by light. *Journal of Biological Rhythms, 20*, 326–338.

Duke, J., Huhman, M., & Heitzler, C. (2003). Physical activity levels among children aged 9–13 years: United States, 2002. *Morbidity and Mortality Weekly Report, 52*, 785–788.

Earls, F., & Carlson, M. (2001). The social ecology of child health and well-being. *Annual Review of Public Health, 22*, 143–166.

Ekman, L. (1996). *On the treatment of traffic safety analysis: A non-parametric approach applied on vulnerable road users* (Bulletin 136). Lund, Sweden: Department of Technology and Society, Lund Institute of Technology.

Elvik, R. (2001). Area-wide urban traffic calming schemes: A meta-analysis of safety effects. *Accident Analysis and Prevention, 33*, 327–336.

Environmental Protection Agency. (2001). *Our built and natural environments: A technical review of the interactions between land use, transportation, and environmental quality* (EPA Publ. No. 231-R-01–002). Washington, DC: Author.

Environmental Protection Agency, Office of Transportation and Air Quality. (2006). Mobile source emissions: Past, present, and future. Retrieved October 17, 2006, from http://www.epa.gov/otaq/invntory/overview/pollutants/index.htm

Epstein, P. R. (2000). Is global warming harmful to health? *Scientific American, 283*, 50–57.

Erdmann, T. C., Feldman, K. W., Rivara, F. P., Heimbach, D. M., & Wall, H. A. (1991). Tap water burn prevention: The effect of legislation. *Pediatrics, 88*, 572–577.

Ernst, M., & McCann, B. (2002). *Mean streets, 2002*. Washington, DC: Surface Transportation Policy Project and Environmental Working Group. Retrieved October 17, 2006, from http://www.transact.org/PDFs/ms2002/MeanStreets2002.pdf

Etzel, R. A., & Balk, S. J. (Eds.). (2003). *Pediatric environmental health* (2nd ed.). Elk Grove Village, IL: American Academy of Pediatrics Committee on Environmental Health.

European Centre for Health Policy. (1999). *Health impact assessment: Main concepts and suggested approach*. Brussels, Belgium: World Health Organization Regional Office for Europe. Retrieved October 17, 2006, from http://www.who.dk/document/PAE/Gothenburgpaper.pdf

Evans, G. W. (2003). The built environment and mental health. *Journal of Urban Health, 80*, 536–555.

Evans, G. W., Lepore, S. J., Shejwal, B. R., & Palsane, M. N. (1998). Chronic residential crowding and children's well-being: An ecological perspective. *Child Development, 69*, 1514–1523.

Evans, G. W., Saegert S., & Harris, R. (2001). Residential density and psychological health among children in low-income families. *Environment and Behavior, 33*, 165–180.

Ewing, R. (1997). Is Los Angeles-style sprawl desirable? *Journal of the American Planning Association, 63*, 107–126.

Ewing, R., Schieber, R. A., & Zegeer, C. V. (2003). Urban sprawl as a risk factor in motor vehicle occupant and pedestrian fatalities. *American Journal of Public Health, 93*, 1541–1545.

Feldman, K. W., Schaller, R. T., Feldman, J. A., & McMillon, M. (1978). Tap water scald burns in children. *Pediatrics, 62*, 1–7.

Fishman, R. (1987). *Bourgeois utopias: The rise and fall of suburbia.* New York: Basic Books.

Flegal, K. M., Carroll, M. D., Kuczmarski, R. J., & Johnson, C. L. (1998). Overweight and obesity in the United States: Prevalence and trends, 1960–1994. *International Journal of Obesity and Related Metabolic Disorders, 22*, 39–47.

Frank, L. D., Andresen, M. A., & Schmid, T. L. (2004). Obesity relationships with community design, physical activity, and time spent in cars. *American Journal of Preventive Medicine, 27*, 87–96.

Frank, L. D., & Pivo, G. (1995). Impacts of mixed use and density on utilization of three modes of travel: Single-occupant vehicle, transit, and walking. *Transportation Research Record, 1466*, 44–52.

French, S. A., Story, M., & Jeffery, R. W. (2001). Environmental influences on eating and physical activity. *Annual Review of Public Health, 22*, 309–335.

Frumkin, H. (2003). Healthy places: Exploring the evidence. *American Journal of Public Health, 93*, 1451–1455.

Frumkin, H. (2004). White coats, green plants: Clinical epidemiology meets horticulture. *Acta Horticulturae, 639*, 15–26.

Frumkin, H., Frank, L. D., & Jackson, R. J. (2004). *Urban sprawl and public health: Designing, planning, and building for healthy communities.* Washington, DC: Island Press.

Gallagher, W. (1993). *The power of place: How our surroundings shape our thoughts, emotions, and actions.* New York: Poseidon Press.

Gannon, J. J., & Musse, M. K. (1989). *E. coli* and enterococci levels in urban stormwater, river water, and chlorinated treatment plant effluent. *Water Research, 23*, 1167–1176.

Garreau, J. (1991). *Edge city: Life on the new frontier.* New York: Doubleday.

Gill, T. M., Williams, C. S., Robison, J. T., & Tinetti, M. E. (1999). A population-based study of environmental hazards in the homes of older persons. *American Journal of Public Health, 89*, 553–556.

Gillham, O. (2002). *The limitless city: A primer on the urban sprawl debate.* Washington, DC: Island Press.

Haines, A., & Patz, J. A. (2004). Health effects of climate change. *Journal of the American Medical Association, 291*, 99–103.

Hall, P. (1998). *Cities in civilization.* London: Weidenfeld & Nicolson.

Halperin, K. (1993). A comparative analysis of six methods for calculating travel fatality risk. *Risk: Health, Safety and Environment, 4*, 15–33.

Handy, S., Boarnet, M., Ewing, R., & Killingsworth, R. (2002). How the built environment affects physical activity: Views from urban planning. *American Journal of Preventive Medicine, 23*(Suppl. 2), 64–73.

Harding, R. W., Morgan, F. H., Indermaur, D., Ferrante, A. M., & Blagg, H. (1998). Road rage and the epidemiology of violence: Something old, something new. *Studies on Crime and Crime Prevention, 7*, 221–228.

Hartley, L., & el Hassani, J. (1994). Stress, violations, and accidents. *Applied Ergonomics, 25,* 221–230.

Hauber, A. R. (1980). The social psychology of driving behavior and the traffic environment: Research on aggressive behavior in traffic. *International Review of Applied Psychology, 29,* 461–474.

Hedley et al. (2004). Prevalence of overweight and obesity among U.S. children, adolescents, and adults, 1999–2002. *Journal of the American Medical Association, 291,* 2847–2850.

Heschong, L. (2003a, October). Windows and Classrooms: A Study of Student Performance and the Indoor Environment. Attachment 7 to Public Interest Energy Research Program. *Integrated Energy Systems: Productivity and Building Science* (Publ. No, 500–03–082-A-08). Sacramento: California Energy Commission. Retrieved October 27, 2006, from http://www.energy.ca.gov/reports/2003–11–17_500–03–082_A-07.pdf

Heschong, L. (2003b, October). Windows and Offices: A Study of Office Worker Performance and the Indoor Environment. Attachment 9 to Public Interest Energy Research Program. *Integrated Energy Systems: Productivity and Building Science* (Publ. No. 500–03–082-A-09). Sacramento: California Energy Commission. Retrieved October 17, 2006, from http://www.energy.ca.gov/reports/2003–11–17_500–03–082_A-09.pdf

Horne, J. A., & Reyner, L. A. (1995). Sleep-related vehicle accidents. *British Medical Journal, 4,* 565–567.

House, J. S., Landis, K. R., & Umberson, D. (1988). Social relationships and health. *Science, 241,* 540–545.

Humpel, N., Owen, N., & Leslie, E. (2002). Environmental factors associated with adults' participation in physical activity: A review. *American Journal of Preventive Medicine, 22,* 188–199.

Institute of Transportation Engineers. (1998). *Design and safety of pedestrian facilities.* Washington, DC: Author.

Istre et al. (2003). Childhood injuries due to falls from apartment balconies and windows. *Injury Prevention, 9,* 349–352.

Jackson, K. T. (1985). *Crabgrass frontier: The suburbanization of the United States.* New York: Oxford University Press.

Jacobsen, P. L. (2003). Safety in numbers: More walkers and bicyclists, safer walking and bicycling. *Injury Prevention, 9,* 205–209.

Jargowsky, P. A. (2002). Sprawl, concentration of poverty, and urban inequality. In G. D. Squires (Ed.), *Urban sprawl: Causes, consequences, and policy responses.* Washington, DC: Urban Institute Press.

Kahn, P. H., Jr., & Kellert, S. R. (Eds.). (2002). *Children and nature: Psychological, sociocultural, and evolutionary investigations.* Cambridge, MA: MIT Press.

Kain, J. F. (1968). Housing segregation, Negro employment, and metropolitan decentralization. *Quarterly Journal of Economics, 82,* 175–197.

Kampert, J. B., Blair, S. N., Barlow, C. E., & Kohl, H. W., III. (1996). Physical activity, physical fitness, and all-cause and cancer mortality: A prospective study of men and women. *Annals of Epidemiology, 6,* 452–457.

Kaplan, G. A., Pamuk, E., Lynch, J. W., Cohen, R. D., & Balfour, J. L. (1996). Income inequality and mortality in the United States. *British Medical Journal, 312*, 999–1003.

Kaplan, R. (1992). The psychological benefits of nearby nature. In D. Relf (Ed.), *The role of horticulture in human well-being and social development*. Portland, OR: Timber Press.

Kaplan, R. (2001). The nature of the view from home: Psychological benefits. *Environment and Behavior, 33*, 507–542.

Kaplan, R., Kaplan, S., & Ryan, R. L. (1998). *With people in mind: Design and management of everyday nature*. Washington, DC: Island Press.

Kaplan, S., Talbot, J. F., & Kaplan, R. (1988). *Coping with daily hassles: The impact of nearby nature on the work environment*. Washington, DC: USDA Forest Service, North Central Forest Experiment Station.

Kawachi, I. (1999). Social capital and community effects on population and individual health. *Annals of the New York Academy of Science, 896*, 120–130.

Kawachi, I., & Kennedy, B. P. (1999). Income inequality and health: Pathways and mechanisms. *Health Services Research, 34*, 215–227.

Kawachi, I., Kennedy, B. P., Lochner, K., & Prothrow-Stith, D. (1997). Social capital, income inequality, and mortality. *American Journal of Public Health, 87*, 1491–1498.

Kemm, J., Parry, J., & Palmer, S. (2004). *Health impact assessment: Concepts, theory, techniques, and applications*. New York: Oxford University Press.

Kennedy, B. P., Kawachi, I., & Prothrow-Stith, D. (1996). Income distribution and mortality: Cross-sectional ecological study of the Robin Hood index in the United States. *British Medical Journal, 312*, 1004–1007.

Knauth, P., & Hornberger, S. (2003). Preventive and compensatory measures for shift workers. *Occupational Medicine (Oxford), 53*, 109–116.

Kockelman, K. M. (1997). Travel behavior as a function of accessibility, land use mixing, and land use balance: Evidence from San Francisco Bay Area. *Transportation Research Record, 1607*, 116–125.

Koplan, J. P., & Dietz, W. H. (1999). Caloric imbalance and public health policy. *Journal of the American Medical Association, 282*, 1579–1581.

Koslowsky, M., Kluger, A. N., & Reich, M. (1995). *Commuting stress: Causes, effects, and methods of coping*. New York: Plenum Press.

Kuczmarski, R. J., Flegal, K. M., Campbell, S. M., & Johnson, C. L. (1994). Increasing prevalence of overweight among U.S. adults: The National Health and Nutrition Examination Surveys, 1960 to 1991. *Journal of the American Medical Association, 272*, 205–211.

Kuller, R., & Lindsten, C. (1992). Health and behavior of children in classrooms with and without windows. *Journal of Environmental Psychology, 12*, 305–317.

Kunstler, J. H. (1993). *The geography of nowhere: The rise and decline of America's man-made landscape*. New York: Simon & Schuster.

Kunstler, J. H. (2005). *Big and blue in the USA*. Retrieved July 14, 2006, from http://www.oriononline.org/pages/oo/curmudgeon/index_BigAndBlue.html

Künzli et al. (1997). Association between lifetime ambient ozone exposure and pulmonary function in college freshmen: Results of a pilot study. *Environmental Research, 72*, 8–23.

Kuo, F. E. (2001). Coping with poverty: Impacts of environment and attention in the inner city. *Environment and Behavior, 33*, 5–34.

Kuo, F. E., & Sullivan, W. C. (2001a). Aggression and violence in the inner city: Effects of environment via mental fatigue. *Environment and Behavior, 33*, 543–571.

Kuo, F. E., & Sullivan, W. C. (2001b). Environment and crime in the inner city: Does vegetation reduce crime? *Environment and Behavior, 33*, 343–367.

Kuo, F. E., & Taylor, A. F. (2004). A potential natural treatment for attention-deficit/hyperactivity disorder: Evidence from a national study. *American Journal of Public Health, 94*, 1580–1586.

Laberge-Nadeau et al. (2003). Wireless telephones and the risk of road crashes. *Accident Analysis and Prevention, 35*, 649–660.

Lack L., & Wright, H. (1993). The effect of evening bright light in delaying the circadian rhythms and lengthening the sleep of early morning awakening insomniacs. *Sleep, 16*, 436–443.

Langdon, P. (1994). *A better place to live: Reshaping the American suburb.* Amherst: University of Massachusetts Press.

Larsen, L., Adams, J., Deal, B., Kweon, B. S., & Tyler, E. (1998). Plants in the workplace: The effects of plant density on productivity, attitudes, and perceptions. *Environment and Behavior, 30*, 261–282.

Leden, L. (2002). Pedestrian risk decreases with pedestrian flow: A case study based on data from signalized intersections in Hamilton, Ontario. *Accident Analysis and Prevention, 34*, 457–464.

Lee, I. M. (2003). Physical activity and cancer prevention: Data from epidemiologic studies. *Medicine and Science in Sports and Exercise, 35*, 1823–1827.

Lee, I. M., & Paffenbarger, R. S., Jr. (2000). Associations of light, moderate, and vigorous intensity physical activity with longevity. *American Journal of Epidemiology, 151*, 293–299.

Lewy, A. J., Kern, H. A., Rosenthal, N. E., & Wehr, T. A. (1982). Bright artificial light treatment of a manic-depressive patient with seasonal mood cycle. *American Journal of Psychiatry, 139*, 1496–1498.

Lienhardt, C. (2001). From exposure to disease: The role of environmental factors in susceptibility to and development of tuberculosis. *Epidemiologic Review, 23*, 288–301.

Local Government Commission. (1991). *Awhahnee principles.* Retrieved July 14, 2006, from http://www.lgc.org/ahwahnee/principles.html

Loo, C. M., & Smetana, J. (1978).The effects of crowding on the behavior and perception of 10-year-old boys. *Environmental Psychology and Nonverbal Behavior, 2*, 226–249.

Lourens, P. F., Vissers, J. A., & Jessurum, M. (1999). Annual mileage, driving violations, and accident involvement in relation to drivers' sex, age, and level of education. *Accident Analysis and Prevention, 31*, 593–597.

Louv, R. (2005). *Last child in the woods: Saving our children from nature-deficit disorder.* Chapel Hill, NC: Algonquin Press.

Lynch et al. (1998). Income inequality and mortality in metropolitan areas of the United States. *American Journal of Public Health, 88*, 1074–1080.

Lynch, J. W., Smith, G. D., Kaplan, G. A., & House, J. S. (2000). Income inequality and mortality: Importance to health of individual income, psychosocial environment, or material conditions. *British Medical Journal, 320*, 1200–1204.

Macera et al. (2003). Prevalence of physical activity, including lifestyle activities among adults: United States, 2000–2001. *Morbidity and Mortality Weekly Review, 52*, 764–769.

Magnusson, M. L., Pope, M. H., Wilder, D. G., & Areskoug, B. (1996). Are occupational drivers at an increased risk for developing musculoskeletal disorders? *Spine, 21*, 710–717.

Marmot, M., & Wilkinson, R. G. (1999). *Social determinants of health.* New York: Oxford University Press.

Marosi, R. (1999, November 28). Pedestrian deaths reveal O.C.'s car culture clash. *Los Angeles Times*, p. A1.

Maxwell, L. E. (2003). Home and school density effects on elementary school children: The role of spatial density. *Environment and Behavior, 35*, 566–578.

Maxwell, L. E. (2006). Crowding. In H. Frumkin, R. Geller, & L. Rubin (with J. Nodvin) (Eds.), *Safe and healthy school environments* (pp. 13–19). New York: Oxford University Press.

Mazzeo, R., Cavanagh, P., & Evans, W. (1998). American College of Sports Medicine position stand: Exercise and physical activity for older adults. *Medicine and Science in Sports and Exercise, 30*, 992–1008.

McConnell et al. (2002). Asthma in exercising children exposed to ozone: A cohort study. *Lancet, 359*, 386–391.

Mizell, L. (1997, March). Aggressive driving. In *Aggressive driving: Three studies*. Washington, DC: AAA Foundation for Traffic Safety. Retrieved July 14, 2006, from http://www.aaafoundation.org/pdf/agdr3study.pdf

Mo, R., & Wilkie, C. (1997). *Changing places: Rebuilding community in the age of sprawl.* New York: Henry Holt.

Mokdad et al. (1999). The spread of the obesity epidemic in the United States, 1991–1998. *Journal of the American Medical Association, 282*, 1519–1522.

Mokdad et al. (2001). The continuing epidemics of obesity and diabetes in the United States. *Journal of the American Medical Association, 286*, 1195–1200.

Mokdad et al. (2003). Prevalence of obesity, diabetes, and obesity-related health risk factors, 2001. *Journal of the American Medical Association, 289*, 76–79.

Moore, E. O. (1981). A prison environment's effect on health care service demands. *Journal of Environmental Systems, 11*, 17–34.

Moore, R. C. (1997). The need for nature: A childhood right. *Social Justice, 24*, 203–221.

Moreno, S., & Sipress, A. (1999, August 27). Fatalities higher for Latino pedestrians: Area's Hispanic immigrants apt to walk but unaccustomed to urban traffic. *The Washington Post*, p. A1.

Morrow, V. (2002). Children's experiences of "community": Implications of social capital discourses. In C. Swann & A. Morgan (Eds.), *Social capital for health: Insights from qualitative research* (pp. 9–28). London: National Health Service, Health Development Agency.

Mumford, L. (1961). *The city in history: Its origins, its transformations, and its prospects.* New York: Harcourt, Brace & World.

Must et al. (1999). The disease burden associated with overweight and obesity. *Journal of the American Medical Association, 282,* 1523–1529.

National Assessment Synthesis Team. (2000). *Climate change impacts on the United States: The potential consequences of climate variability and change.* New York: Cambridge University Press.

National Highway Traffic Safety Administration. (2004). *Traffic safety facts, 2004: A compilation of motor vehicle crash data from the Fatality Analysis Reporting System and the General Estimates System.* (DOT Publ. No. HS 809 919). Washington, DC: Author.

National Safety Council. (2004). *Injury facts* (2004 ed.). Itasca, IL: Author.

Newman, P., & Kenworthy, J. (1999). *Sustainability and cities: Overcoming automobile dependence.* Washington, DC: Island Press.

Noble, C. (1999). Lifeline for a landscape: Baltimore-Washington area. *American Forests, 105,* 37–39.

Novaco, R. (1991). Aggression on roadways. In R. Baenninger (Ed.), *Targets of violence and aggression* (pp. 253–326). Amsterdam: Elsevier.

Novaco, R., Stokols, D., Campbell, J., & Stokols, J. (1979). Transportation, stress, and community psychology. *American Journal of Community Psychology, 7,* 361–380.

Ogden, C. L., Flegal, K. M., Carroll, M. D., & Johnson, C. L. (2002). Prevalence and trends in overweight among U.S. children and adolescents, 1999–2000. *Journal of the American Medical Association, 288,* 728–732.

Oldenburg, R. (1989). *The great good place: Cafés, coffee shops, community centers, beauty parlors, general stores, bars, hangouts, and how they get you through the day.* New York: Paragon House.

Oliver, J. E. (2001). *Democracy in suburbia.* Princeton, NJ: Princeton University Press.

Ossenbruggen, P. J., Pendharkar, J., & Ivan, J. (2001). Roadway safety in rural and small urbanized areas. *Accident Analysis Prevention, 33,* 485–498.

Pack, A. M., Cucchiara, A., Schwab, C. W., Rodgman, E., & Pack, A. L. (1994). Characteristics of accidents attributed to the driver having fallen asleep. *Sleep Research, 23,* 141.

Parker, D., Lajunen, T., & Summala, H. (2002). Anger and aggression among drivers in three European countries. *Accident Analysis and Prevention, 34,* 229–235.

Parry, M. H. (1968). *Aggression on the road.* London: Tavistock.

Patel, I. C. (1992). *Community gardening fact sheet for Rutgers cooperative research and extension.* Retrieved November 15, 2006, from http://www.rcre.rutgers.edu/pubs/publication.asp?pid=FS624

Pietri et al. (1992). Low-back pain in commercial travelers. *Scandinavian Journal of Work and Environmental Health, 18,* 52–58.

Pope et al. (1995). Particulate air pollution as a predictor of mortality in a prospective study of U.S. adults. *American Journal of Respiratory and Critical Care Medicine, 151,* 669–674.

Portes, A. (1998). Social capital: Its origins and applications in modern sociology. *Annual Review of Sociology, 24,* 1–24.

Powell, K. E., Martin, L. M., & Chowdhury, P. P. (2003). Places to walk: Convenience and regular physical activity. *American Journal of Public Health, 93*, 519–521.

Pucher, J., & Dijkstra, L. (2000). Making walking and cycling safer: Lessons from Europe. *Transportation Quarterly, 54*, 25–51.

Pucher, J., & Dijkstra, L. (2003). Promoting safe walking and cycling to improve public health: Lessons from the Netherlands and Germany. *American Journal of Public Health, 93*, 509–516.

Putnam, R. (2000). *Bowling alone: The collapse and revival of American community.* New York: Simon & Schuster.

Randall, K., Shoemaker, C. A., Relf, D., & Geller, E. S. (1992). Effects of plantscapes in an office environment on worker satisfaction. In D. Relf (Ed.), *The role of horticulture in human well-being and social development.* Portland, OR: Timber Press.

Rathbone, D. B., & Huckabee, J. C. (1999, June). *Controlling road rage: A literature review and pilot study.* Washington, DC: AAA Foundation for Traffic Safety.

Redelmeier, D. A., & Tibshirani, R. J. (1997). Association between cellular-telephone calls and motor vehicle collisions. *New England Journal of Medicine, 336*, 453–458.

Retting, R. A., Ferguson, S. A., & McCartt, A. T. (2003). A review of evidence-based traffic engineering measures designed to reduce pedestrian-motor vehicle crashes. *American Journal of Public Health, 93*, 1456–1463.

Roberts, I. (1993). Why have child pedestrian death rates fallen? *British Medical Journal, 306*, 1737–1739.

Roberts, I., Marshall, R., & Norton, R. (1992). Child pedestrian mortality and traffic volume in New Zealand. *British Medical Journal, 305*, 283.

Runyan, C. W., & Casteel, C. (Eds.). (2004). *The state of home safety in America* (2nd ed.). Washington, DC: Home Safety Council. Retrieved October 17, 2006, from http://www.homesafety-council.org/state_of_home_safety/stateofhomesafety.aspx

Runyan et al. (2005). Risk and protective factors for fires, burns, and carbon monoxide poisoning in U.S. households. *American Journal of Preventive Medicine, 28*, 102–108.

Saegert, S. (1982). Environment and children's mental health: Residential density and low-income children. In A. Baum & J. E. Singer (Eds.), *Handbook of psychology and health* (Vol. 2, pp. 247–271). Mahwah, NJ: Erlbaum.

Saelens, B. E., Sallis, J. F., Black, J. B., & Chen, D. (2003). Neighborhood-based differences in physical activity: An environment scale evaluation. *American Journal of Public Health, 93*, 1552–1558.

Saelens, B. E., Sallis, J. F., & Frank, L. D. (2003). Environmental correlates of walking and cycling: Findings from the transportation, urban design, and planning literatures. *Annals of Behavioral Medicine, 25*, 80–91.

Sallis, J. F., Bauman, A., & Pratt, M. (1998). Physical activity interventions: Environmental and policy interventions to promote physical activity. *American Journal of Preventive Medicine, 15*, 379–397.

Sarkar, S., Nederveen, A.A.J., & Pols, A. (1997). Renewed commitment to traffic calming for pedestrian safety. *Transportation Research Record, 1578*, 11–19.

Sattin, R. W., Rodriguez, J. G., DeVito, C. A., & Wingo, P. A. (1998). Home environmental hazards and the risk of fall injury events among community-dwelling older persons. *Journal of the American Geriatric Society, 46*, 669–676.

Schieber, R. A., & Thompson, N. J. (1996). Developmental risk factors for childhood pedestrian injuries. *Injury Prevention, 2*, 228–236.

Serdula et al. (1993). Do obese children become obese adults? A review of the literature. *Preventive Medicine, 22*, 167–177.

Sesso, H. D., Paffenbarger, R. S., Jr., & Lee, I. M. (1998). Physical activity and breast cancer risk in the College Alumni Health Study (United States). *Cancer Causes and Control, 9*, 433–439.

Shaper, A. G., Wannamethee, S. G., & Walker, M. (1997). Body weight: Implications for the prevention of coronary heart disease, stroke, and diabetes mellitus in a cohort study of middle-aged men. *British Medical Journal, 314*, 1311–1317.

Shaw, G. R. (1994, July). Impact of residential street standards on neo-traditional neighbourhood concepts. *Institute of Transportation Engineers Journal, 64*, 30–33.

Shenassa, E. D., Stubbendick, A., & Brown, M. J. (2004). Social disparities in housing and related pediatric injury: A multilevel study. *American Journal of Public Health, 94*, 633–639.

Smart, R., Stoduto, G., Mann, R., & Adlaf, E. (2004). Road rage experience and behavior: Vehicle, exposure, and driver factors. *Traffic Injury Prevention, 5*, 343–348.

Smith, N. A. (2000). *Lighting for health and safety.* Oxford: Butterworth-Heinemann.

Snow, R. W. (2000, January). *1999 National Highway Safety Survey: Monitoring American's attitudes, opinions, and behaviors.* Mississippi State: Social Science Research Center, Mississippi State University.

Spencer, C., & Woolley, H. (2000). Children and the city: A summary of recent environmental psychology research. *Child Care, Health, and Development, 26*, 181–198.

Stanistreet, D., Scott-Samuel, A., & Bellis, M. A. (1999). Income inequality and mortality in England. *Journal of Public Health Medicine, 21*, 205–207.

Staunton, C. E., Frumkin, H., & Dannenberg, A. L. (2006). Injury prevention through environmental design. In L. S. Doll, S. E. Bonzo, J. A. Mercy, & D. A. Sleet (Eds.), *Handbook of injury and violence prevention.* Secaucus, NJ: Springer.

Stokols, D., Novaco, R., Stokols, J., & Campbell, J. (1978). Traffic congestion, type A behavior, and stress. *Journal of Applied Psychology, 63*, 467–480.

Stunkard, A. J., Faith, M. S., & Allison, K. C. (2003). Depression and obesity. *Biological Psychiatry, 54*, 330–337.

Surface Transportation Policy Project. (2002). *High-mileage moms: The report.* Washington, DC: Author. Retrieved October 17, 2006, from http://www.transact.org/report.asp?id=184

Teaford, J. C., & Kilpinen, J. T. (1997). *Post-suburbia: Government and politics in the edge cities.* Baltimore: Johns Hopkins University Press.

Tennessen, C. M., & Cimprich, B. (1995). Views to nature: Effects on attention. *Journal of Environmental Psychology, 15*, 77–85.

Transportation Research Board, Committee on Physical Activity, Health, Transportation and Land Use. (2005). *Does the built environment influence physical activity? Examining the evidence* (TRB Special Report No. 282). Washington, DC: Author. Retrieved October 17, 2006, from http://trb.org/publications/sr/sr282.pdf

Trost, S. G., Owen, N., Bauman, A. E., Sallis, J. F., & Brown, W. (2002). Correlates of adults' participation in physical activity: Review and update. *Medicine and Science in Sports and Exercise, 34*, 1996–2001.

Tuan, Y. F. (1977). *Space and place: The perspective of experience*. Minneapolis: University of Minnesota Press.

Turner, C. W., Layton, J. F., & Simons, L. S. (1975). Naturalistic studies of aggressive behavior: Aggressive stimuli, victim visibility, and horn honking. *Journal of Personality and Social Psychology, 31*, 1098–1107.

Ulrich, R. S. (1984). View through a window may influence recovery from surgery. *Science, 224*, 420–421.

Ulrich, R. S., Simons, R. F., Losito, B. D., & Fiorito, E. (1991). Stress recovery during exposure to natural and urban environments. *Journal of Environmental Psychology, 11*, 201–230.

U.S. Department of Health and Human Services. (1996). *Physical activity and health: A report of the surgeon general*. Atlanta: Author.

U.S. Department of Transportation. (2010). *Transportation's role in reducing U.S. greenhouse gas emissions*. Washington D.C.: Author.

Van Metre, P. C., Mahler, B. J., & Furlong, E. T. (2000). Urban sprawl leaves its PAH signature. *Environmental Science and Technology, 34*, 64–70.

Van Someren, E.J.W., Kessler, A., Mirmirann, M., & Swaab, D. F. (1997). Indirect bright light improves circadian rest-activity rhythm disturbances in demented patients. *Biological Psychiatry, 41*, 955–963.

Wannamethee, S. G., Shaper, A. G., & Walker, M. (1998). Changes in physical activity, mortality, and incidence of coronary heart disease in older men. *Lancet, 351*, 1603–1608.

Wannamethee, S. G., Shaper, A. G., Walker, M., & Ebrahim, S. (1998). Lifestyle and 15-year survival free of heart attack, stroke, and diabetes in middle-aged British men. *Archives of Internal Medicine, 158*, 2433–2440.

Wei et al. (1999). Relationship between low cardiorespiratory fitness and mortality in normal-weight, overweight, and obese men. *Journal of the American Medical Association, 282*, 1547–1553.

Whyte, W. H. (1956). *The organization man*. New York: Simon & Schuster.

Whyte, W. H. (1958, January). Urban sprawl. *Fortune*, pp. 102–109.

Whyte, W. H. (1980). *The social life of small urban spaces*. Washington, DC: Conservation Foundation.

Wilkinson, R. G. (1996). *Unhealthy societies: The afflictions of inequality*. London: Routledge.

Willett, W. C., Dietz, W. H., & Colditz, G. A. (1999). Guidelines for healthy weight. *New England Journal of Medicine, 341*, 427–434.

Zielinski, J. (2000). The benefits of better site design in commercial development. In T. R. Schueler & H. K. Holland (Eds.), *The practice of watershed protection* (pp. 647–656). Ellicott City, MD: Center for Watershed Protection.

12

Creating Healthy Food Environments to Prevent Chronic Disease

Leslie Mikkelsen
Catherine S. Erickson
Juliet Sims
Marion Nestle

LEARNING OBJECTIVES

- Conceptualize the status and health consequences of current dietary trends in the United States.
- Be introduced to the ways in which the agricultural system impacts food choices, nutrition, and the environment.
- Understand how the food environment is affecting food choices.
- Review examples of prevention solutions in several food environments, including schools, workplaces, and communities.

Food is a unique component of life in that it provides the nutrition necessary for our health and survival while also playing a central role in the customs and traditions that add meaning to our lives. Although our need for food is fundamentally biological, we select our diets in the context of the social, economic, and cultural environments in which we live. Our food selections are particularly affected by what and where foods are available, the price of foods, and the advertising and promotion of foods. Taken together, these elements are often referred to as the *food environment.*

Ideally, the food environment would support biological needs, meaning that healthy, nutritious food would be readily available, affordable, and appealing to our palates. Unfortunately, the food environment in the United States today is characterized by a proliferation of heavily marketed snacks and sodas, doughnut shops and fast-food chains, and foods that are highly processed and *supersized.*

This food environment has largely been shaped by the business practices of corporations that dominate the U.S. food industry and by the ways in which these practices interact with consumer preferences. Fierce competition for consumer food dollars has contributed to a proliferation of new foods and beverages formulated to tap into our biological preferences for foods high in calories, especially fat and sugars (Brownell & Horgen, 2004). Social trends, such as women entering the workforce and families moving to distant suburbs (creating longer commutes for parents), have contributed to a demand for quickly consumed convenience and take-out foods. As a result of this interplay between what people want to eat and what the food industry offers, people in the United States are eating more food, more often, in more places. It is increasingly common for people to eat on the go, too, sometimes even in their automobiles.

The impact of this food environment on health is of major concern as the United States faces an epidemic of caloric excess and its health consequences. Primary prevention activities supporting more healthful eating practices are urgently needed. By creating a food environment that encourages and supports diets rich in fruits, vegetables, legumes, and whole grains and balanced in calories, it should be possible to reduce risks in the overall population for high blood pressure, cardiovascular disease, type 2 diabetes, and certain types of cancer.

Although this chapter focuses primarily on the nutritional aspects of the food environment, other aspects of this environment are also important. The dominant industrialized agricultural system that produces cheap raw ingredients for processed food requires heavy use of synthetic pesticides, herbicides, and fertilizers. These kill wildlife and contribute to cancer, birth defects, neurological disorders, and asthma in humans (Sanborn et al., 2004). Concentrated animal feeding operations (CAFOs) are major sources of air and water pollution (International Society for Ecology and Culture, n.d.). The rising prevalence of antibiotic-resistant bacteria has been linked to the routine nontherapeutic use of antibiotics

---

Portions of this chapter are adapted from Nestle, M. (2002). Introduction: The food industry and "eat more." In M. Nestle, *Food politics: How the food industry influences nutrition and health.* University of California Press.

in animal husbandry, which constitutes 70 percent of all antibiotic use in the United States (Mellon, Benbrook, & Lutz-Benbrook, 2001). Furthermore, transportation of produce for an average of 1,500 to 2,100 miles contributes to heavy truck traffic on our highway system and diesel exhausts linked to cancer, asthma, and other respiratory illnesses (Pirog, Van Pelt, Enshayan, & Cook, 2001). Concerns about these issues have increased interest in sustainable food systems and a new social movement focused on production methods that enhance environmental quality, protect natural resources, and provide a livable income and fair working conditions for growers and laborers.

PROMOTING NUTRITION AND SUSTAINABLE FOOD SYSTEMS

Health professionals and nutritionists are increasingly aware of the linkages between nutrition, the food system, and their impact on both public health and the environment. Although nutrition standards and guidelines tend to focus on the nutritional content of foods, there is growing consensus it is not just the nutrient profile that impacts health. Other elements, such as the amount of processing a food undergoes or the farming practices used to produce it, have impacts on nutritional quality, the health of those who work to produce our food, and the environment.

In an effort to create a more holistic definition of healthy food, health and nutrition experts and advocates developed *Setting the Record Straight: Health and Nutrition Professionals Define Healthful Food. Setting the Record Straight* contains a set of healthful food principles that recognize healthful food comes from a food system where food is produced, processed, transported, and marketed in ways that are environmentally sound, sustainable, and just. The principles are intended to be used as a framework for developing programs, shaping community food systems, and advocating for food, nutrition, and agriculture policies that promote health.

Setting the Record Straight's Healthful Food Principles
Healthful Food is wholesome for the following reasons:

- It includes whole and minimally processed fruits, vegetables, whole grains, legumes, nuts, seeds, eggs, dairy, meats, fish, and poultry.
- It contains naturally occurring nutrients (for example, vitamins, minerals, phytonutrients).
- It is produced without added hormones or antibiotics.
- It is processed without artificial colors, flavors, or unnecessary preservatives.

Healthful Food is produced, processed, and transported in a way that prevents the exploitation of farmers, workers, and natural resources and also the cruel treatment of animals. The process of healthful food production adheres to the following principles:

- Upholds the safety and quality of life of all who work to feed us.
- Treats all animals humanely.
- Protects the finite resources of soil, water, air, and biological diversity.
- Supports local and regional farm and food economies.
- Replaces fossil fuels with renewable energy sources.

Healthful Food should be available, accessible, and affordable to everyone in the following ways:

- Distributed equitably among all communities.
- Available and emphasized in children's environments such as childcare, school, and after-school settings.
- Promoted within institutions and workplaces, in cafeterias, vending machines, and at meetings and events.
- Reflective of the natural diversity found in traditions and cultures.

More information is available at www.preventioninstitute.org/sa/settingtherecordstraight.html

For the past several decades, public health efforts to improve dietary intake have been primarily limited to disseminating educational messages about the importance of healthful eating and to building individual skills in food purchasing and preparation. Although nutrition education is always important, it is not sufficient to change eating habits in an environment that promotes consumption of heavily advertised and ever-available processed and fast foods. Given that the current food environment is shaped in large part by food industry practices and government policies, improving health behaviors requires focusing on the very practices and policies of these institutions. People need to know how to make healthful food choices, but it also needs to be easy for them to make such choices.

Transforming the food environment is a multistep process; some aspects of the food environment, such as the busy lives of working families, are not readily altered. It is possible, however, to transform the availability and promotions of food products. Creating food environments that motivate and support individuals to follow nutritional recommendations should make it easier to achieve long-term, broad-based improvements in eating trends.

Furthermore, by adopting more ecologically sustainable production methods, the food system will support both good nutrition and a healthy natural environment.

Recently, public health advocates and practitioners have been working to achieve this type of transformation. They are developing and implementing comprehensive environmental approaches to community nutrition that make healthful foods more widely available in schools, workplaces, and neighborhoods. These strategies derive from those used in other health campaigns (for example, tobacco control to change industry practices, government policies, and community norms).

This chapter describes the current status of nutrition and the food environment in the United States and highlights promising new public health strategies for improving the environment to make healthful food accessible, affordable, and attractive to all Americans.

THE STATUS AND CONSEQUENCES OF CURRENT EATING HABITS

To promote health as effectively as possible, diets must achieve balance. They must provide enough energy (calories) and vitamins, minerals, and other essential nutrients to prevent deficiencies and support normal metabolism. At the same time, they must not include excessive amounts of calories and other nutritional factors that might promote development of chronic diseases.

HEALTHFUL DIETS VERSUS WHAT WE REALLY EAT

Fortunately, the optimal intake range of most dietary components is quite broad. People throughout the world eat many different foods and follow many different dietary patterns that promote excellent health and longevity. As with other behavioral factors that affect health, diet interacts with individual genetic composition as well as with cultural, economic, and geographical factors. On a population basis, the balance between getting enough of the right kinds of nutrients and avoiding too much of the wrong kinds is best achieved by diets that include large proportions of energy from plant foods, such as fruits, vegetables, legumes, and grains, especially whole grains. These diets tend to be relatively low in calories but high in vitamins, minerals, fiber, and other components of plants (phytochemicals) that act together to protect against disease.

Research tells us the American diet is out of balance. On average, people in the United States today are consuming more calories and engaging in less physical activity than in previous decades. This has resulted in caloric imbalances that can lead to weight gain and chronic disease. People are also eating more highly processed, nutrient-poor foods in place of whole plant foods. This has resulted in nutritional imbalances that can lead to deficiencies.

The numbers tell the story. The calories provided by the U.S. food supply increased from 3,200 calories per capita per day in 1980 to 3,900 per capita per day in the late 1990s, an increase of 700 calories per day. These figures tend to overestimate the amounts actually consumed because they do not account for waste, but they give some indication of trends. During the decades from 1971 to 2000, the average daily energy intake for men increased from 2,450 to 2,618 calories and for women from 1,542 to 1,877 calories (Wright, Kennedy-Stephenson, Wang, McDowell, & Johnson, 2004). This suggests a trend toward caloric intakes that exceed the average estimated energy requirements for most adults as recommended by the Institute of Medicine's Food and Nutrition Board (2002).

In the United States, the increased calories come from eating more food in general, especially more of foods high in carbohydrates, such as grain dishes, soft drinks, juice drinks, desserts, and salty snack foods (Wright et al., 2004). At least one-fourth of the calories in the U.S. diet are estimated to come from foods high in refined sugar or fat that contain few micronutrients (Block, 2004). Soft drinks are the single most-consumed food in the American diet, providing 7 percent of all calories (Block, 2004). Heavy soft drink consumption is associated with reduced intake of several important nutrients, including calcium, iron, folate, and vitamin A (Ballew, Kuester, & Gillespie, 2000; Fray, Johnson, & Wang, 2004; Kant, 2000; Kranz, Smicklas-Wright, Siega-Riz, & Mitchell, 2005).

Despite consuming excess calories, most people in the United States are not meeting the nutritional recommendations established by the U.S. Department of Agriculture [USDA], the government agency responsible for developing the MyPyramid food guidance system (USDA, n.d.). The average consumption of whole grain foods is just one serving per day, well below recommended levels. The number of vegetable servings falls short of the recommended five to nine a day, with nearly half the servings (47 percent) coming from just three foods: iceberg lettuce, potatoes (fresh and processed), and canned tomatoes (Wells & Buzby, 2008).

THE HEALTH CONSEQUENCES OF THE CURRENT U.S. DIET

Early in the twentieth century, when the principal causes of death and disability among people in the United States were infectious diseases related in part to the inadequate intake of calories and nutrients, the shared goals of health officials, nutritionists, and the food industry were to encourage people to eat more of all kinds of food. Throughout that century, improvements in the economy affected the diets in important ways: people obtained access to foods of greater variety, their diets improved, and nutrient deficiencies gradually declined. The principle nutritional problems among people in the United States shifted to those of *overnutrition*. In other words, people began eating too much food or too much of certain kinds of food.

This trend has been observed across the globe. It is one of the great ironies of nutrition that the traditional plant-based diets consumed by the poor in many countries are ideally suited to meeting nutritional needs as long as caloric intake is adequate. Once people become more economically advantaged, they enter a nutrition transition in which they abandon traditional plant-based diets and begin eating more meat, fat, and processed foods. By replacing plant foods with nutritionally depleted snacks and treats, people may eat enough or excess calories and yet still not obtain the nutrients necessary for healthy body functioning.

The consequences of this shift are far-reaching. Health experts suggest that the combination of poor diet and sedentary lifestyle contributes to about 365,000 of the 2 million or so annual deaths in the United States, about the same number and proportion affected by cigarette smoking (McGinnis & Foege, 1993; Mokdad, Marks, Stroup, & Gerberding, 2005). The medical costs for just six diet-related health conditions (coronary heart disease, cancer, stroke, diabetes, hypertension, and obesity) exceeded $70 billion in 1995 (Frazão, 1999). The costs of obesity and its consequences were estimated at about $117 billion in 2000 (Office of the Surgeon General, 2001).

Although reversing these trends presents a great challenge, it is worth the attempt; improving eating habits holds great promise for disease prevention. Research has shown that women who follow dietary recommendations display half the rates of coronary heart disease observed among those who eat poor diets, and women who are also active and do not smoke cigarettes have less than one-fifth the risk. Some authorities believe that just a 1 percent reduction in intake of saturated fat across the population would prevent more than thirty thousand cases of coronary heart disease annually and save more than $1 billion in health care costs. Such estimates indicate that even small dietary changes can produce large benefits when their effects are multiplied within an entire population (Stampfer, Hu, Manson, Rimm, & Willett, 2000).

THE FOOD ENVIRONMENT

Every day, most people in the United States make numerous decisions about what to eat. These choices have an important impact on their health and functioning. Unfortunately, so-called junk foods are widely available, heavily advertised, and inexpensive in most people's food environment. Meanwhile, fresh foods are often difficult to find, of poor quality, or prohibitively expensive. The circumstances of work and place also affect individuals' decisions: when time is at a premium, concerns about convenience and cost often outweigh those about health.

Individuals have little direct control over the range of available food choices. Large food corporations are the dominant force that determines the foods we find on grocery store shelves, in convenience stores, and in schools and other institutions. Fast foods that are low in fiber and high in calories have been the primary response to consumers' demand for convenience. In a time of agricultural abundance, the corporate mandate is straightforward: encourage people to eat more food, more often. Although health food remains a niche market, junk food and supersizing are the most effective options for generating profits for shareholders.

To develop comprehensive solutions to address the nation's epidemic of poor nutrition, it is important to understand the complex interaction of the many factors that influence people's choices (and also the choices available to them). This section describes food industry marketing imperatives, how these imperatives influence community food environments, and the context of food choices within the broader food system.

THE U.S. FOOD INDUSTRY AND TODAY'S FOOD SUPPLY

Here we use the term food industry to refer to companies that produce, process, manufacture, sell, and serve foods and beverages. The U.S. food industry is the remarkably successful result of twentieth-century trends that led from small farms to giant corporations, from a society that cooked at home to one that buys nearly half its meals prepared and consumed elsewhere, and from a diet based on *whole* foods grown locally to one based largely on foods that have been processed in some way and transported long distances. Designed for uniformity and long shelf life, many food products are made from highly processed ingredients that have lost their natural taste and nutritional value. Producers rely on added fat, salt, sweeteners, and (frequently) artificial flavors and colors to make these foods palatable.

The U.S. food industry is highly concentrated. In 2002, four companies accounted for 52 percent of the $32 billon total value of shipments in the soft drink industry. Similarly, in the same year, the four largest snack food manufacturers took in 56 percent of the industry's $17 billion in total shipments (U.S. Census Bureau, 2006). In 2003, several U.S. companies, including Philip Morris (Kraft Foods), PepsiCo, and Tyson Foods, ranked among the ten largest food companies in the world (Higgins, 2004). Other U.S. companies, such as ConAgra and Sara Lee, ranked among the top one hundred worldwide companies. These corporations have adopted several techniques to attract customers and maximize profits.

Emphasize Highly Processed Foods and Sweetened Beverages

The food industry produces large numbers of sweet foods and ones that are *energy-dense*, meaning high in calories, fat, and sugar. The human preference for such foods probably has biological origins. For thousands of years, humans had to work hard for their food. It was an evolutionary advantage to consume high-calorie foods during the rare times they were available (Brownell & Horgen, 2004). Such preferences drive the development of new food products, the menus in restaurants, and the allocation of food advertising dollars.

In the United States, food marketers introduce fifteen to twenty thousand new food products every year into a food system that already contains more than three hundred thousand food products. More than two-thirds of new products are condiments, candies and snacks, baked goods, soft drinks, and dairy products (cheese products and ice cream novelties). These products compete for shelf space in supermarkets that stock about fifty thousand products each. Processed, frozen, and baked goods accounted for more than 40 percent of supermarket sales in 2000, while produce represented only 9 percent (Harris, Kaufman, Martinez, & Price, 2002). Most fast-food restaurants follow a similar trend; they feature high-fat meals devoid of fruits, vegetables, and whole grains. Instead, they serve oversized burgers with added cheese or sauces, fried chicken, and pizza.

Supersize It

Marketing methods that encourage people to eat more include substantial increases in the sizes of food packages and restaurant portions (Young & Nestle, 1995). From an industry standpoint, larger portions make good marketing sense. The cost of food is low relative to labor and other expenses, and large portions attract consumers. However, one of the dangers of the increased availability of enlarged portions is *portion distortion*: as portion sizes grow, so do consumers' perceptions of what constitutes a single serving. For example, serving size standards defined by the USDA define a standard serving of grain as one slice of white bread, one ounce of ready-to-eat cereals or muffins, or half a cup of rice or pasta. A marketplace jumbo bakery muffin weighing seven ounces would actually exceed a full day's grain allowances with some left over for the next day, yet a consumer might reasonably believe a single muffin constitutes a single serving.

The practice of *bundling* (adding sides like fries and a soft drink to a fast-food sandwich) is responsible for some of the largest increases in calorie content. Fountain drinks cost the least to add; they provide excess calories along with high profit margins for retailers. Large portions may contribute to weight gain unless people compensate with diet and exercise. Excess calories may also crowd out healthier foods in the diet. Research reveals that adults consume more calories when served larger portion sizes and do not necessarily compensate by decreasing caloric intake at later meals (Diliberti, Bordi, Conklin, Roe, & Rolls, 2004; Ello-Martin, Ledikwe, & Rolls, 2005; Kelly et al., 2009).

Offer Convenience

In the last quarter of the twentieth century, the proportion of women with children who entered the workforce greatly expanded, and many people began to work longer hours and commute longer distances to make ends meet. As a result, many of today's families have less time to shop for, prepare, and serve home-cooked meals (Bowers, 2000).

These societal changes at least partly explain why nearly half of all meals are prepared or consumed outside the home, why fast food is the fastest-growing segment of the food service industry, and why the practice of snacking nearly doubled from the mid-1980s to the mid-1990s (Zizza, Siega-Riz, & Popkin, 2001). The food industry has responded to the demand for convenience by producing heat-and-serve meals; prepackaged sandwiches, salads, entrees, and desserts; "power bars"; yogurt in tubes; prepackaged cereal in a bowl; hot food bars and take-out chicken; and foods designed to be eaten directly from the package. Many such products are high in calories, fat, sugar, or salt but marketed as nutritious because they contain added vitamins.

These food products, and the advertising that promotes them, relegate cooking to a low-priority chore. Even cookbook authors are scaling back their instructions in deference to the growing number of adults who simply do not know how to cook (Sagon, 2006). Nutritionists and traditionalists may lament such developments, but demand for convenience stimulates the food industry to create even more products that can be consumed quickly and with minimal preparation.

Promote Health Benefits

In 1990, the U.S. government passed the Nutrition Labeling and Education Act (NLEA) requiring "nutrition facts" labels on all packaged foods. In return for placing the label on their products, food companies induced Congress to allow them to make two kinds of health claims on product labels: *nutrient content claims* and *claims of health benefits*.

Food manufacturers knew that promotion of nutritional advantages with messages such as "low-fat," "no cholesterol," "high-fiber," or "contains calcium" increased sales, as did the use of health claims ("lowers cholesterol" or "prevents cancer"). They knew that nutrition ranks second after taste as the factor most frequently influencing food purchases (Guthrie, Derby, & Levy, 1999). Because the NLEA allowed companies to say their products were high in vitamins and minerals, the law encouraged the addition of such nutrients to food products. Breakfast cereals, juice drinks, and even candy could bear labels proclaiming "contains 100 percent of ten vitamins" or similar statements, even if most of their energy came from added sugars.

The NLEA allowed claims for health benefits supported by a reasonable degree of scientific substantiation, but FDA efforts to hold such claims to rigorous scientific standards were routinely challenged in court by food companies. Eventually, the FDA was forced to relinquish attempts to require much in the way of scientific substantiation for health claims. In 2009, however, the FDA responded to the outcries of the public and policymakers by addressing the accuracy of a new, standardized *front of package* labeling system.

In the mid-2000s, companies such as PepsiCo and Kraft began to establish their own programs of self-evaluation of the nutritional quality of their products. They set up their own nutrition standards and awarded front of package labels to *better for you* products meeting those standards. Front of package labels of this and other types proliferated. In October 2008, U.S. food producers, including General Mills, Unilever, Coca-Cola, PepsiCo, Kellogg, Con-Agra, Kraft, and Walmart, devised a new front of package labeling system called Smart Choices (Smart Choices Program, 2009) to replace previous industry-specific labeling systems. The labeling system provided a check symbol on the front of packages that passed nutrition criteria developed by the Smart Choices program committee, a coalition of industry, academics, retailers, and other health professionals. Unfortunately, the nutrition standards have been criticized as misleading, allocating Smart Choice checks to products such as Froot Loops, with 12 grams and 44 percent of calories from sugar per serving (Nestle, 2009).

Popular media, academics and government officials were quick to dispute the Smart Choices nutrition criteria for allowing sugar-laden processed foods to make the cut. Richard Blumenthal, Connecticut General Attorney, initiated an investigation of the Smart Choices program in October 2009, while simultaneously requesting the labeling be removed from all products (Blumenthal, 2009). Meanwhile, the popular press reacted in shock that Froot Loops could be marketed as healthy (Nestle, 2009). The FDA was in the spotlight as the public and professionals anticipated their reaction to new multi-industry labels. By late October 2009, the FDA announced they would study consumer responses to front of package labeling to standardize what type of nutritional information is presented on the front of packages (and how) to ensure food labels deliver accurate nutrition information (FDA, 2009). Soon after, the Smart Choices program decided to suspend labeling of new products until the FDA completed its front of package studies and rulemaking (Smart Choices Program, 2009). It appeared as though the FDA, supported by politicians and the public, had begun to exert its authority in regulating the food industry.

Invest in Marketing

The food, beverage, and restaurant industries spend more than $13.4 billion annually on direct media advertising in magazines and newspapers and on billboards, radio, television, and the Internet (Advertising Age, June 22 2009a). In 2008, for example, McDonald's spent $814.5 million, Burger King $326.4 million, Taco Bell $258.4 million, and Coca Cola $253.5 million. Even small products have impressive advertising budgets, as illustrated by expenditures of $103.2 million for M&M'S® candies (Advertising Age, June 22 2009b).

Marketing techniques have now expanded far beyond direct media advertising, with billions of additional dollars spent on *unmeasured media*, such as character licensing, product placement, sponsorship of special events, and school-based campaigns. Although exact expenditures are unavailable, it is clear industry spends tens of billions of dollars on marketing annually; most of this astronomical sum is used to promote the most highly processed and elaborately packaged products. In fact, nearly 70 percent of food advertising is for convenience foods, candy and snacks, alcoholic beverages, soft drinks, and desserts, whereas just 2.2 percent is for fruits, vegetables, grains, or beans (Gallo, 1999). Furthermore, industry disproportionately targets low-income neighborhoods and communities of color (where fruits and vegetables are often less accessible) with its harmful marketing of non-nutritious products (Grier & Kumanyika, 2009; Yancey et al., 2009).

The Federal Trade Commission has estimated advertisers spend $1.6 billion annually marketing food and beverages to children in an effort to encourage lifelong brand loyalty and influence parental purchasing. This number likely underestimates true marketing expenditures because it narrowly defines marketing and does not include industry dollars spent on a number of promotional expenditures, such as supermarket slotting fees or coupon promotions (Federal Trade Commission, 2008). Heavily promoted products are almost universally unhealthy: a recent study found that 97 percent of the industry's child-focused advertisements promote products high in fat, sugar, or sodium (Powell, Szczypka, Chaloupka, & Braunschweig, 2007). Given that most young children cannot comprehend the purpose of advertising or distinguish between television commercials and programming, these statistics are deeply troubling (McGinnis, Grootman, & Kraak, 2006). In fact, despite protestations by industry that marketing plays a minor role in food choice, sales increase with intensity, repetition, and advertising visibility (Novelli, 1990). In its landmark report, *Food Marketing to Children and Youth: Threat or Opportunity?*, the Institute of Medicine concluded that advertising unquestionably influences children's food and beverage preferences, purchase requests, and dietary intake (McGinnis et al., 2006).

THE NEIGHBORHOOD FOOD LANDSCAPE

The U.S. food industry has been highly successful in making snack foods, fast foods, baked goods, and sweetened beverages available at every turn. Many urban areas and suburban malls are dominated by fast-food outlets, making it easy for customers to be attracted by the sights and smells of the latest fad in ice cream, baked goods, or high-calorie coffee drinks. Corporations set specific goals for expanding their presence in new geographical areas and ensuring easy access. For example, Starbucks often places outlets across the street from one another.

Fast-food restaurants deliberately open in areas easily accessed by children and adolescents. Research has found fast-food restaurants to be significantly more clustered in areas within walking distance of schools than would be expected if they were randomly distributed throughout the city (Austin et al., 2005; Simon, Kwan, Angelescu, Shih, & Fielding, 2008). A California study found students with fast-food restaurants located within a half mile of school consumed fewer servings of fruits and vegetables and more servings of soda (Davis & Carpenter, 2009).

Fresh foods are not equally accessible to all neighborhoods. The lack of grocery stores and farmer's markets in neighborhoods where the primary residents are low-income, people of color, or immigrants is well-documented (Chung & Myers, 1999; Larson, Story, & Nelson, 2009; Morland, Wing, Diez, & Poole, 2001; Powell, Slater, Mirtcheva, Bao, & Chaloupka, 2007b). The phenomenon of grocery store flight, which includes the gradual disappearance of grocery stores from inner cities and other low-income neighborhoods during the past forty years, has left the typical low-income neighborhood with 30 percent fewer grocery stores than higher-income areas (Powell, Slater, et al., 2007). This lack of access is compounded by lower household car ownership and nonexistent or cumbersome public transportation options. A number of studies have found that ready access to grocery stores is associated with higher fruit and vegetable consumption (Bodor, Rose, Farley, Swalm, & Scott, 2008; Laraia, Siga-Riz, Kaufman, & Jones, 2004; Larson, Story, & Nelson, 2009; Morland, Wing, & Diez, 2002).

Although grocery stores are the largest purveyors of produce in any neighborhood, they also provide large quantities of junk food. Many grocery stores display junk foods and sodas in high-traffic areas at the ends of aisles or in special displays. Boxes of sweetened cereals featuring toys and popular cartoon characters are placed on low shelves where children can see them. Grocery store chains collect *slotting fees* from product manufacturers to place products in these prime locations (Nestle, 2006).

Schools have not been immune to food industry forces. Formerly relegated to the faculty lounge, vending machines now line the walls of many high schools. Branded fast food is available in many school cafeterias. Those foods and others sold outside the federally funded school breakfast and lunch programs are known as *competitive foods*. Such foods are a source of income for food service departments, school programs, and extracurricular activities. Unlike federally qualified meal programs, competitive foods are not required to meet specific nutritional standards, yet they can be sold in schools as a la carte cafeteria items or through vending machines or school stores and at events elsewhere on school grounds. The most common foods offered are soft drinks, sports drinks, imitation fruit juices, chips, candy, cookies, and snack cakes (Kann, Grunbaum, McKenna, Wechsler, & Galuska, 2005).

Companies, particularly soda companies, have targeted schools for exclusive marketing contracts that prominently feature their products. Most often the corporation donates money or equipment in exchange for the exclusive right to sell its products in schools and to display marketing messages to students.

THE BROADER FOOD SYSTEM CONTEXT

In recent decades, U.S. farm policy has driven down the price of a few farm commodities, including corn and soybeans, through subsidies. The low cost of corn and soybeans, which are used to produce high-fructose corn syrup (a sweetener) and hydrogenated vegetable oil (a fat), has contributed to a proliferation of inexpensive crackers, chips, soda, and candy, among other processed foods, on grocery store shelves. The low cost of corn used for animal feed has also reduced the price of beef and other meats. In the United States, the retail price of fruits and vegetables has increased nearly 40 percent since 1985, while the cost of fats and sugars has declined (Schnoover & Muller, 2006). In this sense, U.S. agricultural subsidy programs are incongruent with the government's nutritional guidelines.

Studies have shown that refined grains, added sugars, and added fats are among the lowest-cost sources of dietary energy in grocery stores, whereas lean meats, fish, and fresh fruit and vegetables generally cost more (Drewnowski & Darman, 2005; Jetter & Cassady, 2005). In restaurants, high-fat, high-sodium fast foods and sugary drinks are relatively inexpensive compared to salads and healthier options. This does not go unnoticed by consumers. In a California survey, about one-third of respondents cited expense as a barrier to eating low-fat foods and fresh fruits and vegetables (California Department of Health and Human Services, 1999). Researchers have shown that reducing the relative price of low-fat snacks and fruits and vegetables stimulates adolescents and adults to purchase healthier products (French, 2003).

This system raises questions of *externalities*, costs that are hidden from consumers. Cheap food has hidden nutritional costs. It stimulates the overconsumption of low-nutrient foods that contribute to chronic disease. Furthermore, cheap food has ecological costs. Government price supports and subsidies for water, fertilizers, and other inputs benefit industrial farms that employ practices that deplete the soil, expose humans and animals to hazardous toxins, and adversely affect health in other ways (Jacobson, 2006).

PREVENTION SOLUTIONS

Although the crises of poor nutrition and caloric imbalance are daunting, there is optimism within the public health community that transformation of the food environment is possible and is indeed beginning to take hold. What is especially promising about the movement for change is that it involves leaders in many fields, including public health, city planning and urban design, sustainable agriculture, transportation, education, and public policy. Pooling expertise and resources, innovative leaders, policymakers, and foundations, as well as advocates, are researching and taking new approaches to address issues. Issues addressed include increased access to healthful and affordable food and decreased availability and marketing of less healthful foods. Leaders are working to identify issues that capture the imagination of the public and methods that will most effectively influence nutrition and physical activity behaviors in a more healthful direction. The following examples describe strategies that hold promise for improving nutrition at the community level.

CREATE MODEL SCHOOL FOOD ENVIRONMENT

To date, much of the energy dedicated to improving the food environment has centered on schools, where 35 to 50 percent of youths' total daily energy is consumed (Neumark-Sztainer, French, Hanna, Story, & Fulkerson, 2005). As parents and policymakers began to understand the scope of childhood obesity and poor nutrition, they started actively pursuing solutions to protect students' short- and long-term health. Though institutional changes generally originated one school at a time through the activism of interested parents and students, early successes inspired broader efforts at the district and state levels. Much room for improvement remains within schools, but progress in the past five years demonstrates food environments can indeed be improved substantially.

In with the Healthy, Out with the Junk

Across the country, individual schools and state and local governments have enacted policies that emphasize offering fresh, nutritious food items to students. For example, changes to meal service in Flagstaff, Arizona, included adding salad bars in secondary schools and fruit and vegetable bars in all elementary schools. The New York City school system is committed to meeting USDA guidelines for all foods sold at mealtimes and in vending machines and is already: serving more fruits and vegetables; limiting beverages to water, milk, and 100 percent juice; and reducing the amount of highly processed foods served (Center for Science in the Public Interest, 2003). To improve capabilities to prepare fresh meals in school cafeterias, communities are remodeling kitchens or passing ordinances stipulating that all new schools must be built with full kitchens (Vallianatos, 2005). In Healdsburg, California, remodeling the kitchen at the local high school was part of an effort to serve fewer branded, prepackaged meals and to prepare more fresh meals on site (California Food Policy Advocates, 2003). Providing adequate time and space for students to eat meals in an unhurried manner has also become a planning priority in some districts (Vallianatos, 2005).

Going hand in hand with efforts to increase the availability of healthy foods are efforts to decrease the availability of junk foods. Many school districts and several states have enacted policies restricting or eliminating the sale of soda and unhealthy snacks in vending machines and cafeterias or reducing the number of hours that vending machines are available. West Virginia was an early pioneer in this effort; it passed comprehensive nutrition standards in 1993 that set limits for the fat and sugar content of all foods sold during the school day (Stuhldreher, Koehler, Harrison, & Deel, 1998). More recently, California passed a bill with stronger standards for fat, sugar, and calorie content that apply to meals and snacks sold anywhere on campus during school hours. A second California law bans the sale of sodas during the school day at elementary, middle, and high schools (California Center for Public Health Advocacy, 2005).

Schools are also making efforts to reduce food marketing and commercialism on campus. The Los Angeles Unified School District, one of the largest districts in California, passed an Obesity Prevention Motion in 2003 that established strict guidelines for the foods and beverages sold during school hours. The motion called for an elimination of contracts and relationships between the district and branded fast-food products. In Mercedes, Texas, the school board has banned all advertising for unhealthy food or beverages on school grounds. In San Francisco, schools are prohibited from using curriculum materials that feature food company brand names (Vallianatos, 2005). Such efforts demonstrate that school districts are finding ways to limit students' exposure to food marketing and to tailor approaches to the specific concerns of their communities.

Bringing the Farm to the Cafeteria Table

Schoolyard gardens and farm-to-school partnerships are emerging as effective strategies for including locally grown, fresh produce in student meals. In addition to introducing students to a variety of fruits and vegetables, many of these programs bridge the gap between cafeteria table and classroom by providing instruction about agriculture and nutrition.

Students participating in schoolyard gardens experience the rewards of watching foods grow and tasting the fruits and vegetables they have tended with their own hands. The *edible schoolyard* at King Middle School in Berkeley, California, provides opportunities for students to grow, harvest, prepare, cook, serve, and eat meals, as well as clean up afterward. Students work while also engaging in conversation with peers and teachers. Teachers of all subject areas use the gardens as a springboard for history, mathematics, language, or other lessons. Today, nearly all of Berkeley's schools have gardens, and a third of these produce vegetables that are included in the preparation of school meals (Finz, 2009).

THE PENNSYLVANIA FRESH FOOD FINANCING INITIATIVE

Recognizing that residents of low-income communities in Philadelphia were experiencing high rates of diet-related chronic disease, the nonprofit Philadelphia Food Trust (PFT) launched an effort to bring grocery stores into low-income areas where access to fresh food and produce was poor. PFT documented the communities' health disparities in the report *Food for Every Child* and concluded the highest-income neighborhoods of Philadelphia had 156 percent more supermarkets than the lowest-income neighborhoods and that the low-income areas of the greater Philadelphia region fell seventy supermarkets short of the number needed. *Food for Every Child* galvanized political support and inspired development of the Food Marketing Task Force.

The leadership task force released another report, *Stimulating Supermarket Development: A New Day for Philadelphia*, with ten recommendations to increase the number of supermarkets in the city's underserved communities by creating a more positive environment for supermarket development. Leaders of the task force, along with two state representatives, pushed for the development of the Pennsylvania Fresh Food Financing Initiative in fall of 2004. A public-private partnership, the initiative serves the financing needs of large and small grocery store operators who plan to operate in these underserved communities, where infrastructure costs and credit needs cannot be accommodated solely by conventional financial institutions.

The first grocery store to be funded under the initiative opened its doors in September 2004. As of June 2009, Pennsylvania Fresh Food Financing Initiative has committed $57.9 million in grants and loans to 74 supermarket projects in 27 Pennsylvania counties. The projects range in size from 900 to 69,000 square feet and are expected to bring or retain 4,854 jobs and more than 1.5 million square feet of food retail across Pennsylvania. In December 2009, U.S. Representative Allyson Schwartz and 32 co-sponsors introduced a National Fresh Food Financing Initiative resolution, based on the Pennsylvania Fresh Food Financing Initiative. The resolution recognizes the need for a national financing program to provide an effective and economically sustainable solution to limited access to healthy foods in underserved communities. It will support private sector efforts to open retail outlets that would provide healthier food options.

The Pennsylvania experience has led to growing interest in fresh food financing among advocates across the country. In 2007, advocates fought to pass a similar bill in California. The bill did not pass due to a lack of state funds. Fresh food financing initiatives are beginning in other parts of the country, including New York State, Louisiana, and Illinois. The Food Trust is currently laying the groundwork for similar initiatives in New Jersey and Colorado and will be expanding this campaign into eight more states across the country during the next several years.

Additional information is available at http://www.thefoodtrust.org

Source: Prevention Institute, with the assistance of Hannah Burton, formerly of the Food Trust.

Schoolyard gardens and farm-to-school partnerships can be as varied as the climates and environments in which they take place. They can also be successfully initiated top-down at the school district level or bottom-up from parents or local farmers.

ENSURE THAT WORKPLACES SUPPORT HEALTHY FOOD NORMS

Just as students need nutritious foods to thrive at school, adults also benefit from the availability of healthy foods and beverages in the workplace. It has long been demonstrated that the physical and social environment of the workplace influences health-related behaviors (Stokols, Pelletier, & Fielding, 1996). As with the enactment of restrictions on smoking, government agencies and health care institutions have taken the lead in improving workplace food environments in the hope that such actions will have a ripple effect, influencing food norms across the community as a whole.

The types of food available in employee cafeterias, in vending machines, and at work-sponsored events frequently determine what people eat throughout the day. Typically, one meal a day is consumed at work, and snacks are often eaten to relieve pressure or during breaks throughout the workday. Applying nutrition standards to all cafeteria meals and vending machine items can provide employees with healthier food options and promote overall well-being. Regulations vary from standards that follow the USDA's nutrition guidelines to those that restrict or completely eliminate junk food.

In Chula Vista, California, for example, the city established nutrition guidelines for all vending machines in city-owned buildings and facilities. These require the machines to be stocked with 100 percent healthy options, including milk, water, juices, and low-calorie snacks (Prevention Institute, 2008). Although vending machines are a logical starting place for many workplaces, a focus on healthy options in cafeterias is equally important. The Cleveland Clinic, one of the nation's top cardiac hospitals, recently revamped its cafeteria menu to include more healthy options and to offer nutritional information to guide purchasing choices.

However, one food source in the workplace is often overlooked for nutritional quality: food provided by an employer at meetings and other gatherings. Often food is used to entice employees to participate in a company event or meeting. Employers can provide healthful, nutritious snacks while still engaging employee participation by substituting healthier food options for high-fat, calorie-dense foods; providing a fruit basket with special, seasonal items; or using nonfood incentives.

ENSURE THE AVAILABILITY OF HEALTHFUL FOOD IN ALL NEIGHBORHOODS

Several aspects of the neighborhood food environment can ultimately influence dietary behavior, including the types of retail outlets present, the product mix offered, the quality and cultural appropriateness of available foods, and the affordability of foods. Community-based efforts to improve neighborhood food environments encompass increasing access to healthy foods while also decreasing the prevalence of unhealthy foods. In today's market economy, improving neighborhood food environments requires the involvement of multiple stakeholders and a long-term outlook.

Attracting Grocery Stores to Underserved Areas

Returning large- and mid-sized grocery stores to underserved neighborhoods is one avenue for increasing access to healthful food. The increased availability of fresh fruits and vegetables is a major factor in increasing consumption, as shown by a landmark study in 2002, which was based on more than 10,000 residents in 221 census tracts and which found that black residents increased fruit and vegetable intake by an average of 32 percent for each grocery store located in their census tract (Morland et al., 2002). In the United Kingdom, a before-and-after comparison demonstrated improvements in dietary behavior following the introduction of a large chain grocery store (Wrigley, Warm, & Margetts, 2003).

Many cities and states are exploring public-private partnerships as a way to meet the public's need for healthy food retailers. Public-private partnerships are agreements between government and private sector organizations that feature shared investments, risks, responsibilities, and rewards. Such arrangements often involve the financing, development, and, operation of food retail outlets (PolicyLink, 2008). Cities such as Philadelphia, Boston, and New York have used public-private partnerships to bring grocery stores into underserved areas (Pothukuchi, 2000). An essential part of establishing grocery stores is developing a strategy to attract retailers and developers to the target community. The city of Chicago markets its development opportunities through Retail Chicago, a program that serves as a single point of contact for retailers and developers, and provides incentives and information about bringing new stores into the City's underserved neighborhoods (Feldstein, Jacobus, & Laurison, 2006).

Although grocery stores and mid-sized stores usually provide quality and variety of foods at affordable prices, they are not a viable solution for all underserved communities. These stores are extremely costly and time-consuming to manage and they often require government subsidies or allowances as well as a suitable building site.

HEALTH CARE WITHOUT HARM

The public health and health care sectors are partnering to bring attention to the links between human health and sustainable food systems. An example of these links can be found in hospital food use. Hospitals and agriculture are not often thought of as being connected, but hospitals feed thousands of patients, staff, and visitors every day and millions every year. It is therefore conceivable hospital food purchasing practices and policies could influence agricultural practices in some of the same ways restaurant practices do. In fact, hospitals can become ongoing and reliable partners in advocating for sustainable agriculture.

Founded in 1996, Health Care Without Harm (HCWH) is a global coalition of more than 450 organizations in more than 50 countries working to transform the health care industry so it is no longer a source of harm to people and the environment. In the United States, HCWH has worked to eliminate the use of thermometers and other medical devices containing mercury and to ensure safer practices for handling medical waste by encouraging hospitals to switch from waste incinerators to safer nonburning waste technologies. HCWH is now applying its success working collaboratively with hospitals to a campaign focused on sustainable food systems. HCWH members encourage hospitals to provide nutritionally improved food for patients, staff, and the general public by adopting food procurement policies that are ecologically sound, economically viable, and socially responsible. By using their buying power to change the ways in which food is produced, health care institutions can demonstrate an understanding of the inextricable links between humans, the public, and ecosystem health.

There are steps health care institutions can take, both small and large, to change their practices and support sustainable agriculture. Many facilities have already switched to purchasing milk produced without using recombinant bovine growth hormone. Hospitals may also consider purchasing foods produced without synthetic chemicals and antibiotics. For example, hospitals can purchase USDA-certified organic foods, which are approved by a government-endorsed certifier to ensure the food has been developed without the use of antibiotics, growth hormones, or most conventional pesticides and synthetic chemicals (USDA, 2002). Saint Luke's Hospital in Duluth, Minnesota, offers certified organic produce at the cafeteria salad bar, serves certified fair-trade coffee, and is in the process of securing antibiotic-free poultry (Marie Kulick, personal communication, July 27, 2006). Buying locally can also become a priority for some facilities: hospitals can work with local farmers or growers' collaboratives to include seasonal and local options on hospital menus. Fletcher Allen Health Care in Burlington, Vermont purchases milk, cheese, and organic produce from area farmers (Kulick, 2005). Other hospitals bring fresh produce to their facilities by hosting regular farmers' markets or creating on-site gardens. For example, Kaiser Permanente's Oakland Medical Center in California instituted the facility's first farmers' market in 2003, providing locally grown organic food as a service to workers and the community. Kaiser now has more than thirty on-site farmers' markets at medical facilities across the country (Kaiser Permanente, 2009). Dominican Hospital in Santa Cruz, California, has its own on-site organic garden that supplies produce for the cafeteria (Kulick, 2005).

By adopting food purchasing policies and practices that support health and sustainable food systems, health care can lead the way in redefining healthy food and increasing U.S. demand for sustainable food products.

More information is available at http://www.noharm.org

Establishing Accessible Farmers' Markets or Farm Stands

Farmers' markets and farm stands are increasingly popular and serve as a valuable source of fresh produce and other goods. Underserved areas particularly benefit from the presence of convenient sources of fresh fruits and vegetables (Conrey, Frongillo, Dollahite, & Griffin, 2003). In addition to supplying fresh produce, farmers' markets and farm stands may offer job training and professional development opportunities for local residents as well as a community space for meetings and entertainment.

Several elements emerge as key to the success of farmers' markets in reaching low-income consumers: price and availability of familiar products, community ownership, transportation to markets, flexible market hours, employment of sales staff from the neighborhood, use of a community organizing approach for outreach, and promotions or sales tailored to the economic level of the community. By supporting small- and mid-range farmers, these farmers' markets help preserve farm lands and promote more sustainable production methods.

To succeed, farmers' markets require a strong customer base. Although such markets have struggled to survive in low-income neighborhoods where the customer base may be limited, they have been more successful on the edges of low-income neighborhoods or in places that draw people of all incomes. Successful markets also depend on Electronic Benefits Transfer (EBT) access for Supplemental Nutrition Assistance Program (SNAP) participants as well as Women, Infants, and Children (WIC) and Senior Farmers' Market Nutrition Program vouchers to pay for produce (Fisher, 1999).

Assisting Small Store Owners in Carrying and Selling Fresh Foods

Families living in underserved communities often rely on small neighborhood stores for much of their daily food. These stores often do not have the space, staff expertise, or equipment to carry fresh produce. As a result, the quality and selection of fresh food offered in small neighborhood stores is often poor. Providing training and incentives to store owners to improve the price, quality, and selection of healthy foods can influence consumption patterns and improve residents' diets.

Strategies have involved identifying ways to help small stores reduce costs and connect with small business development resources, ensuring that small stores are equipped to accept SNAP and WIC benefits, linking stores with local farmers and farmers' markets, and training store owners to purchase and handle produce (Flournoy & Treuhaft, 2005). Training and grants for stores to upgrade storage equipment and enhance store layout and signage and to market changes to neighborhood residents enhance the success of these efforts.

San Francisco high school students participating in a program sponsored by Literacy for Environmental Justice (LEJ), a nonprofit youth organization, launched an effort to improve the availability of fresh foods in the low-income Bayview–Hunters Point neighborhood. After helping one store improve its produce selection to account for 30 percent of overall sales, students, youth, and LEJ staff recruited public and private support for an incentive program for area merchants. The resulting Good Neighbor Project offers benefits to qualifying store owners in energy efficiency, local advertising, business training, cooperative buying, in-store promotions, and participation in branding campaigns. In return, the merchants must agree to stock certain minimum amounts of produce, remove most tobacco and alcohol advertising, and maintain a clean appearance.

The advantages of such programs are that they support small business owners within a neighborhood community. They are also less time-intensive and less costly than programs designed to develop supermarkets. But they require genuine commitments from the store owners to make changes and must address several challenges: it is difficult for small stores to match the low prices, high quality, and selection of larger stores; changing product selection means risking losing profits; and smaller stores are not always valued by community residents.

Partnering with Local Restaurants to Enhance Healthy Food Options

As more and more families consume a greater proportion of their calories away from home, the variety and quality of prepared restaurant menu items increasingly influence consumption patterns. Restaurants are an important element of the neighborhood food environment and have been shown to be potential mediators in patterns of vegetable consumption (Glanz & Hoelscher, 2004). Encouraging local restaurants and carry-out dining establishments to provide healthier dining options, such as offering more selections that include fresh produce and are lower in fat, sugar, and sodium, will expand the ability of families to make healthful food choices.

A number of communities around the country have recognized an opportunity to partner with local restaurants to create healthier dining options. Incentives and technical assistance provided to local restaurants often include the creation of nutritional standards for healthy menu items, assistance with recipe revisions, in-store marketing to highlight healthy items, and broader publicity efforts such as door decals and media attention. The *Steps to a Healthier Salinas* initiative, in Monterey County, California, has successfully collaborated with local taqueria owners to modify menu items and promote healthier options. Since the initiative started, participating taquerias have introduced or begun promoting healthier entrees and sides. Local taqueria owners now see themselves as "gatekeepers for a healthy community" (Hanni, Garcia, Ellemberg & Winkleby, 2009). In Somerville, Massachusetts, the *Shape Up Somerville* program has also prioritized improving healthy options in local restaurants. As of 2009, nineteen restaurants were participating in the Shape Up program, guaranteeing healthy options and benefitting from city-sponsored publicity (Nicole Rioles, personal communication, July 5, 2009).

Limit the Presence of Fast Food Chain Restaurants

In addition to improving access to more healthful foods, advocates and community residents have also sought ways to limit the presence of food retailers that sell predominantly unhealthy foods. Consumption of fast food has been associated with poorer diet quality and increased risk of cardiovascular disease and type 2 diabetes (Smith et al., 2009). Land use and zoning regulations that limit unhealthy food retailers hold particular promise for improving neighborhood food environments. Examples from around the country are as follows:

- Concord, Massachusetts, and Calistoga, California, have attempted to prohibit fast-food outlets and drive-through service restaurants. Warner, New Hampshire has regulated the density of fast-food restaurants by requiring a specific spacing distance between restaurants in its commercial district.
- Detroit, Michigan now requires fast-food restaurants to be located a minimum of 500 feet away from any school site (Mair, Pierce, & Teret, 2005).

The legal basis for these actions is often more to preserve historic town character than to improve health. However, in 2008, Los Angeles, California passed a one-year moratorium on all new fast food chains in the South Los Angeles neighborhood with the express intent to improve community health.

Require Menu Labeling at Fast Food Chain Restaurants

Identifying calorie and nutrition information for items sold at fast food restaurants has long been a challenge, with nutritional brochures often difficult to find or unavailable. Menu labeling laws provide consumers with information they need to make healthier selections, while at the same time motivating restaurants to reformulate their products to be healthier (Center for Science in the Public Interest, 2006).

The Nutrition Labeling and Education Act of 1994 required nearly all packaged foods to display nutrition information; however, that legislation specifically exempted restaurants.

Menu labeling laws address this exemption by requiring chains to post nutrition information on their menu boards where it is clearly visible to customers. Recently, Seattle/King County, Washington, New York City and California have passed nutrition labeling regulations. In addition to the aforementioned policies, numerous other cities and states have introduced or passed menu labeling legislation (National Conference of State Legislators, 2009) and a Federal Menu Labeling Bill passed in 2009 as part of the national health reform legislation.

ELIMINATE ADVERTISING OF LESS HEALTHFUL FOODS TO CHILDREN

Nutrition-related chronic disease is at once serious, widespread, and costly, warranting decisive action to prevent the advertising of less healthful foods and beverages directly to children.

The Institute of Medicine (IOM) has called on food and beverage manufacturers to shift their marketing resources toward significantly healthier items (McGinnis et al., 2006). Historically, however, voluntary industry action has not made a meaningful difference. The Children's Advertising Review Unit (CARU) was established in 1974 to ensure that marketing aimed at children be "truthful, accurate, and sensitive to the special nature of children" (CARU, 2003). In fact, under CARU's watch, during the 1990s, there was a twentyfold increase in spending on children's advertising (Strasburger, 2001). Furthermore, between 1994 and 2004, more than 4,400 new food and beverage products were targeted to children and youth, most of which were high in calories, sugar, or fat and low in nutrients (McGinnis et al., 2006). Given these disturbing trends, IOM now recommends government mandates of necessary changes to industry marketing practices.

Ultimately, the most impactful approaches will include federal legislation or regulation by the Federal Trade Commission. Although there are currently few restrictions in the United States, consumer, public health and parent advocates have recently taken up this issue with renewed interest. Strong policies do already exist in other countries. According to the Center for Science in the Public Interest, more than thirty countries have imposed limitations on television advertising to children, with Australia forbidding advertisements during preschool programming and Norway and Sweden banning advertising during all children's programming. The United Kingdom was the first country in the world to set nutritional standards for food advertised to children on television (Center for Science in the Public Interest, 2007).

Local and state governments can also play an important role in addressing harmful marketing practices aimed at children. Communities across the United States have worked with local retailers to eliminate in-store advertising and ensure that healthier options are actively promoted (Literacy for Environmental Justice Website). Others have successfully removed junk food and junk food marketing from local schools. Nutrition policy advocates are considering new strategies, such as banning cartoon character endorsements of unhealthy products and restricting *giveaways* to nutritious children's meals.

ALIGN AGRICULTURAL POLICY WITH PUBLIC HEALTH GOALS

Although arguments about how best to improve the farm system and the food supply are complex, advocates in agriculture, environmental health, and public health need to explore ways to align government agriculture policies to support more healthful eating patterns and sustainable production methods. The farm bill, which Congress renews every five years, is perhaps the most critical legislation shaping every aspect of our food system (from how foods are produced to what ends up in grocery stores and on our kitchen tables). It presents opportunities to protect farmland, promote production of healthier products, create new market opportunities for farmers, support beginning and minority farmers, and protect the environment. The legislation also includes provisions concerning healthy food retail and federal nutrition programs (for example, the SNAP program). The 2008 Farm Bill benefitted from increased collaboration among advocates who had previously worked in silos to ensure their issues were heard on Capitol Hill. However, opportunities remain to broaden the collaboration, to bring new voices and interests to the discussion, and to shape an agenda that recognizes diverse priorities and reflects our collective stake in food policy.

Beyond the farm bill, opportunities abound to advance regional and sustainable food systems. As communities work to get healthier foods into stores, schools, institutions, and other settings, local and regional farms are an obvious potential source for such foods. For farmers, these markets can serve as an economic lifeline. Local land use decisions are also critical to preserving agricultural land. More local jurisdictions are looking closely at the impact of land use decisions on health. This creates an opportunity to ensure that farmland preservation is at the core of such efforts.

CONCLUSION

The movement to transform the food environment is in its early stages. Public health practitioners, investigative journalists, researchers, policymakers, and other leaders have been making the case that eating habits cannot be changed by information and promotional messages alone. The environment must be changed to facilitate more healthful eating and activity patterns. Many school districts, work sites, government agencies, and health care institutions are making environmental changes to improve access to healthful, sustainably produced food and to decrease the promotion and presence of junk foods. Such local actions constitute the core of a movement to create new social norms in the United States, norms that favor the consumption of fruits, vegetables, whole grains, and legumes, all of which are currently lacking in the American diet. Government regulations as well as voluntary institutional efforts will be needed to propel changes in the food environment that are significant enough to reverse current trends in chronic disease rates related to poor nutrition.

DISCUSSION QUESTIONS

1. Think about what you ate in the last twenty-four hours. What aspects of your food environment do you think affected your food choices? What could be changed about your school, workplace, or community environment that would change your food choices?

2. Do you think you could identify what a standard portion size is? Go to the NHLBI Portion Distortion Quiz and see if you if you have portion distortion (http://hp2010.nhlbihin.net/portion). What do you think motivates food and beverage companies to increase portion sizes?

3. Food and food service companies spend billions marketing their products to children, often with funny, entertaining advertisements and commercials. Do you think the practice of marketing unhealthy foods to children is acceptable? Why or why not? What effects do you think this type of marketing has on children?

REFERENCES

Advertising Age. (June 22 2009a). *Total U.S. measured ad spending by category: 2008*. Retrieved July 14, 2009, from http://adage.com/images/random/datacenter/2009/spendtrends09.pdf

Advertising Age. (June 22 2009b). *Top 200 megabrands: 2008*. Retrieved July 14, 2009, from http://adage.com

Austin et al. (2005). Clustering of fast food restaurants around schools: A novel application of spatial statistics to the study of food environments. *American Journal of Public Health, 95*, 1575–1581.

Ballew, C., Kuester, S., & Gillespie, C. (2000). Beverage choices affect adequacy of children's nutrient intakes. *Archives of Pediatrics & Adolescent Medicine, 154*(11), 1148–1152.

Block, G. (2004). Foods contributing to energy intake in the U.S.: Data from NHANES III and NHANES 1999–2000. *Journal of Food Composition and Analysis, 17*, 439–447.

Blumenthal, Richard. Connecticut Attorney General's Office. (October 29, 2009, updated November 11, 2009). Press Release: Attorney General announces all food manufacturers agree to drop smart choices logo. Retrieved December 18, 2009. Available at: http://www.ct.gov/ag/cwp/view.asp?Q=449880&A=3673

Bodor, J. N., Rose, D., Farley, T. A., Swalm, C., & Scott, S. K. (2008). Neighborhood fruit and vegetable availability and consumption: The role of small food stores in an urban environment. *Public Health Nutrition, 11*(4), 413–420.

Bowers, D. E. (2000). Cooking trends echo changing roles of women. *FoodReview, 23*(1), 23–29.

Brownell, K. D., & Horgen, K. B. (2004). *Food fight: The inside story of the food industry, America's obesity crisis, and what we can do about it*. New York: McGraw-Hill.

California Center for Public Health Advocacy. (2005). *California SB 12 (Escutia): School nutrition standards—summary and California SB 695 (Escutia) healthy beverage bill.* Davis, CA: Author. Retrieved October 18, 2006, from http://www.publichealthadvocacy.org

California Department of Health and Human Services. (1999). *California dietary practices survey: Overall trends in healthy eating among adults, 1989–1997,* Pt. 2. Sacramento: Author.

California Food Policy Advocates. (2003). *Improving meal quality in California's schools: A best practices guide for school meal service.* San Francisco: Author. Retrieved October 18, 2006, from http://www.cfpa.net/obesity/MealQualityReport_May2003.pdf

Center for Science in the Public Interest. (2003, September). *School foods tool kit: A guide to improving school foods and beverages,* Pt. 2: *Case studies.* Washington, DC: Author. Retrieved May 24, 2006, from http://www.cspinet.org/schoolfoodkit/school_foods_kit_part3.pdf

Center for Science in the Public Interest. (2006, January). *Myth vs. reality: Nutrition labeling at fast-food and other chain restaurants.* Retrieved July 13, 2009, from http://www.cspinet.org/nutritionpolicy/Myth_vs_Reality_Nutrition_Labeling.pdf

Center for Science in the Public Interest. (2007, February). *Food marketing in other countries.* Retrieved July 14, 2009, from http://www.cspinet.org/nutritionpolicy/foodmarketing_abroad.pdf

Children's Advertising Review Unit. (2003). *Self-regulatory guidelines for children's advertising.* New York: Council of the Better Business Bureau's Children's Advertising Review Unit. Retrieved June 25, 2006, from http://www.caru.org/index.asp

Chung, C., & Myers, S. L. (Eds.). (1999). Do the poor pay more for food? An analysis of grocery store availability and food price disparities. *Journal of Consumer Affairs, 33,* 276–296.

Conrey, E. J., Frongillo, E. A., Dollahite, J. S., & Griffin, M. R. (2003). Integrated program enhancements increased utilization of farmers' market nutrition program. *Journal of Nutrition, 133,* 1841–1844.

Davis, B. & Carpenter, C. (2009). Proximity of fast-food restaurants to schools and adolescent obesity. *American Journal of Public Health, 99*(3), 505–10.

Dibb, S. (1996). *A spoonful of sugar: Television food advertising aimed at children—an international comparative study.* London: Consumers International.

Diliberti, N., Bordi, P. L., Conklin, M. T., Roe, L. S., & Rolls, B. J. (2004). Increased portion size leads to increased energy intake in a restaurant meal. *Obesity Research, 12,* 562–568.

Drewnowski, A., & Darman, N. (2005). The economics of obesity: Dietary energy density and energy cost. *American Journal of Clinical Nutrition, 82*(Suppl.), 265S–273S.

Ello-Martin, J. A., Ledikwe, J. H., & Rolls, B. J. (2005). The influence of food portion size and energy density on energy intake: Implications for weight management. *American Journal of Clinical Nutrition, 82*(Suppl.), 236S–241S.

Federal Trade Commission. (2008). *Marketing food to children and adolescents: A review of industry expenditures, activities, and self-regulation.* Washington, DC: Author.

Feldstein, L. M., Jacobus, R., & Laurison, H. B. (2006). *Economic development and redevelopment: A toolkit on land use and health.* Oakland, CA: Public Health Law and Policy. Retrieved July 10, 2009, from http://www.healthyplanning.org/toolkit_edrd.html

Finz, S. (2009, May/June). The skinny on school lunches. *California Magazine*. Retrieved July 8, 2009, from http://www.alumni.berkeley.edu/California/main.asp

Fisher, A. (1999). *Hot peppers and parking lot peaches: Evaluating farmers' markets in low-income communities*. Venice, CA: Community Food Security Coalition.

Flournoy, R. & Treuhaft, S. (2005). *Healthy food, healthy communities: Improving access and opportunities through food retailing*. Oakland, CA: Policy Link. Retrieved July 13, 2009, from http://www.policylink.org/

Food and Drug Administration. (2009). Letter to the Smart Choices Program. Retrieved May 3, 2010, from http://www.fda.gov/Food/LabelingNutrition/LabelClaims/ucm180146.htm

The Food Trust. *Grocery store campaign: Improving access to grocery stores in underserved communities*. Philadelphia, PA: Author. Retrieved July 14, 2009, from http://www.thefoodtrust.org/php/programs/super.market.campaign.php

Fray C., Johnson R., & Wang, M. (2004). Children and adolscents' choices of foods and beverages high in added sugars are associated with intakes of key nutrients and food groups. *Journal of Adolescent Health, 34*(1), 56–63.

Frazão, E. (1999). High costs of poor eating patterns in the United States. In E. Frazão (Ed.), *America's eating habits: Changes and consequences* (pp. 5–32). Washington, DC: U.S. Department of Agriculture.

French, S. A. (2003). Pricing effects on food choices. *Journal of Nutrition, 133*(3), 841S–843S.

Gallo, A. E. (1999). Food advertising in the U.S. In E. Frazão (Ed.), *America's eating habits: Changes and consequences* (pp. 173–180). Washington, DC: U.S. Department of Agriculture.

Glanz, K., & Hoelscher, D. (2004). Increasing fruit and vegetable intake by changing environments, policy, and pricing: Restaurant-based research, strategies, and recommendations. *Preventive Medicine, 39*(Suppl. 2), 88–93.

Grier, S. A., & Kumanyika, S. K. (2009). The context for choice: Health implications of targeted food and beverage marketing to African Americans. *American Journal of Public Health, 98*(9), 1616–1629.

Guthrie, J. F., Derby, B. M., & Levy, A. S. (1999). What people know and do not know about nutrition. In E. Frazão (Ed.), *America's eating habits: Changes and consequences* (pp. 243–280). Washington, DC: U.S. Department of Agriculture.

Hanni, K. D., Garcia, E., Ellemberg, C., & Winkleby, M. (2009). Steps to a healthier Salinas: Targeting the taqueria: Implementing healthy food options at Mexican American restaurants. *Journal of Health Promotion Practice, 10*, 91S-99S.

Harris, J. M., Kaufman, P. R., Martinez, S. W., & Price, C. (2002). *The U.S. food marketing system: Competition, coordination, and technological innovations into the 21st century* (Publ. No. AER-811). Washington, DC: U.S. Department of Agriculture. Retrieved July 12, 2006, from http://www.ers.usda.gov/publications/aer811

Higgins, K. (2004, October 4). The world's top 100 food and beverage companies: Diets define profit and loss. *Food Engineering, 76*(10), 58.

Institute of Medicine, Food and Nutrition Board. (2002). *Dietary reference intakes for energy, carbohydrate, fiber, fat, fatty acids, cholesterol, protein, and amino acids.* Washington, DC: National Academies Press.

International Society for Ecology and Culture. (n.d.). *Local food toolkit: Factsheet.* Retrieved July 20, 2006, from http://www.isec.org.uk/toolkit/factsheet.html

Jacobson, M. (2006). *Six arguments for a greener diet.* Washington, DC: Center for Science in the Public Interest.

Jetter, K. M., & Cassady, D. L. (2005, March). *The availability and cost of healthier food items* (Issue Brief No. 29). Davis: University of California Agricultural Issues Center.

Kaiser Permanente. (2009). *Medical center and grocery store.* Oakland, CA: Author. Retrieved July 14. 2009, from http://members.kaiserpermanente.org/redirects/farmersmarkets/

Kann, L., Grunbaum, J. A., McKenna, M. L., Wechsler, H., & Galuska, D. A. (2005). Competitive foods and beverages available for purchase in secondary schools—selected sites, United States, 2004. *Morbidity and Mortality Weekly Report, 54*(37), 917–921.

Kant, A. (2000). Consumption of energy-dense, nutrient-poor foods by adult Americans: Nutritional and health implications. The third National Health and Nutrition Examination Survey, 1988–1994. *American Journal of Clinical Nutrition, 72*(4), 929–936.

Kelly et al. (2009). Increased portion size leads to a sustained increase in energy intake over 4 d in normal-weight and overweight men and women. *British Journal of Nutrition, 16*, 1–8.

Kranz, S., Smicklas-Wright, H., Siega-Riz, A., & Mitchell, D. (2005). Adverse effect of high added sugar consumption on dietary intake in American preschoolers. *Journal of Pediatrics, 146*(1), 105–111.

Kulick, M. (2005). Healthy food, healthy hospitals, healthy communities. *Institute for Agriculture and Trade Policy Food and Health Program.* Minnesota.

Laraia, B. A., Siega-Riz, A. M., Kaufman, J. S., & Jones, S. J. (2004). Proximity of grocery store is positively associated with diet quality index for pregnancy. *Preventive Medicine, 39*, 869–875.

Larson, N. I., Story, M. T., & Nelson, M. C. (2009). Neighborhood environments: Disparities in access to healthy foods in the U.S. *Journal of Nutrition Education and Behavior, 36*(1), 74–81.

Literacy for Environmental Justice. (n.d.). *When it comes to food, what does it mean to be a good neighbor?* San Francisco, CA: Author. Retrieved July 13, 2009, from http://www.lejyouth.org/programs/food.html

Mair, J. S., Pierce, M. W., & Teret, S. P. (2005). *The use of zoning to restrict fast-food outlets: A potential strategy to combat obesity* [Monograph]. Johns Hopkins and Georgetown Universities. Retrieved June 28, 2006, from http://www.publichealthlaw.net/Research/Affprojects.htm#Zoning

McGinnis, J. M., & Foege, W. H. (1993). Actual causes of death in the United States. *Journal of the American Medical Association, 270*, 2207–2212.

McGinnis, J. M., Gootman, A. J., & Kraak, V. I. (Eds.). (2006). *Food marketing to children and youth: Threat or opportunity?* Washington, DC: National Academies Press. Retrieved June 15, 2006, from http://www.nap.edu/catalog/11514.html#toc

Mellon, M., Benbrook, C., & Lutz-Benbrook, K. (2001). *Hogging it: Estimates of antimicrobial abuse in livestock.* Cambridge, MA: Union of Concerned Scientists. Retrieved July 11, 2006, from http://www.ucsusa.org/index.html

Mokdad, A. H., Marks, J. S., Stroup, D. F., & Gerberding, J. L. (2005). Correction: Actual causes of death in the United States, 2000. *Journal of the American Medical Association, 293*, 293–294.

Morland, K., Wing, S., & Diez, R. A. (2002). The contextual effect of the local food environment on residents' diets: The Atherosclerosis Risk in Communities study. *American Journal of Public Health, 92*, 176–177.

Morland, K., Wing, S., Diez, R. A., & Poole, C. (2001). Neighborhood characteristics associated with the location of food stores and food service places. *American Journal of Preventive Health, 22*, 23–29.

National Conference of State Legislators. (July 2009). *Trans fat and menu labeling legislation.* Washington, DC: Author. Retrieved July 13, 2009, from http://www.ncsl.org/default.aspx?tabid=14362

Neumark-Sztainer D., French S., Hanna P., Story M., & Fulkerson J. (2005). School lunch and snacking patterns among high school students: Associations with school food environment and policies. *International Journal of Behavioral Nutrition and Physical Activity, 2,* 14.

Nestle, Marion (2006). *What to eat.* New York: North Point Press.

Nestle, Marion. (December 4, 2009) Food politics blog: Smart Choices. Accessed December 18, 2009. Available at: http://www.foodpolitics.com/tag/smart-choices/

Novelli, W. D. (1990). Applying social marketing to health promotion and disease prevention. In K. Glanz, F. M. Lewis, & B. K. Rimer (Eds.), *Health behavior and health education: Theory, research, and practice* (pp. 342–349). San Francisco: Jossey-Bass.

Office of the Surgeon General. (2001). The Surgeon General's call to action to prevent and decrease overweight and obesity. Rockville, MD: U.S. Department of Health and Human Services.

Pirog, R., Van Pelt, T., Enshayan, K., & Cook, E. (2001). *Food, fuel, and freeways: An Iowa perspective on how far food travels, fuel usage, and greenhouse gas emissions.* Ames, IA: Leopold Center for Sustainable Agriculture, Iowa State University.

PolicyLink. (2008). *Grocery store attraction strategies: A resource guide for community activists and local governments.* Oakland, CA: Author. Retrieved July 10, 2009, from www.policylink.org/

Pothukuchi, K. (2000). *Attracting grocery retail investment to inner-city neighborhoods: Planning outside the box.* Detroit, MI: Wayne State University.

Powell, L. M., Slater, S., Mirtcheva, D., Bao, Y., & Chaloupka, F. J. (2007). Food store availability and neighborhood characteristics in the United States. *Preventive Medicine, 44*, 189–195.

Powell, L. M., Szczypka, B. A., Chaloupka, F. J., & Braunschweig, C. L., (2007). Nutritional content of television food advertisements seen by children and adolescents in the United States. *Pediatrics, 120*(3), 576–583.

Prevention Institute. (2008.). *ENACT local policy database: Public vending machines in city facilities.* Oakland, CA: Author. Retrieved on July 8, 2009, from http://preventioninstitute.org/sa/policies

Sagon, C. (2006, March 18). Cooking 101: Add 1 cup of simplicity—cookbooks simplify terms as kitchen skills dwindle. *Washington Post*, p. A1.

Sanborn et al. (2004). *Pesticides literature review*. Toronto: Ontario College of Family Physicians.

Schnoover, H., & Muller, M. (2006). *Food without thought: How U.S. farm policy contributes to obesity*. Minneapolis, MN: Institute for Agricultural and Trade Policy.

Simon, P. A., Kwan, D., Angelescu, A., Shih, M., & Fielding, J. E. (2008). Proximity of fast food restaurants to schools: Do neighborhood income and type of school matter? *Preventive Medicine, 47*(3), 284–288.

Smart Choices Program. Accessed on December 18, 2009. Available at: http://www.smartchoices-program.com/index.html

Smith et al. (2009). Takeaway food consumption and its associations with diet quality and abdominal obesity: A cross-sectional study of young adults. *International Journal of Behavioral Nutrition and Physical Activity, 6*, 29.

Stampfer, M. J., Hu, M. F., Manson, J. E., Rimm, E. B., & Willett, W. C. (2000). Primary prevention of coronary heart disease in women through diet and lifestyle. *New England Journal of Medicine, 343*, 16–22.

Stokols, D., Pelletier, K. R., & Fielding, J. E. (1996). The ecology of work and health: Research and policy directions for the promotion of employee health. *Health Education Quarterly, 23*, 137–158.

Strasburger, V. C. (2001). Children and TV advertising: Nowhere to run, nowhere to hide. *Journal of Developmental and Behavioral Pediatrics, 22*(3), 185–187.

Stuhldreher, W. L., Koehler, A. N., Harrison, M. K., & Deel, H. (1998). The West Virginia standards for school nutrition. *Journal of Child Nutrition and Management, 22*, 79–86.

U.S. Census Bureau. (2006). *Concentration ratios, 2002: 2002 economic census: Manufacturing, subject series*. Washington, DC: U.S. Department of Commerce. Retrieved October 18, 2006, from http://www.census.gov/prod/ec02/ec0231sr1.pdf

U.S. Department of Agriculture. (2002, April). *Organic food labels and standards: The facts*. Washington, DC: Author. Retrieved July 31, 2006, from http://www.ams.usda.gov/nop/Consumers/brochure.html

U.S. Department of Agriculture. (n.d.). *Steps to a healthier you*. Washington, DC: Author. Retrieved June 13, 2006, from http://www.mypyramid.gov

U.S. Food and Drug Administration (FDA). *Guidance for Industry: Letter Regarding Point of Purchase Food Labeling*. October 2009. Accessed on December 18, 2009. Available at: http://www.fda.gov/Food/GuidanceComplianceRegulatoryInformation/GuidanceDocuments/FoodLabelingNutrition/ucm187208.htm

University of California-Berkeley School of Public Health. (2005, November). Health pitches on packages. *UC-Berkeley Wellness Letter, 22*(2), 6.

Valkenburg, P. M. (2000). Media and youth consumerism. *Journal of Adolescent Health, 27*(Suppl.), 52–56.

Vallianatos, M. (2005, June). *Healthy school food policies: A checklist*. Los Angeles, CA: Center for Food and Justice, Urban and Environmental Policy Institute, Occidental College. Retrieved June 28, 2006, from http://departments.oxy.edu/uepi/cfj/publications/healthy_school_food_policies_05.pdf

Wells, H. F. & Buzby, J. C. (2008, March). Dietary assessment of major trends in U.S. food consumption, 1970–2005, *Economic Information Bulletin No. 33*. Economic Research Service, U.S. Dept. of Agriculture. Retrieved June 30, 2009, from http://www.ers.usda.gov/Publications/EIB33/EIB33.pdf

Wright, J. D., Kennedy-Stephenson, J., Wang, C. Y., McDowell, M. A., & Johnson, C. L. (2004). Trends in intake of energy and macronutrients: United States, 1971–2000. *Morbidity and Mortality Weekly Report, 53*, 80–82.

Wrigley, N., Warm, D., & Margetts, B. (2003). Deprivation, diet, and food-retail access: Findings from the Leeds 'food deserts' study. *Environment and Planning A, 35*(1), 151–188.

Yancey et al. (2009). A cross sectional prevalence study of ethnically targeted and general audience outdoor obesity-related advertising. *Millbank Quarterly, 87*(1), 155–184.

Young, L. R., & Nestle, M. (1995). Portion sizes in dietary assessment: Issues and policy implications. *Nutrition Review, 53*, 149–158.

Zizza, C., Siega-Riz, A. M., & Popkin, B. M. (2001). Significant increase in young adults' snacking between 1977–1978 and 1994–1996 represents a cause for concern! *Preventive Medicine, 32*, 303–310.

13

A Public Health Approach to Preventing Violence

Deborah Prothrow-Stith
Rachel A. Davis
Sidebar Contributors:
Dionne Smith Coker-Appiah,
Mysha R. Wynn, Donald Parker

LEARNING OBJECTIVES

- Define violence, articulate why violence is a public health issue, and reflect upon how violence plays a vital role for the public health field.
- Describe why violence should be prevented before it occurs and the strengths of a population-based approach to violence prevention.
- Explain the role of norms and why preventing violence requires a shift in community norms.
- Use frameworks and tools for planning, implementing, and evaluating community-based violence prevention efforts.

Violence is one of the most serious health threats in the nation today. It is a leading cause of injury, disability, and premature death. It disproportionately affects young people and people of color, and it increases the risk of other poor health outcomes. Violence affects where we live, where we shop, where we walk and where we work; indeed, violence affects whether or not there are shops and jobs in our communities at all.

Most violence is preventable, not inevitable, and we now know what to do to substantially reduce it. There is a strong evidence base, grounded in research, community wisdom and effective practice, showing that prevention works in the following ways:

- Cities with more coordination, communication, and attention to preventing violence have achieved lower violence rates (National Crime Prevention Council, 1999; Prothrow-Stith & Spivak, 2004; Weiss, 2008).
- Schools can reduce violence by 15 percent in as few as six months through universal school-based violence prevention efforts (Hahn, 2007).
- Street outreach and conflict interruption models have shown 41 to 73 percent drops in shootings and killings and 100 percent drops in retaliation murders (Skogan et al., 2008), with the first year of impact regularly showing 25 to 45 percent drops in shootings and killings.

Violence cannot and will not be solved by *after-the-fact* approaches alone. Precedent has framed violence as a criminal justice concern after the fact without also prioritizing what can be done upfront. Increasingly, law enforcement professionals, community activists and others recognize that criminal justice alone has not solved the problem. A prevention approach is needed. Effective prevention involves the collaboration of multiple sectors, looks at environmental factors that contribute to violence, and understands links between the individual and the environment. Given its mandate, skill set, and credibility, the public health field should engage intensively in this work. For example, the public health field can serve as a convener and focal point for community-wide efforts, helping to maintain a fundamental focus on and commitment to identifying programs and policies aimed at preventing violence *before* it occurs. Channeling diverse resources for preventing violence can help ensure the discussion shifts from the historical emphasis on enforcement and suppression to a public health focus on addressing the underlying contributors to violence (see Exhibit 13.1).

Portions of this article by the American Society of Law, Medicine, and Ethics originally appeared in the *Journal of Law, Medicine, and Ethics*. (2004). Reprinted with permission.

EXHIBIT 13.1   VIOLENCE *IS* A PUBLIC HEALTH ISSUE

Violence is a leading cause of injury, disability, and premature death

- 5.5 percent of high school students feel too unsafe to go to school, 18 percent report carrying a weapon on school grounds, 35.5 percent have been in a physical fight, 12 percent report having been forced to have sex, and 14.5 percent report having seriously considered attempting suicide (National Center for Chronic Disease Prevention and Health Promotion, & Centers for Disease Control and Prevention, 2007).
- More than 720,000 young people ages 10 to 24 (Web-based Injury Statistics Query and Reporting System, n.d.) were treated in emergency departments for injuries sustained from violence in 2006 (CDC, n.d.).
- Homicide is the second leading cause of death among youth between the ages of 10 and 24. For each such homicide there are approximately 1,000 nonfatal violent assaults (Bureau of Justice Statistics, 2006).

Violence is a significant disparity, disproportionately affecting young people and people of color

- There are disproportionately high rates of community and street violence in low-income communities and communities of color, and these disparities contribute to overall health inequities in significant ways.
- Among African Americans between the ages of 10 and 24, homicide is the leading cause of death. In this same age range, homicide is the second leading cause of death for Hispanics and the third leading cause of death for American Indians, Alaska Natives, and Asian/Pacific Islanders (CDC, & National Center for Injury Prevention and Control, n.d.). Homicide rates among non-Hispanic, African American males 10 to 24 years of age (58.3 per 100,000) exceed those of Hispanic males (20.9 per 100,000) and non-Hispanic, white males in the same age group (3.3 per 100,000) (CDC, & National Center for Injury Prevention Control, n.d.).

Violence increases the risk of other poor health outcomes

- Violence is a factor in the development of chronic diseases (Feletti, 1998), which account for a majority of premature U.S. deaths, lost productivity, and the majority and fastest growing percentage of our healthcare spending (Thorpe, Florence, & Joski, 2004).
- Violence and safety concerns in some neighborhoods affect other determinants of health, such as whether or not parents will allow their children to be physically active outside or walk to school.
- The consequences of violence for victims and those exposed are severe, including serious physical injuries, post traumatic stress disorder, depression,

anxiety, substance abuse, and other longer-term health problems associated with the biopsychosocial effects of such exposure (Lynch, 2003).

- Many urban youth experience trauma and may have post traumatic stress disorder (PTSD) from exposure to violence. One study found more than 75 percent of urban elementary school children living in high-violence neighborhoods had been exposed to community violence (Hill & Jones, 1997), and other studies have shown that 35 percent of urban youth exposed to community violence develop PTSD.

- A growing body of research confirms the intersection between violence and healthy eating and active living (Loukaitou-Sideris, 2006; Weir, Etelson, & Brand, 2006; Molnar, Gortmaker, Bull & Buka, 2004; Harrison, Gemmell, & Heller, 2007; Sallis, King, Sirard, & Albright, 2008; Eyler et al., 2003; Bennett et al., 2007; Yancey & Kumanyika, 2007; Neckerman, Bader, Purciel & Yousefzadeh, 2009; Rohrer, Arif, Pierce & Blackburn, 2004). Violence, and the fear of it, can undermine attempts to improve nutrition and activity levels, thereby exacerbating existing illnesses and increasing the risk for onset of disease.

UNDERSTANDING VIOLENCE

There are multiple forms of violence, including but not limited to community and street, family, gang, gender, intimate partner, child and elder abuse, sexual, school, structural violence, and violence affecting youth. Although multiple forms of violence are interrelated and share common risk and resilience factors, and although the public health approach provides a framework for addressing these myriad forms of violence, this chapter is focused largely on violence affecting youth, particularly street, community and school violence.

The health consequences for those who are victimized through (or exposed to) violence are severe and can include serious physical injuries, PTSD, depression, anxiety, substance abuse, and other longer-term health problems (Lynch, 2003). In addition, the social impacts of violence (such as diminished academic achievement and worker productivity and the deterioration of families and communities) are substantial and costly, according to Golden and Siegel (Vera Institute of Justice).

Contrary to the stereotype, much of the violence experienced in the United States occurs among people who are not strangers. A typical homicide in the United States involves two people who know each other, are under the influence of alcohol, get into an argument, and have handguns. In homicides of children and adolescents (0–17) in the United States, 22 percent are killed by a parent, 5 percent by another family member, 36 percent by an acquaintance and 11 percent by a stranger (Snyder & Sickmund, 1999). Even in the unlikely situation where all of the 26 percent of the remaining homicides, classified as an *unknown relationship*, were committed by strangers, this means that 74 percent of all homicides are committed by family, friends, and acquaintances.

In the case of violence against women, the acquaintance nature of violent injury is even more compelling. According to the 2000 National Crime Victimization Survey, 62 percent of rapes and sexual assaults came at the hands of a person the female victim called a friend or acquaintance, and 18 percent of attackers were identified as intimate partners (National Institute of Justice, 2000). In the National Violence against Women Survey, 25 percent of women said that current or former spouses, a cohabiting partner, or a date had raped or physically assaulted them during their lifetime (Tjaden & Thoennes, 2000).

INDIVIDUAL RESPONSIBILITY AND THE CRIMINAL JUSTICE LENS

Historically, society has relied almost exclusively on the criminal justice system to respond to violence. This approach has been well-rooted in a few assumptions, such as: (1) violence is an individual's criminal choice, (2) punishment or the threat of punishment is a deterrent to violent acts, and (3) violence is an inevitable aspect of the behaviors of some people. Police, prosecutors, public defenders, judges, probation officers, and prison guards are part of a sophisticated system designed to respond to crimes after they have been committed by identifying, apprehending, prosecuting, punishing, and controlling the violent offender. Those who respond to crimes are not typically working to prevent crimes. The efforts to reduce violence that are a part of the criminal justice system are found in the passage of laws and in the deterrence resulting from enforcement.

Viewed from the perspective of those interested in preventing violence, the criminal justice system's responses have had only limited success. Inherent limitations in the reactive nature of the criminal justice system are partly responsible. *Deterrence*, the mainstay violence reduction strategy, has limited prevention capacity (particularly in the context of the most common forms of violence, which occur among acquaintances and family). *Rehabilitation*, a form of prevention, is offered after a conviction and at variable levels of implementation from state to state.

Although the juvenile justice system was created with a fundamental belief in the potential for prevention and rehabilitation among children, its major responsibility is punishment. Many states are eliminating specialized juvenile justice systems for criminal offenses and incorporating youth into the adult criminal process.

Police activities and many of the laws officers enforce are geared toward predatory violence that occurs among strangers on the street. As a result, the many episodes of violence among family, friends, and acquaintances that emerge from insults, frustrations, and festering disputes and that take place in intimate settings are less well addressed. The significant presence of acquaintances, friends, and family among the perpetrators of violent injury (rape, assaults, and homicides) begs for strategies beyond aggressive traditional efforts that blame and punish. It creates the need for a more comprehensive set of prevention activities as well (for example, changes in social norms, organizational practice, public education, and policy) and creates the context for cooperation between public health, criminal justice, and other partners.

FOSTERING A NEW PARADIGM TO PREVENT VIOLENCE

Traditional views of violence, and the intervention approaches in response, failed to reflect the complexity of violence or to incorporate a perspective that moves beyond individual responsibility and toward a community-centered approach to prevention. Recognizing this gap, the National Center for Injury Prevention and Control (2001) at the United States' Centers for Disease Control and Prevention (CDC) developed a new, expanded definition of violence within the public health profession in 2001. The CDC classifies both *unintentional injuries* (accidents) and *intentional injuries* (violence) as public health problems, as illustrated in Figure 13.1. Figure 13.2 shows that intentional injuries are divided into *self-directed violence* (suicides and suicide attempts) and *interpersonal violence* (assaults and homicides). Violence is defined by the CDC as "the threatened or actual use of physical force or power against another person, against oneself, or against a group or community that either results or is likely to result in injury, death, or deprivation."

The CDC's definition of violence highlights the breadth of behaviors involved, which are not limited to physical violence. This definition also avoids the labels of *perpetrator* and *victim* that have been traditionally assigned based on the outcome of a fight (where the person more injured is often labeled as the victim), and which showed very little regard for the events leading up to the event, the roles of participants, or the situation's environmental contributions. Because public health is concerned with prevention and reduction of risk factors, the labels victim and perpetrator, particularly with regard to youth violence, are less helpful. Behaviors like spanking children, tackling on the football field, and playing rough among peers all illustrate the importance of the interpretation by the recipient of the action.

Figure 13.1   Classification of injury in public health

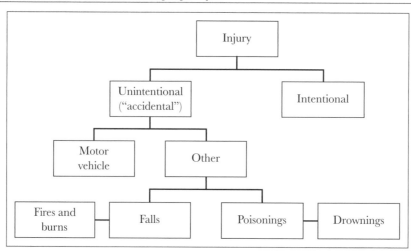

Figure 13.2   Two categories of intentional injuries in public health

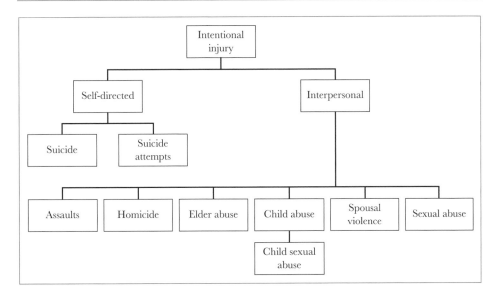

Effectively preventing violence *before* it occurs involves comprehensive and multi-disciplinary efforts to address the complex underlying contributors to violence and builds resilience in youth, families, and communities. This is a *public health approach to preventing violence*. The public health approach to youth violence is similar to the public health approach to all other injuries. It involves data collection and analysis, identifying the populations and locations at greatest risk, identifying risk and protective factors, and developing and using evidence-based strategies and programs to address violence at the individual, family, community and societal levels. The movement to prevent violence is actually broader than public health in concept and in participation, but is based on some fundamental public health tenets, including the following:

- **Prevention orientation**: efforts designed to prevent violence before it occurs, reduce risks, and reduce likelihood of recurrence
- **Resilience-building**: focusing on individual, family, and community strengths
- **Collaborative orientation**: multiple partners from public health, law enforcement, education, recreation, economic development, mental health, substance abuse, business, and other disciplines work together to produce change
- **Data-driven**: approaches based on data that helps identify the nature and location of the problem, contributing risk and resilience factors, and the solutions that have been shown to be effective
- **Population-based**: seeking community-wide or *environmental* solutions and recognizing that community environments can be a key element in shaping behaviors.

THE ROLE OF NORMS IN THE NEW PARADIGM

As stated above, the emphasis on population-based strategies is key for effective prevention. Changing the environment is a mechanism for changing norms and resulting behaviors broadly across communities. Changes in tobacco laws (with public health professionals in a leadership role) changed the community environment and thus reduced the number of smokers. The same environment-changing paradigm can and should be applied to violence. People generally conform to certain behavioral conventions and disapprove of deviance from the norms (Ullmann-Margalit, 1990). Norms are not simply habits. Often based in culture and tradition, they are attitudes, beliefs, and standards we take for granted. In other words, norms pattern our behavior and function as environmental signals that tell people what is okay and not okay to do. Norms describe what actually occurs (that is to say, are descriptive) and also signify a standard of proper behavior (that is to say, are normative or prescriptive) (Margolis, 1990).

A prevention strategy must account for norms because these standards are pervasive, powerful determinants of behavior. If violence is typical, expected, and reinforced by the media, family, community, peers, or school, it is far more likely to occur. It will occur, in fact, with greater frequency and potency. If norms discourage safe behavior and are unsupportive of healthy and safe relationships, then programs focused on change at the individual level will not produce safe behavior unless social norms are changed as well. Thus, changing norms is critical to preventing violence.

NORMS AND VIOLENCE AGAINST WOMEN

There are at least five damaging norms that contribute to violence against women:

1. Narrow male roles, where society promotes domination, exploitation, objectification, control, oppression, and dangerous, risk-taking behavior in men and boys, often victimizing women and girls.

2. Limited female roles, where from a young age females are often encouraged, through subtle and overt messages, to act and be treated as objects, used and controlled by others.

3. Power, where value is placed on claiming and maintaining control over others.

4. Violence, where aggression is tolerated and accepted as normal behavior and can be used as a way to solve problems and get what one wants.

5. Privacy and secrecy, where notions of individual and family privacy foster secrecy and silence, and certain topics (such as child sexual abuse) are considered taboo and thus not discussed.

A PREVENTION CONTINUUM

Devising conceptual frameworks can alleviate interprofessional tension, facilitate definitions of roles in addressing the problem, and assist in developing a broader perspective on programmatic strategies involved in breaking the spectrum of violence into levels that reflect different points of intervention. This framework, used frequently in public health circles, structures approaches to problems into three stages: primary prevention, secondary prevention (or early intervention), and tertiary prevention (or treatment and rehabilitation). These distinctions have proved valuable in thinking about intervention efforts even though their boundaries are not discrete. In this discussion, it might be best to think of these distinctions in terms of concentric circles that widen out in space and time from a central point, which is the occurrence of some violent event.

In a prevention planning process focused on community street violence, Philadelphia youth renamed the prevention elements as *Upfront, In the Thick*, and *Aftermath*, respectively.

Upfront, or primary prevention, explicitly focuses on action *before* there are symptoms and includes strategies every community or everyone needs. Examples include developing positive social connections in neighborhoods; committing to economic development; reducing the availability of firearms; providing quality early care and education, parenting skills, and after-school programming; and training youth in conflict resolution and leadership.

In the Thick, or secondary prevention, relies on the presence of risk factors to determine action, focusing on the more immediate responses *after* symptoms or risks have appeared. Secondary prevention is aimed at those communities and individuals who may be at increased risk for violence. Examples include street outreach and violence interruption, family support services, and mentoring.

Aftermath, or tertiary prevention, focuses on *longer-term* responses to deal with the consequences of violence after it has occurred to reduce the chances it will reoccur. Examples include successful reentry, restorative justice, and mental health services (for example, therapeutic foster care, functional family therapy, and multisystemic therapy).

UNITY STRATEGIES TO PREVENT VIOLENCE

As part of a national initiative to prevent violence entitled UNITY (Urban Networks to Increase Thriving Youth), city representatives and young people identified a set of key strategies throughout the prevention continuum that would support violence prevention efforts in cities and that should be prioritized nationally to strengthen violence prevention resources and policies. Key strategies are summarized in Table 13.1, and the UNITY RoadMap follows.

Table 13.1   Prioritized Strategies to Prevent Violence

Primary Prevention: Upfront	Secondary Prevention: In the Thick	Tertiary Prevention: Aftermath
Positive early care and education	Mental health services**	Mental health services
Positive social and emotional development	Family support services	Successful reentry
Parenting skills	Street outreach and conflict interruption	
Mentoring		
Quality after school programming		
Conflict resolution		
Youth leadership		
Social connections in neighborhoods		
Quality education* (including universal school-based violence prevention strategies and bullying prevention)		
Economic development*		

* For broad categories that are largely under the purview and mandate of specific agencies, the focus should be on delineating the elements within that category that will specifically address violence.
** For example, therapeutic foster care

THE UNITY ROADMAP: A FRAMEWORK FOR OUTCOMES

The UNITY RoadMap is a framework for mapping out solutions to effectively and sustainably prevent violence. It was developed after the UNITY City Assessment—conducted with mayors, police chiefs, public health directors, and school superintendents—revealed that although youth violence is a serious concern, cities generally characterize their responses as inadequate. The RoadMap builds on similarly complex tools that have been effective for other challenging issues. In fact, many of the categories were drawn from the AIDS Program Efforts Index (API) developed by The POLICY project, USAID, and UNAIDS to measure the effort put into national HIV/AIDS programs throughout the world. Various components of the UNITY RoadMap have undergone a literature review and/or been informed by interviews with violence prevention practitioners and city representatives. The RoadMap has been reviewed by city representatives and refined accordingly.

The UNITY RoadMap highlights key components of an urban approach to effectively and sustainably prevent violence before it occurs. These elements are reflected in the UNITY Urban Agenda and in the work of members of the UNITY City Network. Organized by partnerships, prevention, and strategy, the RoadMap comprises nine elements, each selected for its importance in affecting and sustaining efforts to prevent violence before it occurs.

Partnerships (Who)

- *High-level leadership.* The mayor and other local leaders insist that the violence stops, provide necessary supports and resources, and hold people accountable.
- *Collaboration and staffing.* There is a formal structure for multidisciplinary collaboration to coordinate priorities and actions across multiple jurisdictions, and there is dedicated staffing in place to support collaboration and implement priorities.
- *Community engagement.* Members of the community—youth and adults, community-based organizations, the faith community, the business sector, and survivors—are actively engaged in setting priorities and participating in ongoing activities.

Prevention (What)

- *Programs, organizational practices, and policies.* There are effective and far-reaching efforts in place to prevent violence, particularly in highly affected neighborhoods.
- *Training and capacity building.* Participants, practitioners, and policymakers have the skills and capacities necessary to work across multiple disciplines and in partnership with communities to implement effective prevention programs, policies, and practices.
- *Communication.* The case has been made for preventing violence before it occurs, and people are aware of what's being done to prevent it.

Strategy (How)

- *Strategic plan.* There is a plan in place that prioritizes prevention, is well known, and informs priorities and actions for multiple departments, agencies, jurisdictions, and community groups.

- *Data and evaluation.* Efforts are informed by data and continuously improved through ongoing evaluation.
- *Funding.* Adequate resources support collaboration and staffing; community engagement; the implementation of programs, policies, and practices; skills development and capacity building; communications; strategic planning; and data and evaluation.

For more information, visit http://preventioninstitute.org/component/jlibrary/article/id-30/288.html

PRIMARY PREVENTION IN ACTION

Using primary prevention approaches to preventing violence requires addressing the multiple risk factors associated with violence, including poverty, unemployment, discrimination, substance abuse, educational failure, fragmented families, domestic abuse, internalized shame, and felt powerlessness. Preventing violence requires shifting community norms, some of the most powerful societal and community influences in shaping behavior. Efforts to prevent violence build on resilience in individuals, families, and communities and are distinct from violence containment or suppression. Preventing violence contributes to empowerment, educational and economic progress, and improved life management skills, while fostering healthy communities in which people can grow in dignity and safety. Finally, efforts shift policies and realign institutions to be more inclusive and receptive in responding to community needs. Key elements of putting primary prevention in action include: prioritizing key risk and resilience factors, convening community partners, and developing a multifaceted plan.

Prioritizing Key Risk and Resilience Factors

Underlying risk and resilience factors contribute to violence or its prevention. *Risk factors* are community, family, or individual characteristics or circumstances that increase the likelihood violence will occur. *Resilience factors* are community, family, or individual characteristics or circumstances that reduce the likelihood violence will take place, in spite of the presence of risk factors. Research shows that, like risk, the effects of resilience factors accumulate; those with more factors are less likely to engage in violence and other high-risk behaviors. Having more resilience factors also increases the chances young people will have positive attitudes and behaviors, such as good health, success in school, self-control, and value for diversity (Search Institute, 2002). As shown in Table 13.2, a growing body of research demonstrates the interrelationship between risk and resilience (Pollard, Hawkins, & Arthur, 1999), the ability of resiliency to mitigate the effect of some risks (Bradley et al. 1994; Smith, Lizotte, Thornberry, & Krohn, 1995), and the importance of focusing on both sets of factors (Smith, Lizotte, Thornberry, & Krohn, 1995). Indeed, building community resilience factors can counteract the negative effects of risk factors.

Table 13.2   Risk and resilience factors for violence and preventing violence

	Risk Factors	Resilience Factors
Community	Diminished economic opportunities, including economic disparity, poverty, and high concentrations of poverty Low levels of community participation Discrimination and oppression Firearms Availability of alcohol and other drugs Community deterioration, including blight, graffiti, vacant buildings and lots Housing issues, including high levels of transiency Incarceration and reentry Low levels of community participation	Economic capital, including living wage opportunities and ability to access capital Social capital, including strong social networks and trust and willingness of the community to act on its own behalf Meaningful opportunities for participation Positive ethnic, racial, and intergroup relations Built environment, including absence of blight and graffiti, good lighting, and community design that fosters interaction Artistic and creative opportunities
School	Illiteracy School system failure Truancy Bullying	High graduation rates Positive school climate School connectedness High expectations
Family	Negative family dynamics, such as poor family functioning, high level of family disruption, and family violence Poor discipline practices, such as authoritarian childrearing attitudes and harsh, lax, or inconsistent disciplinary practices Parental substance abuse or mental illness Parental criminality and/or incarceration Unengaged parents, as reflected by low parental involvement in educational and other activities and poor monitoring and supervision of children	Positive parenting skills Engaged family members, including frequent shared activities with parents and consistent presence of parent during at least one of the following events: when awakening, when arriving home from school, during evening meal, or when going to bed Strong attachments, including connectedness to family or adults outside the family Structured home environments that offer predictable consequences

Table 13.2   (*Continued*)

	Risk Factors	Resilience Factors
Individual	Mental illness and trauma, including experiencing and witnessing violence and high emotional distress Substance use or abuse, including involvement with drugs, alcohol, or tobacco Peer relations, including association with delinquent peers and social rejection by peers Lack of involvement in conventional activities School problems, including poor academic performance, school failure, and low commitment to school Antisocial beliefs and attitudes	Mental health Positive attachments and relationships (including with family and peers) and ability to discuss problems with parents Emotional and cognitive competence, including the ability to regulate emotions and impulses and to have empathy for others Involvement in social activities Religiosity, including participation in organized religion

SAMPLE COMMUNITY-LEVEL STRATEGIES TO PREVENT VIOLENCE

- *Alcohol availability*. Decrease the density of alcohol outlets and advertising in neighborhoods afflicted with high crime and violence.
- *Conflict resolution*. Create proactive dispute resolution structures and support at the neighborhood level.
- *Economic opportunity and employment*. Enhance economic development opportunities in communities most impacted by violence and for individuals and families most at risk for violence, including those individuals reentering the community. Implement *Ban the Box* policies so formerly incarcerated individuals are not restricted from employment opportunities. Expand the involvement of local businesses to create employment services such as job skills training, placement programs for youth and formerly incarcerated individuals, and assistance in the reentry process. Tie job training and placement programs for community residents to neighborhood beautification and maintenance. Expand meaningful employment opportunities for youth, including those within local government, churches, businesses, and community organizations through career fairs, information sharing, career clubs, mentoring

programs, vocational training, widespread internships, and apprenticeships. Expand the availability of job training opportunities, including the incorporation of job skills training into high school curricula with linkages to internships and mentors.

- *Firearms.* Reduce the availability and usage of firearms through policy and norms change.
- *Physical appearance.* Improve the physical appearance of neighborhoods by fostering arts programs and community gardens, improving park and neighborhood maintenance, and removing graffiti and blight.
- *Restorative justice.* Implement restorative justice programs with community organizations and the justice system.
- *Reentry.* Create more viable connections between communities and inside detention facilities, provide incentives for hiring ex-felons, and support transition from detention to the community through mental health services, substance abuse treatment, job training and employment services, and support for family members.
- *Social connectedness.* Support communities to foster strong social connections and to heal from community violence, while translating fear and anger into action to prevent future violence. Strengthen ties among neighbors and community members. Strong ties are characterized by trust, concern for one another, and a willingness to take collective action for the community good, including increased social sanctions against violent behaviors.
- *Street outreach.* Reduce violence, injury, and lethality through detection, interruption, and de-escalation with help from street outreach workers in highly impacted neighborhoods; outreach workers can help change the thinking and behaviors of the highest-risk people.

Sample School-Level Strategies to Prevent Violence

- *Bullying.* Intervene in early bullying behavior and address underlying causes. Effective bullying prevention includes a focus not only on aggressors but also on victims, bystanders, and the climate in which bullying could occur.
- *School climate.* Foster safe and positive school climates for all students and school staff by valuing safety, academic achievement, and positive youth development. Examples of desirable features of schools include physical and psychological safety, appropriate structure, supportive relationships, opportunities to belong, positive social norms, support for efficacy and mattering, opportunities for skill building, and integration of family, school, and community efforts; enhancing trust and communication between adults on campus and youth; and increasing adult involvement and presence on

school campuses (for example, school resource officers, social workers, and counselors).

- *School connectedness.* Foster school connectedness through opportunities for parental and caregiver involvement within a welcoming environment; provide meaningful activities that appeal to multiple interests and skills, and support constructive engagement rather than exclusion and punishment.
- *School-linked services.* Link community services through school sites to increase opportunities for participation by providing services where young people and their families are and to reduce duplication.
- *Universal school-based violence prevention.* Teach all students in a school (or in a grade in school) about the problems of violence and its prevention or about one or more of the following topics or skills intended to reduce aggressive or violent behavior: emotional self-awareness, emotional control, and self-esteem; positive social skills; social problem solving; conflict resolution; and teamwork.

CONVENING COMMUNITY PARTNERS

Encouraging collaboration among community partners early in a planning process will serve to build a common understanding and language, forge a shared vision, and enhance buy-in for selected strategies. Prioritization of key risk and resilience factors can indicate which partners to further involve in planning and implementation. Potential partners can be drawn from local government (such as law enforcement, probation, schools, and public health), community organizations (such as businesses, community-based organizations, faith institutions, health care providers, media, and youth development organizations), and members of the community (such as youth, families, caregivers, former gang members, formerly incarcerated individuals, and survivors of violence).

It is vital that collaborative efforts garner strong community participation. Community members—particularly youth and adults from neighborhoods highly affected by violence—should help define and prioritize the problems, design and implement a strategic plan, and advance collaborative efforts. Community engagement, input, and leadership are critical in ensuring that planning, programming, and policies will best meet community needs and that they will encourage equitable outcomes. Meaningful community engagement can help build the capacity of individuals, organizations, and communities to forge solutions for their community (Hambleton, Clark, Sumaya, Weissman, & Horner, 1997; Bowen, Gwiasda, & Brown, 2004).

DEVELOPMENT OF A MULTIFACETED PLAN

Because violence is complex, it requires a comprehensive approach. A critical aspect of a comprehensive approach is having a multifaceted strategy, meaning multiple complementary activities affecting individuals, communities, organizations, and policies. Traditional methods have focused solely on individual or educational approaches, but a public health approach necessitates addressing broader environmental and systems-level issues as well. Developing multiple strategies that build on one another maximizes the results of each activity and produces a more effective strategy than would be possible by implementing a single initiative or program in isolation. Each community will develop a unique approach that addresses its own risks and builds on its existing strengths.

COMMUNITY EXAMPLES OF PREVENTING VIOLENCE

The City of Minneapolis has documented significant decreases in juvenile crime since implementing its four-point, public health-based *Violence Prevention Blueprint for Action*. In the Minneapolis precinct that includes four neighborhoods targeted in the *Blueprint*, juvenile crime dropped 43 percent from 2006 to 2008 (Minneapolis Police Department, 2008). This measured success is in part the byproduct of the totality of strategies, relationships, and efforts undertaken by city, community and law enforcement entities.

The *CeaseFire Chicago* model has been replicated sixteen times and has been validated by a three-year U.S. Department of Justice study conducted by four universities. The study shows 41 to 73 percent drops in shootings and killings and 100 percent drops in retaliation murders (Skogan, Harnett, Bump, & Dubois, 2008). The first year of impact regularly shows 25 to 45 percent drops in shootings and killings. The return of businesses have been seen in these neighborhoods (Skogan, Harnett, Bump, & Dubois, 2008).

Through targeted outreach, the Boys and Girls Clubs of America's Gang Prevention Program has markedly impacted community violence. Other community groups refer at-risk boys to the program, who are then recruited. Early evaluations of these programs showed promise: data indicated that 39 percent of the boys did better at school and 93 percent of those who completed the program had not been further involved with the juvenile justice system (Arbreton & McClanahan, n.d.). These types of interventions reflect an important interface between the criminal justice and public health professions. With further attention, with the dedication of resources of the public health system to this issue, and with the broadening vision of criminal justice, a more reasonable balance between prevention and treatment can be achieved.

Boston, Massachusetts, with its dramatic and sustained decline in youth violence, serves as a model of multilevel programmatic activity with exemplary integration between public health and policing strategies (Prothrow-Stith & Spivak, 2004). Two decades of activities within public health and criminal justice, and most important within the broader community of parents, teens, and survivors of violence, have resulted in the creation of an extensive set of programs for youth throughout the city. Boston's efforts reflect the range needed to reduce the extent of violent behavior and to respond to the violence that does occur. It is not only an example for elected officials and community activists, it is also a model for public health and criminal justice professionals.

USING LOVE TO PREVENT ADOLESCENT DATING VIOLENCE

Dionne Smith Coker-Appiah, Mysha R. Wynn, and Donald Parker

Adolescent dating violence (ADV) occurs at an alarming rate among teens from all backgrounds, particularly among those who are African American (Howard, Qiu & Boekeloo, 2003; Malik, Sorenson & Aneshensel, 1997; Raiford, Wingood & Diclemente, 2007; Rickert, Vaughan, & Wiemann, 2002; Watson, Cascardi, Avery-Leaf, O'Leary, 2001) and live in rural communities (Spencer & Bryant, 2000). Dating violence doesn't just affect young people; nor is its cause their responsibility alone. Still, prevention efforts often focus on youth as the *problem* and fail to address the multiple factors that contribute to violence (and that should and could contribute to its prevention). *Project LOVE: Letting Our Voices Empower* changes the focus of ADV approaches by incorporating the expertise and perspectives of community partners and simultaneously bringing attention to the complicated, related issues that must play a role in true prevention efforts.

Project LOVE is a research project funded by the Kellogg Foundation that explores knowledge, perceptions, and beliefs about ADV and the implications for sexual and mental health among twenty African American adolescents, aged 18 to 21 years old, living in a rural county in Eastern North Carolina. Project LOVE combines the documented efficacy of community-based participatory research (CBPR) (Connolly & Friedlander, 2009; Flicker, 2008) as a preventive approach (see Chapter Ten for a description of CBPR) and the multi-level framework that is the basis of the Social-Ecological Model (SEM) (Dahlberg & Krug, 2002). Together, CBPR and SEM encourage collective ownership of and collective responsibility for prevention efforts to address adolescent dating violence.

What LOVE Looks Like

Project LOVE grew out of an academic and community partnership between a major public university located in North Carolina and the several community-based individuals and organizations and partners representing sectors integral to the prevention of ADV (for example, ADV, adolescent health, family and school, sexual health, mental health, and policy). Through our use of a community-based participatory research approach, we learned that involving community partners can achieve the following positive results:

1. *Enable collaborative decision making, incorporating research topics that are of importance to the community.* The decision to focus our research on ADV, an issue in which both community and academic partners were interested and invested, developed through a collaborative discussion on community needs, assets, and resources.

2. *Encourage better conceptualization of research projects.* Project LOVE partners were active in all aspects of the research process. Together we designed research questions, interview protocols, recruitment procedures, data collection and analysis methods, and dissemination methods that were culturally appropriate, sensitive, effective, and attractive to our target population. The level of trust and respect that developed out of our process allowed honest communication about the utility, or lack thereof, of particular components of research design; our process included discussion and negotiation of methods.

3. *Highlight the importance of youth advisory boards.* Peer groups play a critical role in shaping attitudes about ADV, and creating partnerships with young people ensures their input is integrated throughout the research process (Connolly & Friedlander, 2009). We did not have a youth advisory board in phase one of Project LOVE, but we quickly recognized the necessity of such a board and have taken steps to create and integrate a youth advisory board in phase two. The youth advisory board will explore similar ADV issues with younger adolescents.

4. *Support the design and implementation of projects that benefit the community.* CBPR builds academic and community capacity and powerfully informs prevention strategies that are attractive and effective. The Project LOVE intervention will have a better chance of being an effective program because it integrates the voices, beliefs, culture, and interests of the community throughout.

From Individuals to Communities, with LOVE

Project LOVE also used a multi-level approach to addressing and preventing ADV within their community. This approach incorporates the *Social Ecological Model* (Dahlberg & Krug, 2002), emphasizing the significance of multiple contexts (such as individual, relationship, community, and societal) within communities and the importance of understanding these contexts before creating community-level prevention strategies.

Project LOVE participants believed communities played negative roles in ADV prevention by not intervening to prevent domestic and other forms of violence. We also found important relationships between adolescents and some community stakeholders had been either nonexistent (for example, politicians), strained (for example, clergy), or negative (for example, law enforcement and juvenile justice). Our findings speak to the need for prevention researchers and practitioners to engage in the following activities:

1. Understand the role of individual and interpersonal factors in the prevention of ADV.
2. Explore the positive and negative impact of community and societal-level responses to ADV.
3. Acknowledge that law enforcement, juvenile justice, and political figures play important roles in ADV prevention, and begin to design strategies to build and rebuild relationships with adolescents.
4. Garner political support for ADV prevention efforts and remain aware of the political implications of ADV prevention research.

The *LOVE* model as we conceptualize it incorporates knowledge, lessons learned, and research findings in an effort to prevent ADV among rural African American youth. LOVE is all-inclusive, understands a diverse group of people need to be present to affect sustainable change, is honest and open-minded, and is willing to right previous wrongs. LOVE also respects and accepts multiple perspectives, beliefs, and cultures and scans the community to better understand the needs, assets, and resources of individuals, agencies, organizations, and institutions. Ultimately, LOVE garners the support of each.

We believe LOVE has preventive properties and when conceptualized and implemented appropriately, it can play a tremendous role in preventing ADV among our rural youth.

THE ROLE OF THE PUBLIC HEALTH FIELD IN PREVENTING VIOLENCE

Although the need for prevention is critical and increasingly recognized and, although the approach of public health is vital, public health as a field has yet to put its full weight and expertise behind the violence issue. A national assessment of activities geared toward preventing violence among youth revealed public health was not seen as a partner in preventing violence by those outside the field and that the *public health community did not see itself as part of the solution* (Weiss, 2008). Still, public health leaders and practitioners who understand effective, quality prevention have the theoretical and practical expertise needed to enrich efforts to reduce violence. Public health leaders and practitioners can help bring about a comprehensive solution in the following ways:

- *The public health field has a track record in addressing threats to the public's health.* By definition, public health is charged with addressing serious threats to health and safety in the population, and it has a track record of doing so. Although its history lies in addressing acute conditions, public health has increasingly taken on more chronic and persistent epidemics and pandemics. It has a track record of improving the health of populations. Public health can bring to bear the same kinds of skills, approaches, and methods that have proven effective in addressing other threats to the public's health.
- *Public health improves the health and safety of a population.* Overall levels of violence cannot be prevented by targeting one person at a time. The most effective and sustainable strategies for preventing violence are community or population-based and address the complex interplay of social, behavioral, and environmental contributors to violence, such as poverty, homelessness, school failure, lack of activities, oppression, mental health problems, substance abuse, victimization history, and others. Preventing violence requires changing environments and norms within communities. Other disciplines have a clear role to play in providing different pieces of the solution; yet, as a discipline, public health seeks community-wide or *environmental* solutions that are critical for effective prevention.
- Furthermore, the field of public health has discipline-defined tools and skill sets that will strengthen approaches to preventing violence and clearly demarcate advocacy roles
- *Public health can measure the problem and progress in addressing it.* A science-based public health approach has considerable strengths, including, for example, the capacity to describe the nature of the problem, as well as to contribute risk and resilience factors. Effective efforts for preventing violence must be firmly grounded in evidence and conscious of unique community perceptions and conditions. Such collated statistics allow useful conclusions to be drawn about those conditions that are conducive to violence. Furthermore, a multitude of efforts have been implemented across the nation and their impacts have also been evaluated. Such research can guide program and policy development to maximize health and safety and prevent violence before it occurs. Bringing this data together is a public health imperative.
- *Public health can play a key role in coordinating the range of needed efforts.* Preventing violence requires coordination among many partners, including public, private, and multiple disciplines and sectors. Most solutions span many providers and sectors and

many are not within the purview of a specific sector. There is a need for a focal point to hold the range of strategies and foster collaborative efforts. Public health brings a tradition of integrative leadership, which can organize a broad array of scientific disciplines, organizations, and communities to work together to prevent violence. The public health field is equipped to coordinate, convene, and catalyze a combination of diverse and multidisciplinary perspectives and resources. By unifying the various scientific disciplines relevant to preventing violence, public health can engender comprehensive knowledge that is more useful than the separate, discipline-specific parcels of information often provided.

- Indeed, as defined by the Institute of Medicine (1988), public health is "what we as a society do *collectively* to assure the conditions in which people can be healthy." Furthermore, public health, rather than being a single discipline, includes professionals from many fields with the collective purpose of protecting the health of a population (American Public Health Association, n.d.). To prevent duplication of effort, major gaps are being addressed and scarce resources are being coordinated and leveraged. Someone (or some collaborative group) needs to coordinate these efforts; public health can play this coordinating role. Public health can also advise on models for coordination.

- *Public health can build capacity among multiple players to prevent violence.* The reach and influence of the public health community can serve as a powerful force to unite and strengthen prevention work. Public health can serve as a clearinghouse or hub for vital prevention efforts. It can convene stakeholders from schools, law enforcement, social services and other potential partners in economic development (such as public works, zoning, recreation and parks, and many other public and private sectors). Public health can provide the big tent to help ensure all understand their own stake in and contributions to the solutions. Public health has the ability to increase capacity and integrate disparate sectors, building on the contributions and strengths of each stakeholder, and creating a more unified, strategic, and effective movement in the process.

- *Public health can develop data-informed strategies.* Building on its capacity to measure a problem and assess what's contributing to the problem, public health can develop strategies to address the root causes of violence.

- *Public health can be an invaluable advocate for prevention of violence.* Because health and public health practitioners see the end result of unnecessary death, injury, and disability, they can build on their empathy for victims to advocate powerfully for prevention. By speaking up in public meetings, serving as experts to the media, and testifying to legislators, public health providers can shape issues, influence the debate, and challenge public and political discourse. Examples include advocating for decreases in the portrayal of violence in the media and supporting state and national legislative efforts to change policy and norms.

TIMELINE OF VIOLENCE AS A PUBLIC HEALTH ISSUE (CDC)

1979. The United States Surgeon General's Report, *Healthy People*, identified stress and violent behavior among the key priority areas for public health. *Healthy People* emphasized that "the healthy community cannot ignore the consequences of violent behavior in efforts to improve health."

1980. A landmark Department of Health and Human Services report, *Promoting Health/Preventing Disease: Objectives for the Nation*, established goals for preventing violence.

1983. CDC established the Violence Epidemiology Branch to focus its public health efforts on violence prevention.

1985. The Surgeon General's Workshop on Violence and Public Health focused the attention of the public health world on violence and encouraged all health professionals to become involved.

1985. The Report of the Secretary's Task Force on Black and Minority Health was released. It underscored the importance of addressing interpersonal violence as a public health problem and identified homicide as a major contributor to health disparities among African Americans.

1990. "Violent and abusive behavior" was included as one of twenty-two public health priority areas in *Healthy People 2000*, the national disease-prevention and health-promotion strategy. *Healthy People 2000* called for "cooperation and integration across public health, health care, mental health, criminal justice, social service, education, and other relevant sectors."

1992. A landmark issue of the *Journal of the American Medical Association* addressed violence as a public health issue.

1993. CDC published *The Prevention of Youth Violence: A Framework for Community Action* to mobilize communities to effectively address the epidemic of youth violence sweeping the nation.

1996. The World Health Organization declared that "violence is a leading worldwide public health problem."

2000. WHO created the Department for Injuries and Violence Prevention.

2001. The U.S. Surgeon General released a report on youth violence.

2002. WHO released the World Report on Violence and Health.

2002. The National Violent Death Reporting System launched in six states. This was the first state-based surveillance system to link data from multiple sources with the goal of enhancing violence prevention efforts.

2004. The National Violent Death Reporting System expanded to include seventeen states.

2007. CDC published a study that estimated the cost of violence in the United States exceeds $70 billion each year.

2008. The U.S. Conference of Mayors declared violence to be a public health crisis.

CONCLUSION

With the help of new prevention efforts, the tide is turning in how violence is perceived and how it is being addressed. Viewing the prevention of violence through a public health lens reveals the potential to see a decrease in violence and also a simultaneous increase in the overall health and resilience of our families and communities. The continued application of a preventive approach to the understanding of violence is essential to further progress, and these approaches will be assured greater success with concerted and coordinated involvement, leadership, and guidance from the public health field.

The interface between public health, criminal justice, schools, and other sectors must be continually explored to ensure that strategies and activities are complementary. Although examples of collaboration exist, more effort must be placed on overcoming obstacles to create and fund a joint research and action agenda. Public health also has the potential to go beyond and unify the various scientific disciplines relevant to preventing violence; public health can engender comprehensive knowledge that is more useful than the separate, discipline-specific parcels of information often provided. It's time to treat violence as the major threat to the public's health that it is: we need a sustained investment in *preventing* violence in the United States.

DISCUSSION QUESTIONS

1. Using what you have learned about coalition building in Chapter Five ("Working Collaboratively to Advance Prevention"), what are some strategies to enhance collaboration between public health and other sectors concerned with preventing violence?

2. How is violence related to other public health issues (for example, chronic disease prevention)? How would you design a comprehensive strategy that incorporates a focus on preventing violence into other public health approaches (for example, enhancing access to healthy food and physical activity)?

3. Using what you learned in Chapter Three ("Individual, Family, and Community Resilience"), how would you incorporate resiliency in the public health strategies to prevent violence in families and communities?

REFERENCES

American Public Health Association. (n.d.). What is public health? Retrieved November 15, 2006, from http://www.apha.org/NR/rdonlyres/C57478B8-8682-4347-8DDF-A1E24E82B919/0/what_is_PH_May1_Final.pdf

Arbreton, A.J.A., & McClanahan, W. S. (n.d.). Targeted outreach: Boys & Girls Club of America's approach to gang prevention and intervention. Retrieved November 15, 2006, from http://www.ppv .org/ppv/publications/assets/148_publication.pdf

Bennett et al. (2007). Safe to walk? neighborhood safety and physical activity among public housing residents. *PLoS Medicine, 4*(10), E306.

Bowen, L. K., Gwiasda, V., & Brown, M. M. (2004). Engaging community residents to prevent violence. *Journal of Interpersonal Violence, 19*, 356.

Bradley et al. (1994). Early indications of resilience and their relation to experiences in the home environments of low birth weight, premature children living in poverty. *Child Development, 65*, 346–360.

Bureau of Justice Statistics. (2006). Criminal victimization in the United States, 2003: statistical tables. Retrieved December 30, 2009, from http://www.ojp.usdoj.gov/bjs/pub/pdf/cvus03.pdf

Centers for Disease Control and Prevention, and National Center for Injury Prevention and Control. (n.d.). Youth violence. Retrieved from http://www.cdc.gov/ncipc/dvp/YV_DataSheet.pdf

Centers for Disease Control and Prevention. (2002, June 28). Youth risk behavior surveillance. United States, 2001. *Morbidity and Mortality Weekly Report, 51*(SS-4).

Centers for Disease Control and Prevention. (n.d.). A timeline of violence as a public health issue. Retrieved October 7, 2009, from http://www.cdc.gov/ncipc/dvp/timeline.htm

Centers for Disease Control and Prevention. (2005). Web-based Injury Statistics Query and Reporting System (WISQARS). National Center for Injury Prevention and Control, Centers for Disease Control and Prevention (producer). [Cited April 10, 2008].

Connolly, J. & Friedlander, L. (2009). Peer group influences on adolescent dating aggression. *The Prevention Researcher 16*, 8–11.

Dahlberg, L. L., & Krug, E. G. (2002). Violence—a global public health problem. In E. Krug, L. L. Dahlberg, J. A. Mercy, A. B. Zwi, & R. Lozano (Eds.), *World Report on Violence and Health* (pp. 1–56). World Health Organization: Geneva, Switzerland.

Eyler et al. (2003). Quantitative study of correlates of physical activity in women from diverse racial/ethnic groups: The women's cardiovascular health network project summary and conclusions. *American Journal of Preventative Medicine, 25*(3Si), 93–103.

Feletti, V. J. (1998). Relationship of childhood abuse and household dysfunction to many of the leading causes of death in adults: the adverse childhood experiences (ACE) study. *American Journal of Preventive Medicine, 14*(4), 245–258.

Flicker, S. (2008). Who benefits from community-based participatory research? A case study of the Positive Youth Project. *Health Education & Behavior, 35*, 70–86.

Hahn R. (2007). Effectiveness of Universal School-Based Programs to Prevent Violent and Aggressive Behavior. *American Journal of Preventive Medicine, 33*(2S), S114–S129.

Hambleton, B. B., Clark, G., Sumaya, C. V., Weissman, G., & Horner, J. (1997). HRSA's strategies to combat family violence. *Academic Medicine, 72*, S110–S115.

Harrison, R. A., Gemmell, I., & Heller, R. F. (2007). The population effect of crime and neighbourhood on physical activity. *Journal of Epidemiology and Community Health, 61*, 34–39.

Hill, H. M., & Jones, L. P. (1997). Children's and parents' perceptions of children's exposure to violence in urban neighborhoods. *Journal of the National Medical Association, 89*, 270–276.

Howard, D., Qiu, Y., & Boekeloo, B. (2003). Personal and social contextual correlates of adolescent dating violence. *Journal of Adolescent Health, 33*, 9–17.

Institute of Medicine. (1988). The future of public health. Washington, DC: National Academies Press.

Institute of Medicine. (2003). Who will keep the public healthy? Washington, DC: National Academies Press.

Loukaitou-Sideris, A. (2006). Is it safe to walk?: Neighborhood safety and security considerations and their effects on walking. *Journal of Planning Literature, 20*(3), 219–232.

Lynch, M. (2003). Consequences of children's exposure to community violence. *Clinical Child and Family Psychology Review, 6*(4), 265–274.

Malik, S., Sorenson, S. B., & Aneshensel, C. S. (1997). Community and dating violence among adolescents: perpetration and victimization. *Journal of Adolescent Health, 21*, 291.

Margolis, H. (1990). Equilibrium norms. *Ethics, 100* (4), 821–837.

Minneapolis Police Department. (2008). *2008 Fourth Precinct Juvenile Crime Suspect & Arrest Statistics.*

Molnar, L. A., Gortmaker, S. L., Bull, F. C., Buka, S.L. (2004). Unsafe to play? neighborhood disorder and lack of safety predict reduced physical activity among urban children and adolescents. *American Journal of Health Promotion, 18*(5), 378–386.

National Center for Chronic Disease Prevention and Health Promotion, and Centers for Disease Control and Prevention. (2007). Youth risk behavior surveillance system. Retrieved December 30, 2009, from http://www.cdc.gov/HealthyYouth/yrbs/pdf/yrbs07_us_violence_trend.pdf

National Center for Injury Prevention and Control. (2001). *Injury fact book, 2001–2002.* Atlanta: Centers for Disease Control and Prevention.

National Crime Prevention Council. (1999). *Six Safe Cities: On the Crest of the Crime Prevention Wave.* Washington, D.C.

National Institute of Justice. (2000). *Criminal victimization 2000: Changes, 1999–2000, with Trends, 1993–2000.* Washington, DC: U.S. Department of Justice.

Neckerman, K.M., Bader, M., Purciel, M., Yousefzadeh, P. (2009). *Measuring food access in urban areas.* National Poverty Center Working Paper 2009. Retrieved July 30, 2009, from http://www.npc.umich.edu/news/events/food-access/index.php

Pollard, J. A., Hawkins, J. D., & Arthur, M. W. (1999). Risk and protection: Are both necessary to understand diverse behavioral outcomes in adolescence? *Social Work Research, 23*, 145–158.

Prothrow-Stith, D., & Spivak, H. R. (2004). *Murder is no accident: Understanding and preventing youth violence in America.* San Francisco: Jossey-Bass.

Public opinion about public health, California and the United States 1996, 1998. (1998, February 6). *Morbidity and Mortality Weekly Report, 47*(4), 69–73. Retrieved November 15, 2006, from http://www.cdc.gov/mmwr/preview/mmwrhtml/00051341.htm

Raiford, J. L., Wingood, G. M. & Diclemente, R. J. (2007). Prevalence, incidence, and predictors of dating violence: A longitudinal study of African American female adolescents. *Journal of Women's Health, 16*, 822–832.

Rickert, V. I., Vaughan, R. D., & Wiemann, C. M. (2002). Adolescent dating violence and date rape. *Current Opinions in Obstetrics and Gynecology, 14*, 495–500.

Rohrer, J. E., Arif, A. A., Pierce, J. R., Blackburn, C. (2004). Unsafe neighborhoods, social group activity, and self-rated health. *Journal of Public Health Management and Practice, 10*(2), 124–129.

Sallis, J. F., King, A. C., Sirard, J. R., & Albright, C. L. (2008). Perceived environmental predictors of physical activity over 6 months in adults: Activity counseling trial. *Health Psychology, 27*(2), 214.

Search Institute. (2002). *The power of assets.* Retrieved March 22, 2002, from http://www.search-institute.org/power-assets

Skogan, W., Hartnett, S., Bump, N., & Dubois, J. (2008). *Executive summary: Evaluation of CeaseFire-Chicago.* (Conducted with the support of Grant Number 2005-MU-MU-003, National Institute of Justice, Office of Justice Programs).

Smith, C., Lizotte, A. J., Thornberry, T. P., & Krohn, M. D. (1995). Resilient youth: Identifying factors that prevent high-risk youth from engaging in delinquency and drug use. In J. Hagan (Ed.), *Delinquency and disrepute in the life course: Contextual and dynamic analyses* (pp. 217–247). Greenwich, CT: JAI Press.

Snyder, H., & Sickmund, M. (1999). *Juvenile offenders and victims: 1999 national report.* Washington, DC: Office of Juvenile Justice and Delinquency Prevention.

Spencer, G. A., & Bryant, S. A. (2000). Dating violence: a comparison of rural, suburban, and urban teens. *Journal of Adolescent Health, 27*, 302–305.

Thorpe, K. E., Florence, C. S., & Joski, P. (2004). Which medical conditions account for the rise in health care spending? *Health Affairs, W4*, 437–445. Retrieved April 15, 2009, from http://content.healthaffairs.org/cgi/content/abstract/hlthaff.w4.437v1

Tjaden, P., & Thoennes, N. (2000). *Full report of the prevalence, incidence and consequences of violence against women: findings from the National Violence Against Women survey.* Washington, DC: National Institute of Justice.

Ullmann-Margalit, E. (1990). Revision of norms. *Ethics, 100*, 756–767.

Vera Institute of Justice. (n.d.). *Cost benefit analysis of LA's gang prevention efforts.* Retrieved April 15, 2009, from http://www.advancementprojectca.org/doc/p3_cost.pdf

Watson, J. M., Cascardi, M., Avery-Leaf, S. & O'Leary, K. D. (2001). High school students' responses to dating aggression. *Violence and victims, 16*, 339.

Web-Based Injury Statistics Query and Reporting System (WISQARS). (n.d.). *National Center for Injury Prevention and Control Web site.* Retrieved August 1, 2006, from http://www.cdc.gov/ncipc/wisqars

Weir, L. A., Etelson, D., & Brand, D. A. (2006). Parents' perceptions of neighborhood safety and children's physical activity. *Preventive Medicine, 43*(3), 212–217.

Weiss, B. (2008, June). *An assessment of youth violence prevention activities in USA cities*. Los Angeles: Southern California Injury Prevention Research Center, UCLA School of Public Health.

World Health Organization (WHO). (n.d.). *Violence*. Retrieved March 21, 2009, from http://www .who.int/topics/violence/en

Yancey, A. K., & Kumanyika, S. K. (2007). Bridging the gap: Understanding the structure of social inequities in childhood obesity. *American Journal of Preventive Medicine, 33*(4S1), S172–S174.

14

The Limits of Behavioral Interventions for HIV Prevention

Dan Wohlfeiler
Jonathan M. Ellen

LEARNING OBJECTIVES

- Describe the epidemiology of HIV in the United States and the roots of HIV prevention.
- Learn the limitations of behavioral interventions to reduce HIV infection rates.
- Articulate the role and importance of structural-level interventions as a prevention strategy.
- Identify five principles of sexual network-level interventions for HIV prevention.

For the past twenty-five years, prevention of HIV has relied heavily on behavioral interventions aimed at reducing individual risk behaviors that have been found to lead to infection and that include unprotected sex and sharing contaminated needles. Although numerous studies have been conducted that demonstrate the effectiveness of behavioral interventions in increasing knowledge, changing attitudes, and reducing risky behaviors, few studies have demonstrated the impact of behavioral interventions on reducing HIV infections. This is significant because reducing infections is ultimately the goal of primary prevention efforts.

Behavioral interventions are a necessary but insufficient component of HIV prevention. This is due to their moderate success in reducing risky behaviors, their minimal success at decreasing infections, and sadly, their lack of demonstrated effectiveness at altering the course of HIV epidemics. Structural factors such as economic and racial disparities fuel the HIV epidemic. They often act by affecting *sexual networks* (the web of sexual partnerships).

In this chapter, we argue that reducing HIV infections requires more than relying on individual behavior change. We suggest two new directions for HIV prevention. The first is to take cues from other fields of public health, most notably injury prevention and tobacco control, where professionals have used policy as an integral part of the strategy to achieve desired outcomes. These fields, with more years of experience than HIV's quarter-century, have achieved greater success at developing economic, policy, environmental, and technological strategies that allow their prevention efforts to be more self-sustaining and less reliant on a constant infusion of public health resources (including staff and financial support). This approach requires public health professionals to be facilitators of change in addition to service providers. Second, as part of a strategy that relies heavily on structural interventions and policies, we suggest developing interventions that will directly affect the sexual networks that facilitate viral transmission.

Most of this chapter will draw upon examples from the United States. This is not meant to diminish the importance of interventions in other countries. The relatively numerous resources available for behavioral interventions in the United States, the rich diversity of behavioral interventions, and the epidemiological and sociopolitical context of the HIV epidemics in the United States make many aspects of the U.S. epidemic unique.

EPIDEMIOLOGY OF HIV IN THE UNITED STATES

By the end of 2007, 998,255 people had been diagnosed with AIDS in the United States and 562,793 (56 percent) had died (Centers for Disease Control and Prevention [CDC], 2009a). Gay men and African Americans are the two communities most profoundly affected by HIV in the United States (Valleroy et al., 2000). However, the experiences of the gay and African American communities in confronting HIV are very different from each other.

Gay men and men who have sex with men (MSM), including MSM who also report injection drug use, continue to make up the largest segment of infections (53 percent of all infections in 2007; data are from thirty-four states with confidential name-based HIV infection reporting since at least 2003), even though the percentage of men who have sexual contact with other males is estimated at between 3 and 9 percent of the general population (Anderson & Stall, 2002; Laumann, Gagnon, Michael, & Michaels, 1994; Sell, Wells, & Wypij, 1995).

The AIDS epidemic, much like other diseases and other sexually transmitted diseases (STDs), is increasingly marked by profound racial disparities. The CDC (2009) reported that non-Hispanic African Americans, who represent 13 percent of the U.S. population, accounted for 51 percent of the HIV/AIDS cases diagnosed in 2007. Among African American men diagnosed with AIDS in 2007, more than half had been exposed through male-male sexual contact. Hispanics, who represent 12 percent of the adult population, account for 18 percent of the infections. Among adolescents diagnosed during 2007, 72 percent of those infected are African American, even though only 17 percent of adolescents are African American (Centers for Disease Control and Prevention, 2009b).

ROOTS OF HIV PREVENTION

Shortly after the first cases were reported in the United States in 1981, HIV quickly spread through gay communities and through networks of injection drug users. By the mid-1980s, approximately one-half of the gay men in San Francisco and one-half of injection drug users in New York City were infected. Many of these people began developing illnesses rarely seen in young, otherwise healthy adults. By studying the characteristics of those who were first affected by these illnesses, epidemiologists were quickly able to determine the disease was being transmitted sexually (Auerbach, Darrow, Jaffe, & Curran, 1984) and through injecting needles (CDC, 1982).

Many gay men quickly reduced their high-risk behavior. Most notably, they reduced the number of partners with whom they had unprotected sex (McCusick et al., 1985; Winkelstein et al., 1987). This was demonstrated both by numerous survey studies and through epidemiologic surveillance and modeling. In fact, the rates of infection plummeted almost as quickly as they had increased initially.

A careful examination of the history of HIV/AIDS, particularly among gay men, reveals that profound behavior changes took place before any governmental support and funding became available. Early organizers used grassroots mobilizing and information distribution through the press, brochures, and posters to provide people at risk with the information they lacked about this new disease. For example, in San Francisco, reductions in risk behavior occurred as the gay community formed organizations and later engaged in more formal education efforts. Although many contemporary community-based interventions attempt to replicate the strategies used in these early community mobilizations, it is unlikely they will ever have the impact or reach the scale of the early mobilizations, primarily because it is impossible to replicate the social context in which they occurred. In particular, it is unrealistic to hope to mobilize communities to the same extent as when HIV first took hold, when HIV had no known etiology or treatment.

TYPES OF BEHAVIORAL INTERVENTIONS AND THEIR SUCCESS

The following sections describe behavioral interventions at the individual, group, and community levels and then discuss their strengths and weaknesses.

INDIVIDUAL-LEVEL INTERVENTIONS

HIV testing to date has for the most part been accompanied by brief pretest and posttest counseling sessions that aim to inform an individual as to what the HIV test will and will not reveal, what strategies can reduce risk, and what sources of medical and social support are available in case of a positive result. This ambitious scope for brief sessions has long served as a mainstay of HIV prevention. Meta-analyses of multiple studies have demonstrated the impact of counseling and testing is greatest for HIV-positive individuals, most of whom will take significant measures not to expose anyone else to the virus. The impact on HIV-negative individuals, however, is less pronounced (Weinhardt, Carey, Johnson, & Bickham, 1999).

Client-centered counseling offered by well-trained staff has been shown to help reduce STD transmission. A key study, Project Respect, demonstrated that client-centered counseling was more effective than either interactive counseling or didactic messages in reducing new STD infections (Kamb et al., 1998).

One of the most intensive and broad-based individual-level interventions, Project Explore, recruited more than four thousand high-risk gay and bisexual men to ten one-time counseling sessions. The intervention also included quarterly sessions aimed at maintaining the effect of the counseling sessions (Koblin, Chesney, & Coates, 2004). This is a level of intensity and scale that is much higher than the vast majority of HIV interventions have been able to offer. Nevertheless, although the infection rate was lower in the intervention group than in the standard comparison group, the difference was not statistically significant.

GROUP-LEVEL INTERVENTIONS

Group workshops have long been used in public health to promote healthy behaviors and provide social support. AIDS prevention programs have relied on group-level interventions to reduce risk of infection in gay men and in MSM of all ethnicities who participate in the workshops (Carballo-Dieguez et al., 2005; Peterson et al., 1996; Valdiserri et al., 1989), in women (Kelly et al., 1994), injection drug users (el-Bassel & Schilling, 1992), and in adolescents (Jemmott, Jemmott, & Fong, 1992; Rotheram-Borus et al., 2003). These programs have been used to convey information, to promote norms favoring risk reduction, and to recruit volunteers for further educational efforts. Both professional and volunteer facilitators have led these sessions. Studies have demonstrated that group workshops have been effective at reducing both sexual and drug-related risk behavior. Some group interventions convene only once; others may continue for weeks or months. Many of these interventions have recruited individuals who did not know each other previously and are unlikely to meet again except by chance after the intervention. Others recruit members of social networks, with the hope the conversations and dynamics that emerge during the formal intervention will be more easily sustained afterward.

One example of a group-level intervention provided four group sessions lasting four hours each to sexually experienced African American girls aged fourteen to eighteen. Compared to a control group, participants reported more condom use and fewer new vaginal sex partners. The study also found small but promising declines in chlamydia infections and self-reported pregnancies (DiClemente et al., 2004).

Although many interventions have succeeded in reducing risk, there is less evidence of their effectiveness in reducing the incidence of HIV infections.

COMMUNITY-LEVEL INTERVENTIONS

Community-level interventions often include both individual- and group-level interventions. These interventions are effective because they support community-wide norms that favor risk reduction, even among individuals who do not participate in the most intensive one-on-one and group-level interventions. These interventions have relied heavily on *diffusion models*. Diffusion describes the processes whereby messages and norms are conveyed throughout a community. Rather than having to reach every individual, practitioners aim to reach a segment of the population, often popular opinion leaders who can then diffuse the message or norm throughout the rest of the community (Rogers, 1962). In some cases, these programs have been generated by the community itself (Wohlfeiler, 1997). Other programs, such as Mpowerment, have been launched by university researchers (Kegeles, Hays, & Coates, 1996). Mpowerment organized gay men aged eighteen to twenty-nine to conduct small group workshops, formal and informal outreach, and media and social events. Participants decreased rates of unprotected anal intercourse. No biological outcomes were measured, however.

FORCES PROMOTING ONE-ON-ONE INTERVENTIONS

Multiple forces working together have pushed the field of HIV prevention to emphasize one-on-one interventions. As the importance of care and treatment increased, it became harder to mobilize volunteers for prevention. Pressures to be accountable to funders also resulted in the creation of programs that were easier to plan, implement, and measure. Finally, the need to constantly seek additional funding has driven many organizations, both governmental and nongovernmental, to choose interventions that did not conflict with economic or political interests (Wohlfeiler, 2002).

THE LIMITS OF BEHAVIORAL INTERVENTIONS

Behavioral interventions often require substantial resources to decrease the odds of risk behavior by approximately 25 percent (Herbst et al., 2005), which is the level reached by the more successful interventions (Johnson et al., 2002). As the Institute of Medicine (IOM) observes, "A program that achieves statistically significant social and behavioral changes still may not avert large numbers of new infections" (2001, p. 26). For behavioral interventions to succeed in reducing infections within a population, they need to reach a broad sector of the population, be of sufficient intensity, and reach the right individuals. In addition, interventions need to occur in supportive social environments and contexts.

Some of the largest-scale interventions do, in fact, reach significant percentages of their populations. However, most of these interventions are relatively low-intensity, such as one-on-one outreach interventions. These may be as simple as handing out information and condoms or as in-depth as conducting risk assessments, recruiting to more in-depth interventions, and testing for STDs or HIV (or both). These interventions may not reach individuals at the highest risk, often referred to as the *core group*. Even if these individuals are reached, it is unlikely a brief intervention will make an impact on their risk behavior, since many of these people have psychosocial needs that are not easily addressed by a workshop, a counseling session, or even by ongoing counseling.

A further limitation of many interventions, particularly at the community level, is that they often offer the same *dose* of prevention, regardless of an individual's risk level. For example, outreach workers may offer condoms and workshop invitations to an individual who has occasional unprotected sex with one partner; they may offer these same services to an individual who has a new unprotected partner each week.

One of the largest-scale community-level interventions carried out that targeted the entire gay community, the *STOP AIDS Project*, has been very successful in recruiting large numbers of men. However, the numbers have decreased over the years. In the mid-1980s, STOP AIDS was able to mobilize three hundred volunteers and recruit some seven thousand men (approximately 15 percent of the gay community) annually to workshops. This was a period marked by widespread fear and numerous individuals were getting sick, visibly deteriorating, and dying. By the early 1990s, when the infection rate had fallen (but before new treatments had become available) STOP AIDS was able to mobilize only half that many volunteers and recruit only twelve hundred men to workshops (Wohlfeiler, 2002).

As the lethality of the threat of HIV infection and its sequelae diminishes, thanks to more effective treatment, it becomes less likely that individuals will be motivated to take an active role in community-level interventions. Furthermore, behavioral interventions typically do not directly address the social contexts in which behavior occurs. Behavioral interventions typically recruit individuals to interventions, increase their knowledge, and. in many cases, identify triggers to risk behavior; triggers include situations where risk behavior is the most likely to occur (for example, going to a bar or socializing with peers who engage in high-risk behavior). Many of these contexts are difficult to alter, since they may require a change in social environments and in peer groups. In addition, individuals may have to contend with corporate practices that lead to environments that promote high-risk behaviors.

Corporate practices, including the products sold and promoted in particular neighborhoods, play an important role in shaping the context in which behavioral interventions occur. These practices often overwhelm and contradict behavioral interventions. For example, alcohol abuse and overconsumption are associated with STD acquisition (Cook & Clark, 2005), yet promotion of alcohol is a multimillion-dollar industry and bars and other purveyors of alcohol are widespread. Considerable variation also exists in the commitment of the adult film industry (CDC, 2005b) and of businesses that facilitate partners meeting one another (for example, Internet companies, bathhouses and sex clubs, and large circuit parties) to support risk reduction (Wohlfeiler & Potterat, 2005).

Beyond legitimate questions regarding their effectiveness, behavioral interventions also have faced numerous obstacles related to infrastructure, political barriers, and network- and social-level contextual issues that further hamper their efficacy. Investment in public health and STD prevention has always been insufficient. The IOM summarizes difficulties in preventing STDs as follows:

> Effective STD prevention efforts are hampered by biological characteristics of STDs, societal problems, unbalanced mass media messages, lack of awareness, fragmentation of STD-related services, inadequate training of health care professionals, inadequate health insurance coverage and access to services, and insufficient investment in STD prevention [1997, p. 2].

In HIV prevention, government agencies have relied heavily on community-based organizations because these organizations may be more effective than the government at using culturally appropriate interventions to reach communities. Community-based organizations are also able to mobilize community support and gain access to communities that may distrust government agencies. However, with few exceptions, most of these agencies pay prevention managers and line staff low salaries. This creates high turnover rates among staff, which consequently creates a constant need to train new staff in both the theory and the skills necessary to design and implement effective interventions.

Political forces have also hampered scientifically based behavioral interventions. Support for abstinence-only education has increased, although these programs have been found to contain numerous inaccuracies and to have little, if any, benefit in reducing incidence of STDs and HIV (Bruckner & Bearman, 2005). Meanwhile, prevention advocates spend considerable time and energy defending behavioral interventions from conservative forces, which means they have less time to spend on prevention efforts themselves.

PREVENTING HIV THROUGH NEEDLE EXCHANGE

The nation's first needle exchange program began as a form of civil disobedience in 1986. Incensed by a professor's comment that addicts should not be the focus of HIV prevention efforts because their behaviors could not be changed, Jon Parker, a public health student at Yale University and former heroin addict, began distributing and later exchanging needles and syringes on the streets of New Haven, Connecticut, and Boston, Massachusetts (Lane, 1993).

Parker's belief that addicts' behaviors could and must be changed was particularly relevant in New York City, where as early as 1983 as many as 50 percent of the city's two hundred thousand drug users were infected with HIV (Susman, 2001). New York City was infamous for its *shooting galleries*, where large groups of people shared needles, meaning that preventing the spread of HIV was intrinsically linked to the behavior of a large population of intravenous drug users (Drucker, n.d.). New York City's health department attempted to institute a needle exchange program as early as 1985, but the idea was met with immediate protest from law enforcement and from some prominent members of the African American community (Drucker, n.d.).

Many people believed such a program would encourage drug use in the midst of a *war on drugs*, and others expressed concern about the location of needle exchange facilities. Even many of the people who agreed with the concept of needle exchange did not want (and still do not want) needle exchanges taking place in their own back yards. To address both concerns, the New York City Department of Health opened an experimental exchange program in 1988 (Lane, 1993).

Injection drug users were accepted into the program only if they agreed to enter treatment; drug users could participate in exchanges only until a treatment slot became available (Lane, 1993). Each participant received one syringe imprinted with a health department logo and a photo identification card that exempted him or her from a law prohibiting the possession of drug paraphernalia. Participants were allowed to exchange only one syringe on each visit. Because there were difficulties housing the exchange program, it was located in the health department headquarters, far from most clients' neighborhoods and near the courthouse and police department (Lane, 1993).

These adaptations to earlier proposals won the support of the current mayor Edward Koch but were not supported by his successor David Dinkins, who in response to vocal community leaders closed the program in 1990, shortly after his election (Lane, 1993).

Subsequently, activists concerned about rising rates of HIV infection attempted to build community consensus for needle exchange programs. Their efforts were aided by Yale Professor Edward Kaplan's evaluation of the exchange program, which concluded the program had succeeded in reducing HIV transmission and in linking needle exchange with drug treatment and housing. Prevention policy shifted toward needle exchange and won the cautious support of the Dinkins administration (Lane, 1993).

According to Dr. Don Des Jarlais of the Beth Israel Medical Center, before the initiation of the needle exchange program, about 4 to 5 percent of drug users were becoming infected each year (Susman, 2001). The rate was reduced to about 1 percent per year after the exchange program started (Des Jarlais et al., 2000). Although still controversial, needle exchange programs in several cities now receive local, state, and even federal funding (Lane, 1993) because of ample evidence programs are effective in preventing the spread of HIV among intravenous drug users, which also helps prevent the spread of HIV in the greater community (Satcher, 2000). According to Des Jarlais, "Large-scale syringe exchange and voluntary HIV counseling and testing programs appear to have 'reversed' the HIV epidemic among injecting drug users in New York City" (2000, p. 358).

Source: Prevention Institute.

ADDRESSING HIV IN THE U.S. PRISON SYSTEM

The Bureau of Justice Statistics confirmed that in 2008, the overall rate of confirmed HIV/AIDS cases among the prison population (0.46 percent) was more than 2½ times the rate in the U.S. general population (0.17 percent) (Bureau of Justice Statistics, 2008). Hammett explains this disparity.

> Correctional inmates engage in drug-related and sexual risk behaviors, and the transmission of HIV, hepatitis, and sexually transmitted diseases occurs in correctional facilities. . . . Whether infection was acquired within or outside correctional facilities, the prevalence of HIV and other infectious diseases is much higher among inmates than among those in the general community, and the burden of disease among inmates and releases is disproportionately heavy [2006, p. 974].

Congress has recently recognized the correlation between prisons and rates of HIV in its work on the Stop AIDS in Prison Act of 2009. The bill, passed in the House of Representatives in March 2009, stipulates routine testing, protection of inmate confidentiality, more comprehensive counseling and medical treatment, and improvement of HIV/AIDS awareness and inmate education. However, the bill fails to recognize the importance of prevention and does not mention access to condoms and clean needles.

Development of prevention programs is slow, even though such programs could save millions in health care costs. For example, it costs about $25,000 per year to provide medical care to one HIV-positive inmate, whereas the provision of condoms costs a fraction of that (Lowe, 2009). Yet in the United States, only two state prison systems and five county jail systems make condoms available to inmates (Mississippi, Vermont, Washington DC, San Francisco, Los Angeles, New York, and Philadelphia) (National Minority AIDS Council, 2006).

Most recently, a condom-distribution program is in progress at the California State Prison in Solano, where the HIV rate among inmates is at least five times higher than that of the general population (Center for Health Justice, 2008). Concerns that condoms would be used as weapons or as a hiding place for drugs have not borne out in practice since the one-year pilot began in November 2008 (Lowe, 2009).

Currently no syringe exchange program for prisons exists in the United States. However, extensive research is available to support the implementation of syringe exchange programs for prisons in all countries. Evidence overwhelmingly shows that these programs reduce HIV and hepatitis C risk, prevent disease transmission, and increase referrals to substance abuse treatment. Furthermore, they neither result in increased drug use nor pose problems with security or violence (Harm Reduction Coalition, 2007).

Source: Prevention Institute

NEW TREATMENTS

Biomedical advances, in particular the discovery and widespread use of new treatments, far extend the lives of HIV-infected individuals. Many in the HIV prevention field have feared that *treatment optimism* has so substantially decreased the threat of HIV as to make prevention even more difficult. However, the relationship between optimism about treatment effectiveness and risk behavior is more complex and may not be unidirectional; risk behavior may both predict and be predicted by such treatment optimism (Huebner, 2005). Regardless of the individual perceptions of new treatment options, it is harder to mobilize community members around a *chronic*, if still ultimately fatal, disease.

New treatments reduce individuals' infectiousness and, if widely used, can do so on a population level (Porco et al., 2004). HIV virulence (ease of infection) in a newly infected individual is high, and treatment can significantly decrease infectivity. In an effort to increase the number of individuals who know their HIV status and can then seek treatment, the CDC launched the Advancing HIV Prevention Initiative in 2003, which also aims to increase the integration of prevention and medical care (CDC, 2003).

STRUCTURAL-LEVEL SOLUTIONS TO PREVENTING HIV

Structural interventions aim to modify the social, economic, and political structures and systems in which we live. These may affect legislation, media, health care, and the marketplace. They may include policy, technology, environmental, and economic interventions. Ideally, structural interventions should rely as little as possible on continued support from the public health sector's scarce resources. Thus, rather than solely relying on outreach workers to surf the Web to answer questions, public health may be better served by working with Internet providers to provide links to factually correct information and resources. Many HIV behavioral practitioners are aware of the numerous contextual factors that contribute to HIV infection. However, similar to practitioners in other fields of public health, they often continue to pursue individual-level interventions (Millett, Peterson, Wolitski, & Stall, 2006; Wohlfeiler, 2002). As Trostle (2004) points out, behavioral interventions often accept the status quo of existing social dynamics and structures.

Structural interventions often take longer and may not yield immediately measurable benefits in the short term and perhaps not even in the generation in which they are implemented (Fenton & Imrie, 2005). However, given their effectiveness in other areas of public health, they represent a promising area for innovative efforts in HIV prevention.

Structural interventions have a long history of success in areas of public health such as violence prevention, tobacco control, and regulation of alcohol consumption. Structural interventions have not typically been associated with HIV prevention, however. Although many structural interventions have yet to be evaluated in HIV prevention, some have proved effective.

Legalizing syringe exchange programs (SEPs), through which injection drug users (IDUs) may exchange used syringes for sterile ones, is one example of a structural intervention. A study of eighty-one cities around the world compared HIV infection rates among IDUs in cities that had SEPs with cities that did not have SEPs. HIV infection rates *increased* by 5.9 percent per year on average in the fifty-two cities without SEPs and *decreased* by 5.8 percent per year in the twenty-nine cities with SEPs. The study concluded that SEPs appear to lead to lower levels of HIV infection among IDUs (Hurley, Jolley, & Kaldor, 1997).

Bathhouses and sex clubs have long been important institutions in the gay community, providing gay men and MSM an opportunity to meet sexual partners in a venue free from harassment. Considerable debates have taken place within the gay community and even within public health as to what role these institutions may play in facilitating HIV or STD transmission. Bathhouses and sex clubs also provide a good way to compare and contrast two approaches. Individual-level outreach happens in many bathhouses and sex clubs across the country. Structural changes have been attempted in some jurisdictions by instituting policies prohibiting unprotected sex and removing private rooms to enforce these policies. Although there are no data to compare effects on infection rates, researchers at the University of California in San Francisco (UCSF) found that men in four cities (San Francisco, Chicago, Los Angeles, and New York) who went to bathhouses and sex clubs all had the same level of unprotected sex overall. But men in San Francisco, where owners have removed the private rooms and enforced rules regarding unprotected sex, reported having less unprotected sex in the clubs themselves (Woods et al., 2003). As will be discussed later, this might have important implications for transmission of STDs and HIV through a community's sexual networks. This is an example of how public health practitioners may gain more ground by modifying environments and policies rather than seeking to modify individuals' behaviors.

In the Dominican Republic, researchers randomized brothels to two different arms of a study. In one arm, they encouraged *voluntary strategies*, such as group workshops and education, to promote condom use. In another arm they used voluntary strategies as well as the threat of enforcement through *legal strategies*. Rather than relying exclusively on reports of changes in rates of condom use, researchers were able to document changes in the incidence of sexually transmitted infections. These researchers found the two-pronged approach that used voluntary and policy strategies through mobilizing community and governmental will had a bigger impact than voluntary strategies alone (Kerrigan et al., 2006).

THE STRUCTURE OF SEXUAL NETWORKS

Many behavioral interventions assume an individual's risk is the result of his or her individual psychosocial factors. This is partially true. However, the risk to an individual is also determined by his or her sexual partners' levels of risk. Thus an individual's total risk is determined by the patterns and networks of sexual relationships among lower- and higher-risk individuals he or she is partnered with (Ellen, 2003; Klovdahl, Potterat, Woodhouse, Muth, & Muth, 1992; Morris, 1997; Morris & Kretzschmar, 1997). This has been documented in both young gay males and young African American females (Harawa et al., 2004). For example, young gay men who have partners older than thirty are at even greater risk than those who report having multiple younger partners or who inject drugs, simply because their older partners are more likely to be infected (Blower & Service, 1997).

There is even stronger evidence among heterosexual adolescents that individual sexual behaviors are not associated with HIV in the United States. Adolescents at greatest risk for HIV are young men who have sex with men and young minority women who have sex with men (Wilson et al., 2001). Studies comparing HIV-infected adolescent women to uninfected young women from the same community and similar household structure found no differences in number of recent sex partners (Ellen, Aral, & Madger, 1998). In fact, consistent condom use was higher among HIV-infected girls. Studies of acquisition of other STDs also suggest individual factors have a limited impact on infection among adolescent women. STDs such as chlamydia and gonorrhea show a similar racial and sex distribution as HIV. A national study of adolescents found that risk factors such as consistency of condom use and alcohol use with sex do not mitigate the risk correlated with ethnicity, age, or gender, which are each in turn associated with sexual norms and sexual networks (Ellen et al., 1998). Interventions that focus on individuals, therefore, are unlikely to substantially alter the relationship between higher- and lower-risk individuals or the structure of risk-taking networks.

As we have already explained, racial disparities in infection rates cannot be explained by differences in risk behavior between different races alone. Differences do exist, however, in the patterns and network structure of relationships, with higher rates of mixing between higher- and lower-risk individuals taking place among African Americans, for example, than among other ethnicities (Laumann & Youm, 1999). This may be related, in part, to mixing patterns among ethnicities and also to a shortage of African American males relative to females, due to males' disproportionate involvement in the criminal justice system and higher rates of mortality (Thomas & Sampson, 2005). AIDS rates have been found to be correlated with incarceration rates (Johnson & Raphael, 2005). Behavioral interventions that attempt to change individual behaviors while ignoring these factors are unlikely to succeed in reducing such disparities. Differences in network structure have been hypothesized to account for racial differences in both heterosexuals and gay men and MSM (Millett et al., 2006).

Focusing a new generation of structural interventions on sexual networks may hold substantial promise. One area of structural interventions likely to be the most promising is to focus on sexual network-level interventions in terms of both feasibility and impact (Johnson & Raphael, 2005; Laumann & Youm, 1999; Millett et al., 2006; Thomas & Sampson, 2005). Network-level interventions may be more cost-effective for a variety of populations, including injection drug users (Neaigus, 1998). The following five principles of sexual network-level interventions may help guide practitioners (Wohlfeiler, 2005):

1. *Consider altering sexual network structures.* Many interventions promote social norms and facilitate communication of risk reduction messages (see, for example, Kelly, 1992; Latkin, Sherman, & Knowlton, 2003; Valente & Saba, 2001) while leaving networks intact. However, given that network structure itself confers risk (Klovdahl et al., 1992; Potterat, Rothenberg, & Muth, 1999; Rothenberg et al., 1998), practitioners should consider altering network structures to gain an epidemiologic advantage. For example, providing *safe sex only* Internet sites or commercial sex venues may help reduce contact between high- and low-risk individuals.

2. *Focus on institutions that either facilitate partner mixing or disrupt ecologies of communities.* Institutions that facilitate mixing between high- and low-risk individuals and that also link different networks together (De, Singh, Wong, Yacoub, & Jolly, 2004) are particularly important for HIV prevention efforts. These include bars, Internet sites, bathhouses, and circuit parties. Although a number of behavioral interventions exist within these settings, these have not been evaluated and are likely to be subject to the same limitations described earlier in this chapter.

As noted previously, the criminal justice system also has a profound impact on the natural ecology of the African American community. Because such a high percentage of African American men are removed from communities, a lower number of men than women remain; this may significantly contribute to the higher rates of concurrency among African Americans (Adimora & Schoenbach, 2005). *Concurrency*, which is defined as having multiple sexual partners at one time (Morris, 1997), increases the likelihood of HIV infection because earlier sexual partners can be infected through later encounters with the same sexual partners (Wohlfeiler & Potterat, 2003). (*Serial monogamy*, in contrast, implies no risk for an individual who ends a relationship with a partner before that partner gets infected.) These patterns of concurrency facilitate HIV transmission more efficiently than monogamy or even serial monogamy. Thus programs that focus on prisoners' transition to outside communities, conjugal visits, and efforts to further diminish the impact of prisons on communities may be particularly important in reducing transmission.

3. *Reduce the odds that low-risk individuals inadvertently partner with highest-risk individuals*. Networks connect high- and low-risk individuals, and the potential exists to reduce transmission throughout the entire community. Creating Web sites and venues that attract specific segments may help. The marketplace is already doing this to some extent; for example, separate Internet sites exist for high- and low-risk gay men (Wohlfeiler & Potterat, 2005). Furthermore, the creation of sites that cater to HIV-positive individuals is an example of a *pulling* strategy that violates no individual rights, gives HIV-positive individuals an opportunity to meet partners without having to risk stigma from disclosing status, and may help reduce transmission to HIV-negative individuals.

4. *Help people make informed choices about their sexual partners*. The Internet may be making it easier for people to find sexual partners, but it also provides public health with a unique opportunity. Disclosing HIV status is often an awkward process, and HIV-positive individuals often risk rejection from prospective partners. On the Internet, profile screens enable individuals to reveal their HIV-status once without having to disclose to a prospective partner each and every time. Web site profiles may also help individuals with low and high risk be more explicit about expressing their risk preferences, even at a site where high- and low-risk individuals mix. Encouraging more Web sites to adopt such practices is likely to become increasingly effective as the Internet becomes a more important means for people to meet partners.

5. *Maintain basic human rights and freedom of choice*. Risk behavior is ultimately a matter of individual choice, regardless of how it affects other people in a community. All of us may choose to smoke in our own homes and eat foods that jeopardize our health. As other chapters in this book attest, public health has sought to protect these individual rights while reducing the likelihood of harm to others (for example, by restricting smoking in public places) and increasing informed choices (for example, through menu labeling). These same principles may help public health practitioners as they seek to complement their behavioral interventions with network- and other structural-level interventions as they apply to HIV prevention.

CONCLUSION

Behavioral interventions will continue to play a strong and necessary role in the prevention of HIV. As new generations become sexually active and consider drug use and other high-risk behaviors, it is imperative for them to have access to scientifically accurate and correct medical information that encourages risk reduction.

However, practitioners must also realize the inherent limitations of behavioral interventions in their depth, breadth, sustainability, and effectiveness. HIV practitioners will need to balance behavioral interventions with biomedical interventions that seek to reduce the virulence of HIV-infected individuals; practitioners also need to understand the complex relationship between these types of interventions. Although many tools exist to help practitioners understand the effectiveness of different interventions, few tools exist to help practitioners allocate adequate resources to different interventions (Cohen, Wu, & Farley, 2004). There also remains a lack of understanding as to which of these interventions may have greater or lesser effectiveness in different populations or at different phases of the epidemic (Wasserheit & Aral, 1996).

Public health practitioners should look for new ways of reducing transmission that are cost-effective, that promote truly informed choice, and that maintain a respect for basic human rights. We contend that structural-level interventions, particularly those that affect the structure of sexual networks, hold particular promise for HIV prevention efforts.

DISCUSSION QUESTIONS

1. The text describes the politics of political support in the section entitled "Preventing HIV Through Needle Exchange". One mayor supports needle exchange, whereas his successor does not and terminates the program. Knowing that political whims can determine the fate of prevention programs, what strategies would you use to promote a sustainable needle exchange program and related structural-level interventions?

2. Using what you learned in Chapter Six ("The Power of Local Communities to Foster Policy"), what strategies might you suggest to empower communities to support and enact a structural-level change or policy initiative? What initiative would you suggest?

REFERENCES

Adimora, A. A., & Schoenbach, V. J. (2005). Social context, sexual networks, and racial disparities in rates of sexually transmitted infections. *Journal of Infectious Diseases, 191*(Suppl. 1), S115–S122.

Anderson, J. E., & Stall, R. (2002). Increased reporting of male-to-male sexual activity in a national survey. *Sexually Transmitted Diseases, 29,* 643–646.

Auerbach, D. M., Darrow, W. W., Jaffe, H. W., & Curran, J. W. (1984). Cluster of cases of the acquired immune deficiency syndrome: Patients linked by sexual contact. *American Journal of Medicine, 76,* 487–492.

Blower, S., & Service, S. (1997). Calculating the odds of HIV infection due to sexual partner selection. *AIDS and Behavior, 1,* 273–274.

Bruckner, H., & Bearman, P. (2005). After the promise: The STD consequences of adolescent virginity pledges. *Journal of Adolescent Health, 36,* 271–278.

Bureau of Justice Statistics. (2008). *HIV in prisons, 2006 and medical problems of prisoners.* Retrieved October 13, 2009, from http://bjs.ojp.usdoj.gov/index.cfm?ty=pbdetail&iid=418

Bureau of Justice Statistics. (2008). *HIV in Prisons, 2007–08.* Retrieved October 13, 2009, from http://www.ojp.usdoj.gov/bjs

Carballo-Dieguez et al. (2005). A randomized controlled trial to test an HIV-prevention intervention for Latino gay and bisexual men: Lessons learned. *AIDS Care, 17,* 314–328.

Center for Health Justice. (2008). *A novel condom distribution program for county jail prisoners.* Retrieved May 4, 2010, from http://www.caps.ucsf.edu/pubs/reports/pdf/PrisoncondomS2C.pdf

Centers for Disease Control. (1982). Pneumocystis pneumonia. *Morbidity and Mortality Weekly Report, 30,* 250–252.

Centers for Disease Control and Prevention. (2003). Advancing HIV prevention: New strategies for a changing epidemic, United States, 2003. *Morbidity and Mortality Weekly Report, 52,* 329–332.

Centers for Disease Control and Prevention. (2005a). *HIV/AIDS surveillance report, 2004.* Atlanta: U.S. Department of Health and Human Services.

Centers for Disease Control and Prevention. (2005b). HIV transmission in the adult film industry—Los Angeles, California, 2004. *Morbidity and Mortality Weekly Report, 54,* 923–926.

Centers for Disease Control and Prevention. (2009a). *HIV/AIDS Surveillance Report, 2007.* Vol. 19. Atlanta: U.S. Department of Health and Human Services, Centers for Disease Control and Prevention. http://www.cdc.gov/hiv/topics/surveillance/resources/reports/

Centers for Disease Control and Prevention. (2009b). *HIV/AIDS Surveillance in Adolescents and Young Adults (through 2007).* Retrieved May 4, 2010, from http://www.cdc.gov/hiv/topics/surveillance/resources/reports/

Cohen, D. A., Wu, S. Y., & Farley, T. A. (2004). Comparing the cost-effectiveness of HIV prevention interventions. *Journal of Acquired Immune Deficiency Syndrome, 37,* 1404–1414.

Cook, R. L., & Clark, D. B. (2005). Is there an association between alcohol consumption and sexually transmitted diseases? A systematic review. *Sexually Transmitted Diseases, 32,* 156–164.

De, P., Singh, A. E., Wong, T., Yacoub, W., & Jolly, A. M. (2004). Sexual network analysis of a gonorrhoea outbreak. *Sexually Transmitted Infections, 80,* 280–285.

Des Jarlais et al. (2000). HIV incidence among injection drug users in New York City, 1992–1997: Evidence for a declining epidemic. *American Journal of Public Health, 3,* 352–359.

DiClemente et al. (2004). Efficacy of an HIV prevention intervention for African American adolescent girls: A randomized controlled trial. *Journal of the American Medical Association, 292*, 171–179.

Drucker, E. (n.d.). *New York, through the eye of the needle: Notes from the drug wars.* Retrieved July 25, 2006, from http://www.drugtext.org/library/articles/89112.htm

el-Bassel, N., & Schilling, R. F. (1992). Fifteen-month follow-up of women methadone patients taught skills to reduce heterosexual HIV transmission. *Public Health Report, 107*, 500–504.

Ellen, J. M. (2003). The next generation of HIV prevention for adolescent females in the United States: Linking behavioral and epidemiologic sciences to reduce incidence of HIV. *Journal of Urban Health, 80*(4 Suppl. 3), iii40–iii49.

Ellen, J. M., Aral, S. O., & Madger, L. S. (1998). Do differences in sexual behaviors account for the racial/ethnic differences in adolescents' self-reported history of a sexually transmitted disease? *Sexually Transmitted Diseases, 25*, 125–129.

Fenton, K. A., & Imrie, J. (2005). Increasing rates of sexually transmitted diseases in homosexual men in western Europe and the United States: Why? *Infectious Disease Clinics of North America, 19*, 311–331.

Fullilove, R. E. (1998). Race and sexually transmitted diseases. *Sexually Transmitted Diseases, 25*, 130–131.

Fullilove, R. E., Green, L., & Fullilove, M. T. (2000). The Family-to-Family program: A structural intervention with implications for the prevention of HIV/AIDS and other community epidemics. *AIDS, 14*(Suppl. 1), S63–S67.

Hammett, T. M. (2006). HIV/AIDS and other infectious diseases among correctional inmates: Transmission, burden and an appropriate response. *American Journal of Public Health, 96*(6), 974–978.

Harawa et al. (2004). Associations of race/ethnicity with HIV prevalence and HIV-related behaviors among young men who have sex with men in 7 urban centers in the United States. *Journal of Acquired Immune Deficiency Syndrome, 35*, 526–536.

Harm Reduction Coalition. (2007). *Syringe exchange in prisons: The international experience.* Retrieved October 13, 2009, from http://www.harmreduction.org/article.php?id=418

Herbst et al. (2005). A meta-analytic review of HIV behavioral interventions for reducing sexual risk behavior of men who have sex with men. *Journal of Acquired Immune Deficiency Syndrome, 39*, 228–241.

Huebner, D. M. (2005). Is optimism really the enemy? New research on treatment optimism. *Focus, 20*(7), 5–6.

Hurley, S. F., Jolley, D. J., & Kaldor, J. M. (1997). Effectiveness of needle-exchange programmes for prevention of HIV infection. *Lancet, 349*, 1797–1800.

Institute of Medicine. (1997). *The hidden epidemic: Confronting sexually transmitted diseases.* Washington, DC: National Academies Press.

Institute of Medicine. (2001). *No time to lose: Getting more from HIV prevention.* Washington, DC: National Academies Press.

Jemmott III, J. B., Jemmott, L. S., & Fong, G. T. (1992). Reductions in HIV risk-associated sexual behaviors among black male adolescents: Effects of an AIDS prevention intervention. *American Journal of Public Health, 82,* 372–377.

Johnson et al. (2002). HIV prevention research for men who have sex with men: A systematic review and meta-analysis. *Journal of Acquired Immune Deficiency Syndrome, 30*(Suppl. 1), S118–S129.

Johnson, R. C., & Raphael, S. (2005). *The effects of male incarceration dynamics on AIDS infection rates among African-American women and men.* Unpublished manuscript.

Kamb et al. (1998). Efficacy of risk-reduction counseling to prevent human immunodeficiency virus and sexually transmitted diseases: A randomized controlled trial. *Journal of the American Medical Association, 280,* 1161–1167.

Kegeles, S. M., Hays, R. B., & Coates, T. J. (1996). The Mpowerment Project: A community-level HIV prevention intervention for young gay men. *American Journal of Public Health, 86,* 1129–1136.

Kelly et al. (1994). The effects of HIV/AIDS intervention groups for high-risk women in urban clinics. *American Journal of Public Health, 84,* 1918–1922.

Kelly, J. A. (1992). HIV risk behavior reduction following intervention with key opinion leaders of population: An experimental analysis. *American Journal of Public Health, 82,* 1483–1489.

Kerrigan et al. (2006). Environmental-structural interventions to reduce HIV/STI risk among female sex workers in the Dominican Republic. *American Journal of Public Health, 96,* 120–125.

Klovdahl, A. S., Potterat J. J., Woodhouse, D. E., Muth, J., & Muth, S. Q. (1992). HIV infection in an urban social network: A progress report. *Bulletin de Methodologie Sociologique, 36, 24*–33.

Koblin, B., Chesney, M., & Coates, T. J. (2004). Effects of a behavioural intervention to reduce acquisition of HIV infection among men who have sex with men: The EXPLORE randomised controlled study. *Lancet, 364,* 41–50.

Lane, S. D. (1993). *Needle exchange: A brief history.* Menlo Park, CA: Henry J. Kaiser Family Foundation. Retrieved July 25, 2006, from http://www.aegis.com/law/journals/1993/HKFNE009.html

Latkin, C. A., Sherman, S., & Knowlton, A. (2003). HIV prevention among drug users: Outcome of a network-oriented peer outreach intervention. *Health Psychology, 22,* 332–339.

Laumann, E. O., & Youm, Y. (1999). Racial/ethnic group differences in the prevalence of sexually transmitted diseases in the United States: A network explanation. *Sexually Transmitted Diseases, 26,* 250–261.

Laumann, E. O., Gagnon, J. H., Michael, R. T., & Michaels, S. (1994). *The social organization of sexuality.* Chicago: University of Chicago Press.

Lowe, S. (2009, February 12). California: Prison condom program reports no major problems. *The Reporter* (Vacaville). Retrieved June 9, 2009, from http://www.aegis.com/news/ads/2009/AD090267.html

McCusick et al. (1985). Reported changes in the sexual behavior of men at risk for AIDS, San Francisco, 1982–84: *The AIDS Behavioral Research Project. Public Health Reports, 100,* 622–629.

Millett, G. A., Peterson, J. L., Wolitski, R. J., & Stall, R. D. (2006). Greater risk for HIV infection of black men who have sex with men: A critical literature review. *American Journal of Public Health, 96*, 1007–1019.

Morris, M. (1997). Sexual networks and HIV. *AIDS, 11*(Suppl. A), S209–S216.

Morris, M., & Kretzschmar, M. (1997). Concurrent partnerships and the spread of HIV. *AIDS, 11*, 641–648.

National Minority AIDS Council. (2006). *African Americans, health disparities and HIV/AIDS: Recommendations for confronting the epidemic in black America*. Retrieved October 13, 2009, from http://www.nmac.org/index/grpp-publications

Neaigus, A. (1998). The network approach and interventions to prevent HIV among injection drug users. *Public Health Reports, 113*(Suppl. 1), 140–150.

Peterson et al. (1996). Evaluation of an HIV risk reduction intervention among African-American homosexual and bisexual men, *AIDS, 10*, 319–325.

Porco et al. (2004). Decline in HIV infectivity following the introduction of highly active antiretroviral therapy. *AIDS, 18*, 81–88.

Potterat, J. J., Rothenberg, R. B., & Muth, S. Q. (1999). Network structural dynamics and infectious disease propagation. *International Journal of Sexually Transmitted Diseases and AIDS, 10*, 182–185.

Rogers, E. M. (1962). *Diffusion of innovations*. New York: Free Press.

Rothenberg et al. (1998). Social network dynamics and HIV transmission. *AIDS, 12*, 1529–1536.

Rotheram-Borus et al. (2003). Reductions in HIV risk among runaway youth. *Prevention Science, 4*, 173–187.

Satcher, D. (2000). *Evidence-based findings on the efficacy of syringe exchange programs: An analysis of the scientific research completed since April 1998*. Washington, DC: U.S. Department of Health and Human Services.

Sell, R. L., Wells, J. A., & Wypij, D. (1995). The prevalence of homosexual behavior and attraction in the United States, the United Kingdom, and France: Results of national population-based samples. *Archives of Sexual Behavior, 24*, 235–248.

Susman, E. (2001, August 13). New York needle exchange "reverses" AIDS. *United Press International Science News*. Retrieved July 25, 2006, from http://www.encyclopedia.com/doc/1P1-46236931.html

Thomas, J. C., & Sampson, L. A. (2005). High rates of incarceration as a social force associated with community rates of sexually transmitted infection. *Journal of Infectious Diseases, 191*(Suppl. 1), S55–S60.

Trostle, J. A. (2004). *Epidemiology and culture*. New York: Cambridge University Press.

Valdiserri et al. (1989). AIDS prevention in homosexual and bisexual men: Results of a randomized trial evaluating two risk reduction interventions. *AIDS, 3*, 21–26.

Valente, T. W., & Saba, W. P. (2001). Campaign exposure and interpersonal communication as factors in contraceptive use in Bolivia. *Journal of Health Communication, 6*, 303–322.

Valleroy et al. (2000). HIV prevalence and associated risks in young men who have sex with men. *Journal of the American Medical Association, 284*, 198–204.

Wasserheit, J. N., & Aral, S. O. (1996). The dynamic topology of sexually transmitted disease epidemics: Implications for prevention strategies. *Journal of Infectious Diseases, 174*(Suppl. 2), 201–213.

Weinhardt, L. S., Carey, M. P., Johnson, B. T., & Bickham, N. L. (1999). Effects of HIV counseling and testing on sexual risk behavior. *American Journal of Public Health, 89*, 1397–1405.

Wilson, C. M., Houser, J., Partlow, C., Rudy, B. J., Futterman, D. C., & Friedman, L. B. (2001). The REACH (Reaching for Excellence in Adolescent Care and Health) project: Study design, methods, and population profile. *Journal of Adolescent Health, 29*(Suppl. 3), 8–18.

Winkelstein et al. (1987). The San Francisco Men's Health Study: III. Reduction in human immunodeficiency virus transmission among homosexual/bisexual men, 1982–86. *American Journal of Public Health, 76*, 685–689.

Wohlfeiler, D. (1997). Community organizing and community building among gay and bisexual men. In M. Minkler (Ed.), *Community organizing and community building for health* (pp. 230–243). New Brunswick, NJ: Rutgers University Press.

Wohlfeiler, D. (2002). From community to clients: The professionalisation of HIV prevention among gay men and its implications for intervention selection. *Sexually Transmitted Infections, 78*(Suppl. 1), i176–i182.

Wohlfeiler, D. (2005). Network-level interventions as feasible structural-level interventions with potentially high impact. In *Prevention strategies for STD and HIV prevention: What, where and when.* Amsterdam: International Society for Sexually Transmitted Diseases Research.

Wohlfeiler, D., & Potterat, J. J. (2003, April). *How do sexual networks affect HIV/STD prevention?* Center for AIDS Prevention Studies Fact Sheet No. 50E. Retrieved July 28, 2006, from http://www.caps.ucsf.edu/pubs/FS/networks.php

Wohlfeiler, D., & Potterat, J. J. (2005). Using gay men's sexual networks to reduce sexually transmitted disease (STD)/human immunodeficiency virus (HIV) transmission. *Sexually Transmitted Diseases, 32*(10 Suppl.), S48–S52.

Woods et al. (2003). Public policy regulating private and public space in gay bathhouses. *Journal of Acquired Immune Deficiency Syndrome, 32*, 417–423.

15

Mental Health in the Realm of Primary Prevention

Anita M. Wells
GiShawn A. Mance
M. Taqi Tirmazi
Sidebar contributor:
Joseph P. Gone

LEARNING OBJECTIVES

- Understand that social determinants influence mental health and that, as a result, many mental health problems are preventable.
- Describe various elements of a primary prevention approach to mental health that promotes positive mental health and that prevents negative health outcomes.

MENTAL HEALTH IN THE UNITED STATES

The World Health Organization (WHO) defines *mental health* as "a state of well-being in which every individual realizes his or her own potential, can cope with the normal stresses of life, can work productively and fruitfully, and is able to make a contribution to her or his community" (WHO, 2007). Keyes (2002) describes the presence of mental health as "flourishing" and the absence of mental health as "languishing." These definitions speak to a strength-based model of mental health rather than to a model that views mental health simply as the absence of illness. A strength-based understanding of mental health opens a pathway to explore strategies for primary prevention.

Although mental health is critical to our overall health and well-being, it is often peripheral to or missing entirely from wide-ranging conversations and policy discussions about preventive health in the United States. Mental health is perhaps most readily associated with secondary and tertiary prevention, that is, with detection and treatment of an already existing illness. This association, however, overshadows the fact that many mental health concerns are indeed preventable.

It is easy to overlook the value of mental health until problems surface. Just as society must promote physical health and address illness through awareness, preventive models, and policy, so, too, must society promote mental health. Mental health is indispensable to personal well-being, family and interpersonal relationships, and contributions to community and society. To fully understand the integral role of mental health, it is important to delineate the continuum of mental health and mental illness. *Mental Health: A Report of the Surgeon General* (U.S. Department of Health and Human Services, 1999) defined *mental health* as "a state of successful performance of mental function, resulting in productive activities, fulfilling relationships with other people, and the ability to adapt to change and to cope with adversity." Alternately, *mental illness* refers collectively to all diagnosable mental disorders, which are health conditions characterized by alterations in thinking, mood, or behavior (or some combination thereof) associated with distress and/or impaired functioning. (This chapter will use the term *mental health problems* for signs and symptoms of insufficient intensity or duration to meet the criteria for any mental disorder.) Poor mental health, not at either end of the continuum, can be characterized by mental distress and by difficulty coping with and adapting to change.

Mental health concerns are often viewed as problems of the individual, primarily genetic or chemical in nature, and the purview of the few, society's most recognizably ill (Üstün, 1999). In reality, the prevalence rate in the United States for lifetime mental illness (those illnesses meeting the criteria for a mental disorder according to the most widely used source for psychiatric diagnoses, the *Diagnostic and Statistical Manual for Mental Disorders-IV*) is roughly 50 percent (Kessler et al., 2008). In other words, at some time in their lives, half of the people in the United States will experience psychological distress significant enough to cause impairment in one or more areas of functioning (for example, work, school, and interpersonal relationships). Estimates of the incidence of mental illness among the U.S. adult population are 26 percent, or approximately one in four; estimates of adults with serious mental illness are 6 percent, or one in seventeen (National Institute of Mental Health, 2009). The incidence of mental illness that impairs children and adolescents is currently estimated at one in ten (U.S. Public Health Service, 2000). Those suffering from mental illness, particularly those receiving no treatment or sporadic treatment, tend to have increased rates of physical illness, a high absentee rate from work, and a pattern of social isolation (Department of Health & Human Services (DHHS) Office of the Surgeon General Substance Abuse and Mental Health Services Administration, 2001). According to the National Academies of Health report (O'Connell, Boat, & Warner, 2009), the financial cost of mental health problems, including treatment and loss in productivity to society, is $247 billion annually.

STRENGTH-BASED MODEL OF MENTAL HEALTH

Research dating back to the 1930s suggests that researchers and practitioners have been interested in the prevention of mental illness for some time (Felix & Kramer, 1952). Felix and Kramer in 1952 suggested that examining the environment's impact on mental illness could shift psychiatry from a focus on treatment to a focus on prevention. Primary prevention in concert with treatment efforts has been described as playing a key role in diminishing the tremendous public health burden of depression (Cuijpers, Van, Smit, Mihalopoulos, & Beekman, 2008). Recent mental health research examining depression (Cuijpers et al., 2008; Schoevers et al., 2006) and *post traumatic stress disorder* (PTSD) (Feldner, Monson, & Friedman, 2007) concluded that primary prevention of these mental disorders is indeed possible.

The community mental health movement of the 1970s prompted practitioners to consider poverty and other social ills as potential root causes of mental illness and, consequently, to view mental illness as preventable (Wagenfield, 1972). The Institute of Medicine (IOM) Committee on Prevention of Mental Disorder published a report in 1994 that defined prevention as primary prevention only; the definition was restricted to interventions occurring before initial onset of an illness. The report referenced some of the social determinants of health (for example, poverty) as risk factors for mental illness, but did not relate poverty or any other social determinant to prevention priorities or strategies. Recent studies have concluded that common mental illnesses like depression and rare mental illnesses like schizophrenia are linked to poverty, unemployment, institutional racism, community violence, limited access to resources, and other social determinants of health (Jenkins et al., 2008; Jones, Gallagher III, Pisa, & McFalls Jr., 2008).

Today the world's population is facing an economic crisis. This crisis has had a severe detrimental impact on many people, including those who have lost jobs, those unable to find work, those attempting to return to work after years of retirement, and those living on fixed incomes. Financial insecurity can be a strong catalyst for anxiety, hopelessness, anger, depression, and new or increased substance use (Jayakody, Danziger, & Pollack, 2000); debt in and of itself has been found to be independently associated with poor mental health (Jenkins et al., 2008). Even after researchers accounted for income level, having a high amount of debt was linked to a greater likelihood of poor mental health (Jenkins et al., 2008). Financial strain, a social determinant of health, has been linked to poor mental health and mental illness. Jones and colleagues (2008) found that the socioeconomic status of the family of origin of a person with schizophrenia was associated with *deficit schizophrenia*, a form of the disease characterized by a dearth of emotional responsiveness, initiative, and enjoyment in life. In essence, deficit schizophrenia was more often found in those who came from backgrounds of low socioeconomic status (Jones et al., 2008).

The disparities created by the social factors that impede physical and psychological well-being have garnered the attention of scholars worldwide. For example, the WHO tasked the Commission on Social Determinants of Health (CSDH) with supporting initiatives that tackle the social causes of poor health and avoidable health inequalities. People's daily living conditions have a strong influence on health equity. The CSDH proposed that access to quality housing, clean water, and sanitation are human rights (Commission on Social Determinants of Health, 2008). Thus, the CSDH called for the following:

- Greater availability of affordable housing by investing in urban slum upgrades that prioritize the provision of water, sanitation and electricity
- Healthy and safe behaviors to be promoted equitably, including encouraging physical activity and healthy eating, and reducing violence and crime through good environmental design and regulatory controls (limiting sales of alcohol, for example)
- Sustained investment in rural development
- Economic and social policy responses to climate change and other environmental degradation that take health equity into account

The assertions of the CSDH highlight the need to move beyond a reactive framework to a preventive model of health. With specific regards to mental health and mental illness, we, as a society, have moved toward a model increasingly focused on genetics and chemical etiology (Kendler, Prescott, Myers, & Neale, 2003); these aspects of mental health and illness are, without question, important to study and understand. However, it remains critical that we keep sight of the social determinants of health that operate in the public sphere. If we do not address the social determinants of mental illness, our efforts to prevent mental illness and promote mental health will ultimately be unsuccessful.

ORGANIZATION OF THIS CHAPTER

We have four primary aims for this chapter: (1) to foreground mental health in the primary prevention discussion; (2) to examine mental illness and strategies for primary prevention in three distinct U.S. populations linked by a common vulnerability to poor mental health and mental illness; (3) to identify shared determinants of mental illness among these populations; and (4) to encourage dialogue about psychological well-being and its place in the landscape of public health. Our approach to mental health in this chapter primarily uses a social determinants framework and, as such, includes environmental and systemic factors that influence the development of mental illness that can be addressed in strategies for primary prevention.

Veterans of the wars in Iraq and Afghanistan, immigrant youth, and urban youth bear a disproportionate burden of mental illness and poor mental health compared to the rest of the U.S. population. We begin with a discussion of mental health among veterans of the wars in Iraq and Afghanistan and then examine mental health among immigrant and urban youth. Each section includes an exploration of strategies for primary prevention. We conclude by offering a social justice analysis of the primary prevention of mental illness.

A PRIMARY PREVENTION FRAMEWORK FOR SUBSTANCE ABUSE AND MENTAL HEALTH IN SAN MATEO COUNTY, CALIFORNIA

San Mateo County, California, has emerged as an innovator in the landscape of primary prevention and mental health. Acknowledging the importance of *primary prevention* for both mental health and alcohol and other drug services, San Mateo County Health System Behavioral Health & Recovery Services (BHRS) devised an interdisciplinary planning process in 2008 to determine strategies that emphasize primary prevention and complement existing treatment services.

A primary prevention approach means taking action *before* mental health problems have occurred, rather than intervening after symptoms have appeared or incidents have occurred. This approach can prevent certain conditions, such as depression, anxiety, and (PTSD), and can reduce or delay onset, reduce severity of symptoms, and support treatment outcomes for those with mental health problems. For instance, creating strong social networks in communities not only supports prevention outcomes, but supports people experiencing mental health problems by reducing social isolation. By focusing on treating those in need and by reducing those who may need services in the first place, BHRS aims to ensure that all San Mateo County residents can live as fully contributing and successful members of their families and communities.

This approach requires looking at the role that the social, physical, economic, and cultural environments play in contributing to mental health problems and at how those environments can be changed to prevent some behavioral health problems from occurring in the first place.

The BHRS Primary Prevention Framework process identified four overarching prevention strategies to reduce the number of people who need intensive behavioral health services:

Enhancing place improves the places people live, work, play, attend school, worship, and socialize, to support mental health, reduce substance abuse, and decrease exposure to violence. Focusing on place helps to ensure that all people live in safe neighborhoods, have access to affordable quality housing, and that their neighborhoods are designed to promote social interaction.

Connecting people strengthens positive social-emotional development, enhances social connections, and reduces isolation and exposure to violence. The policies and programs of neighborhoods, schools, work sites and other community settings can foster social connection and positive social development. For instance, work sites can support positive behavioral health among all employees and schools and other children's settings can provide quality learning environments to support the development of positive assets.

Fostering prosperity reduces stigma and enhances economic opportunity and self-sufficiency, especially for those most at risk for mental health problems and substance abuse. Securing a flourishing business community and providing job opportunities and training services to *all* residents helps ensure financial independence, self-efficacy, and neighborhood stability.

Expanding partnerships engages multiple government sectors, businesses, and community members—including people receiving behavioral health services and their families—to promote mental well-being, reduce substance abuse, and decrease exposure to violence through their actions, decisions, practices, and policies. This strategy acknowledges that the underlying contributors to preventable mental illness and addiction (for example, place, people, and prosperity) expand well beyond the authority and influence of behavioral health and recovery services. The plan recognizes the essential need to collaborate with various sectors within government, the business community, and community groups and residents to ensure that each stakeholder contributes to and understands how their role can help promote community mental health.

By integrating these four primary prevention strategies into the practices and policies of BHRS, other departments within government and the social, physical, economic, and cultural sectors within the community can be modified to improve behavioral health outcomes and quality of life for people in San Mateo County. BHRS's prevention framework can serve as a model for counties throughout the country to advance primary prevention.

For more information on San Mateo's Primary Prevention Framework, see http://preventioninstitute.org/component/jlibrary/article/id-53/127.html

Source: Prevention Institute.

VETERANS

Among the nation's populations most severely and disproportionately affected by poor mental health are veterans returning from the wars in Iraq (Operation Iraqi Freedom, or OIF) and Afghanistan (Operation Enduring Freedom, or OEF) and their family members (Cozza, Chun, & Polo, 2005; Hoge et al., 2004; Huus, 2007). As a result of firsthand exposure to trauma and violence, many OIF and OEF veterans are returning home with serious mental health problems, including PTSD, depression, and substance abuse (Cozza et al., 2005). The exposure to trauma and violence has also resulted in the return of many veterans who have no diagnosable mental illness but who are at risk of developing poor mental health due to stressors they encounter upon their return, such as job loss, difficulty in accessing medical care, and families who are unprepared to provide support during the difficult period of reentry.

One of the distinctions of the wars in Iraq and Afghanistan is that there is no true front line; consequently, both infantry and combat support troops are exposed to trauma, thus increasing the number of veterans at risk of poor mental health or of being burdened by mental disorders (Wynn, 2007). Although the majority of veterans with mental health problems are infantrymen and women, health care workers and combat support troops are also negatively affected (Kolkow, Spira, Morse, & Grieger, 2007). Other hallmarks of OIF and OEF are multiple deployments, extended deployments, and insufficient downtime between deployments; these practices have increased the psychological distress and overall stress of service members and their families (Shanker, 2008). As of this writing, more than 1.7 million troops have been deployed to Iraq and Afghanistan, and nearly half of these troops have been deployed more than once (Associated Press, 2009).

According to Sammons and Batten (2008), OIF and OEF are the first instances of war on record from which psychological injury associated with war is expected to exceed physical injury among survivors. Results from a study of 103,788 OIF & OEF veterans seen at Veterans Administration (VA) facilities showed that 25 percent were diagnosed with a mental disorder (Seal, Bertenthal, Miner, Sen, & Marmar, 2007). Completed suicides among OIF and OEF veterans ages twenty to twenty-four have reached rates four times as high as their peers who have never served in the armed services (twenty-two to thirty-two out of 100,000 and eight out of 100,000, respectively) (Keteyian, 2007a). Family members of OIF and OEF veterans, too, are experiencing mental health problems, including depression and substance abuse (Sayers, Farrow, Ross, & Oslin, 2009).

Given the inevitability of veterans returning home changed, some in severe mental distress, is it appropriate to consider primary prevention as it relates to poor mental health and mental illness of veterans? One could argue that primary prevention of mental health problems among OIF and OEF veterans is impossible, as it would ultimately entail men and women in the armed forces would avoid a war zone. Although the abolition of violent conflict is perhaps the ultimate primary prevention of war-related psychological problems, in the presence and reality of war, we must think broadly about the meaning of primary prevention and about the relationships between primary and secondary prevention.

In doing so we must consider what can be done to prevent the development of poor mental health in members of this population who do not yet have a mental illness.

Primary prevention may occur without abolishing war. Review of and adjustment to military policy regarding multiple deployments is one such avenue. In addition, maladjustment and enduring poor quality of life following reentry, two measurable outcomes that contribute to poor mental health, must be among the targets of primary prevention. Put another way, primary prevention must focus on eliminating those factors that can lead to difficulty coping with life's everyday stressors and to stunted potential and lifetime impairment in social and emotional functioning. For example, interventions can be made to prepare families before deployment and after the return of a loved one. The primary prevention of mental distress is a measurable outcome of mental health promotion. In order to be effective, mental health promotion requires an examination of multiple factors, including social determinants of health such as employment, housing, health care coverage, interpersonal relationships, and stigma associated with mental distress.

SOCIAL DETERMINANTS OF HEALTH

As noted in the introduction to this chapter, social determinants of health inform both physical and mental health outcomes. Two of those determinants, employment and housing, are key concerns for many OIF and OEF veterans (Wynn, 2007). The process of reentry is arduous for many service members (Sayers et al., 2009). Some experience difficulty in finding or maintaining jobs. Some become homeless (Wynn, 2007). For many OIF and OEF veterans who become homeless, their path to homelessness is short and swift compared to veterans of past wars; some become homeless within eighteen months after returning home (O'Keefe & Franke-Ruta, 2009). Documentary filmmaker Lohaus found that veterans across the country are experiencing homelessness and that their lives provide evidence of the direct relationship between homelessness and poor mental health (Lohaus, 2006).

FAMILIAL RELATIONSHIPS

Many military families will experience trauma as a result of a loved one's deployment and will recover (Sammons & Batten, 2008). For others, however, the road to readjustment following a loved one's deployment is rocky (Renshaw, Rodrigues, & Jones, 2009). Relationship difficulties among military families are one indication of the need for increased attention to quality-of-life issues and mental health and well-being in this population (Milliken, Auchterlonie, & Hoge, 2007). Sammons and Batten (2008) suggest that "relationship conflict, occupational dysfunction, depression, and substance abuse" are among the most common and challenging problems for families. News reports have highlighted partner physical abuse by recently returned service members. This consequence of deployment can have dire implications for families, sometimes with tragic results.

Gibbs and colleagues (2007) found that neglect and physical abuse of children by the at-home parent was higher when the enlisted parent was deployed. Reasons for the maltreatment are not fully understood, although it was hypothesized that lack of preparation for the familial experience of deployment and the accompanying stress to the at-home parent are likely to be responsible. Literature on the mental health of children of deployed military parents has emphasized both their vulnerability and their resilience (Lincoln, Swift, & Shorteno-Fraser, 2008).

Many military families experience a sense of loss, whether from a veteran's death or from the ways in which their family members have changed as a result of participating in OIF and OEF (Keteyian, 2007b). The personal loss of familial intimacy and economic stability can be devastating to family members. The loss to communities and society as a whole is also great and may include the following: loss of productive workers, breakdown of families, homelessness, and an increased burden borne by the health care and legal systems (Burnam, Meredith, Tanielian, & Jaycox, 2009; Ritchie, Benedek, Malone, & Carr-Malone, 2006). An additional consequence of OIF and OEF for military families has been a sense of social isolation (Huus, 2007). This feeling is often exacerbated for families of Reserve and National Guard members, most of whom do not live on a base or in an organized military community where they could receive support (Huus, 2007; Lilley, 2007; Renshaw et al., 2009).

STIGMA

The stigma associated with mental health problems and concerns about the detrimental effects of that stigma prevent veterans from seeking help (Stecker, Fortney, Hamilton, & Ajzen, 2007). A study of 6,200 OEF and OIF soldiers and Marines showed that concern about stigma was twice as high among those whose survey responses indicated the presence of poor mental health (Hoge et al., 2004). Stigmatization is seen as embarrassing and potentially damaging to one's career in the military (Hoge et al., 2004; Rand Corporation, 2008). Fear of stigmatization could be a disincentive to honestly report psychological distress, given the concern that a record of mental health problems could result in denial of promotion within the military or could delay the return home following deployment.

ADDRESSING PRIMARY PREVENTION

There are clear primary prevention strategies for poor mental health in veteran populations, some of which will be discussed here. In order to maximize primary prevention, however, it is important to understand strategies for secondary prevention, as well as the synergy between primary and secondary prevention that will ultimately result in greater overall primary prevention. For example, openly addressing the stigma associated with seeking treatment for mental illness in the military—a secondary prevention strategy—can increase the number of people struggling with psychological disorders who seek help. This secondary prevention tactic assists the primary prevention work of shifting the paradigm from one that understands the expression of distress as weakness to one that understands the expression of distress as essential to the promotion of and preservation of mental health and well-being. This combination of strategies is a one-two punch that recognizes the need to proactively prevent poor mental health and be promptly reactive when mental health has been compromised.

Primary prevention must include a focus on the many servicemen and servicewomen who will return home with no measurable mental illness but who will be confronted with: the stress of a job lost while serving, ill-preparedness for civilian employment, gaps in health care coverage when separating from the military and entering the VA health care system, and families unprepared for the ways in which servicemen and servicewomen have changed. These conditions can lead to poor coping, limited productivity, increased isolation, and impaired relationships (in essence, poor mental health), which can, in turn, result in increased experiences of anxiety, depression, and substance abuse.

Here we offer a brief exploration of four considerations for primary prevention, including the following: military deployment policy, social determinants, stigma, and family services. These are followed by related secondary prevention considerations, including mental disorders common among OIF and OEF veterans in need of treatment and changes in health care for those veterans experiencing mental health problems.

MILITARY DEPLOYMENT POLICY

A prudent avenue for primary prevention of mental illness in this population is the revision of military policy to restrict the number of multiple deployments, extended deployments, and *stop-lossing* of service members (the involuntary extension of a service member's active duty, which delays his or her end of term of service)—and to increase the time between deployments. This prevention strategy is supported by research on the detrimental mental health impact of these types of deployments on servicemen and servicewomen (Shanker, 2008). More than 35 percent of those deployed to OIF were deployed more than once, and more than 10 percent were deployed three times or more. Rates of post traumatic stress, anxiety, and depression symptoms, including insomnia, were positively linked to number of deployments (Shanker, 2008). Increased time between deployments (at least twelve months), reliable deployment end dates, a limit on the number of deployments, and fewer deployments overall would likely decrease the psychiatric symptoms in service members and would allow military personnel time to replenish their mental and emotional reserves potentially averting the development of poor mental health.

EMPLOYMENT AND HOUSING

Housing and financial stability are both factors that affect quality of life during reentry (Wynn, 2007). Effective job training and placement programs that specifically target and reach returned veterans are essential. Job training and placement for those able to work will relieve financial strain on veterans and their families and will help to ensure that veterans do not lose their housing.

One program that addresses homelessness and job retraining, as well as mental health concerns, is the Maryland Center for Veterans Education and Training (MCVET, 2009). MCVET is a residential job training and educational rehabilitation program in Baltimore, Maryland that offers safe, clean transitional housing and employment and educational opportunities to any homeless veteran. The program primarily serves those who are experiencing homelessness complicated by substance use and/or a psychiatric or medical illness. Approximately ten percent of MCVET's residents—its students—do not have a comorbid substance abuse problem. MCVET works in conjunction with the Maryland Job Service, the Maryland State Department of Vocational Rehabilitation, and the Veterans Affairs Maryland Health Care System to provide training and preparation for higher-paying jobs than those typically held by students prior to entry into MCVET (MCVET, 2009).In addition, the Post-9/11 GI Bill, effective August 1, 2009, offers educational assistance for college and also vocational training to those who have served ninety or more active-duty days since September, 2001. A unique feature of this program is that it was designed to offer the same benefits to Reserve and National Guard members (Military.com, 2009) who have typically received disparate benefits from their active duty and veteran counterparts. In early November, 2009, at the National Summit on Homeless Veterans, VA Secretary Eric Shinseki announced a five-year-plan to end homelessness among veterans. A major focus of this plan is that it includes a primary prevention emphasis rather than solely a secondary prevention goal of finding housing for those already homeless. The plan acknowledges and plans to confront some of the risk factors for homelessness among veterans, including joblessness (Levine, 2009).

MINIMIZING STIGMA

Hoge and his colleagues (2004) proposed that fear of stigma could best be prevented through outreach to veterans and reassurances of confidentiality. Post-deployment mental health screening of all troops by the VA may aid in decreasing stigmatization and openness regarding mental health problems (Seal et al., 2007). These approaches are valid; however, we must recognize that culture has a profound effect on our understanding of mental health (Link, Mirotznik, & Cullen, 1991). Education of both the military and civilian public and of all health care practitioners about mental health and illness is essential to changing widespread-cultural perceptions of mental illness as weakness and madness. A study with OIF and OEF veterans (Pietrzak, Johnson, Goldstein, Malley, & Southwick, 2009) revealed that those who perceived they had the support of their units were more likely to seek mental health care. In addition, public enforcement of policies in military and civilian employment that prevent tacit dismissal, demotion, or career stagnation due to mental illness could more effectively reduce stigmatization for seeking treatment and, ultimately, help to prevent poor mental health post-deployment. If an individual knows that his or her acknowledgment of stressors and their impact will be received positively and supportively—this goes back to culture—that individual may be more likely to use already existing social supports in his or her environment before the difficulties progress into significant stress and poor mental health. We know from prior research that perceived social support is associated not only with more veterans seeking treatment (Pietrzak et al., 2009) but also with greater health overall, including mental health (Ren, Skinner, Lee, & Kazis, 1999).

FAMILY SERVICES

Services for preparation and care of the family must be provided before deployment and during and following deployment. Additional preparation of families during these phases of service is a primary prevention strategy likely to prevent long-term social and emotional impairment among military families. In fact, psychoeducation and receipt of accurate information will be sufficient to keep some families from developing clinically significant distress (Sammons & Batten, 2008).

Reintegration requires adjustment on the part of all family members (Sammons & Batten, 2008). It is critical to recognize the needs of service members, as well as of families (Sammons & Batten, 2008). Huebner and colleagues (2007) found that understanding the concept of *ambiguous loss*, a combined feeling of uncertainty and loss, is essential to prevention and intervention efforts to forestall the development of poor mental health in children of deployed parents (Huebner, Mancini, Wilcox, Grass, & Grass, 2007). Lincoln, Swift, and Shorteno-Fraser (2008) and Erbes, Westermeyer, Engdahl, and Johnsen (2007) suggest that treatment for veterans that integrates the family is likely to be the most beneficial. Interventions for the entire family prior to, during, and after deployment have the potential to intercept or diminish anxiety, anger, despondency, and isolation—all related to poor mental health.

Two programs that have had success in helping military families manage the stress of deployment and the reintegration of service members are Families OverComing Under Stress (FOCUS) and SOFAR: Strategic Outreach to Families of All Reservists. Both of these programs engage families during and following deployment and work with families to increase communication and understanding of how each member was affected by deployment. The FOCUS program, which has thirteen sites across the United States, was developed in response to the Defense Health Board Task Force on Mental Health's recognition of the need for preventive services to assist military families in fostering positive and adaptive skills for managing stress and emotions. The program describes itself as a *resiliency-training program* (FOCUS Project, 2009). Its mission is to help the entire family (especially children) with the inevitable changes in feelings, routines, and role responsibilities that take place with deployment and reintegration (FOCUS Project, 2009). SOFAR, with branches in four states, emphasizes helping children and is also focused on prevention and building resiliency among military families. Among SOFAR's primary goals are "to prepare the family for the return of the soldier and to work with the reunited family when the soldier has returned . . . and to help the family negotiate the difficult process of reintegration" (SOFAR, 2009). SOFAR provides free psychological support and prevention services through a variety of mental health professionals to families of National Guard and Reservists deployed in or who have returned from OIF or OEF (Darwin & Reich, 2006).

CONCERNS UNIQUE TO PTSD

The most commonly diagnosed mental disorders among returning troops are PTSD and depression (Hoge et al., 2004). PTSD is an anxiety disorder a person can develop after seeing or living through an event that caused or threatened serious harm or death. PTSD causes significant distress and/or impairment in social, occupational, or other important areas of functioning (American Psychiatric Association, 1994).

Reports of PTSD among OIF and OEF service members range from 13 percent to 30 percent. (Hoge, Terhakopian, Castro, Messer, & Engel, 2007; Jakupcak, Luterek, Hunt, Conybeare, & McFall, 2008). Those with PTSD are at increased risk for medical illnesses and additional psychiatric illness (Friedman, 2006; Hoge et al., 2007). PTSD among OIF and OEF veterans has been found to relate directly to health symptoms (Vasterling et al., 2008), frequency of medical visits for sickness, physical-health complaints, days missed from work, poor self-perception of general health (Hoge et al., 2007), and poor health functioning (Jakupcak et al., 2008). PTSD has also been independently associated with impaired social functioning and emotional well-being and with decreased energy and overall quality of life (Erbes et al., 2007), each of which affects interpersonal relationships and ability to work. Veteran PTSD, in particular, is associated with difficulty in reintegration and familial problems, including with children feeling afraid of their veteran parents (Sayers et al., 2009). Thus, the availability of health care providers and prompt access to those providers is key to the mental health and well-being of the veteran. Health care availability also serves as a primary prevention against diminished familial relationships and the potential development of poor mental health among family members.

HEALTH CARE

A large survey of OIF and OEF veterans revealed that 60 percent of those being seen for mental health problems received their initial diagnoses in primary care clinics and not mental health offices. These data suggest a need for funding for appropriately prepared staff among both civilian and VA non-mental health facilities (Seal et al., 2007). Accurate diagnoses are critical to ensuring that a veteran receives the right kind of treatment. The large numbers of Iraq War veterans seeking and using mental health services indicates a significant need for providers (Hoge, Auchterlonie, & Milliken, 2006) that is likely to increase. Non-military health care providers must be trained to recognize symptoms of mental distress in veterans, particularly those returning from OIF and OEF, so that early intervention can take place. Those who do not receive prompt treatment often experience unremitting impairment at a cost to the individual, to his or her family, and to society as a whole (Rand Corporation, 2008). Accurate diagnosis and availability of mental health treatment are factors in the secondary prevention of long-term mental health problems among veterans. Increased and long-term funding for mental health care is essential, as is increased public awareness of the War's impact on its veterans' mental health and well-being. Many veterans who are experiencing mental health problems are not assessed as meeting requisite disability ratings criteria to enable them to receive disability benefits for their mental health. Access to the health care veterans often need immediately—to give them the best chance at stable mental health and well-being—is inadequate. Many still face long wait times to see a mental health professional and establish treatment (Wynn, 2007). The VA system must continue to increase its efforts to move quickly in assessing OIF and OEF veterans and in processing their benefits claims. To err in favor of immediate treatment for veterans seems preferable and less costly in the long run than to err in the opposite direction and later approve benefits for a veteran whose quality of life and ability to contribute to society may have deteriorated in the interim.

AN AMERICAN INDIAN ILLUSTRATION OF PRIMARY PREVENTION

Joseph P. Gone

Given the urgent need to address prevalent mental health problems, it is easy to over-look cultural diversity in the perceived characteristics, causes, courses, and cures for disabling emotional distress. I was reminded of this when I explored depression and drinking on the Fort Belknap Indian reservation in Montana (Gone, 2007, 2008). There I met a middle-aged cultural traditionalist named Traveling Thunder who explained to me why many community members struggled with substance abuse and associated distress. In his view, the primary problem was that, "We never was happy living like a Whiteman." As it turned out, this simple observation captured an entire rationale about reservation mental health that reappears everywhere I go in Indian country.

Traveling Thunder outlined four historical epochs in recounting his communi-ty's past. In the era of Pre-Colonial Paradise, he described indigenous North America as a utopia in which "there was no alcohol, no drugs" because people lived accord-ing to strict aboriginal custom. Once the Whiteman arrived in the era of Colonial Incursion, Euro-American domination changed everything, decimating the customs that had suited Native life for millennia. This Euro-American suppression of cultural practices led to an era of postcolonial anomie in which community members could no longer make sense of who they were and of what their futures might be.

Here Traveling Thunder explicitly referenced mental health problems: "If people ain't proud of who they are, then they're . . . doing alcohol, drugs. Once you're into alcohol and drugs, you're gonna probably get into a depression. . . . And you're gonna want to kill yourself." Fortunately, Traveling Thunder also recognized a fourth epoch, the contemporary era of Post-Colonial Revitalization. He specifically credited the return to ceremonial practice starting in the 1970s with the potential to restore "an alcohol- and drug-free mind" to distressed tribal members. Thus, in contrast to consulting psychiatrists who threaten to "brainwash me forever so I can be like a Whiteman," Traveling Thunder recommended "putting up" a ceremony for people contending with serious emotional distress.

Attention to this *discourse of distress* offers important lessons for the cross-cultural prevention of mental health problems. First, such discourses make plain that "mental health" might be experienced and expressed quite differently in diverse cultural settings. For example, Traveling Thunder's emphasis on history, identity, and spirituality contrast markedly with the professional emphasis on broken brains or unexpressed emotions. Second, such discourses implicate broad-based antecedent conditions (Felner & Felner, 1989) rather than classic disease analogies in tracing the developmental trajectories of emotional distress. For example, Traveling Thunder's post-colonial anomie sets the stage for any number of maladaptive conditions—including substance abuse, educational failure, and interpersonal violence—such that prevention of any one outcome is likely also to forestall others.

Third, such discourses reveal the promise of preventive interventions that originate locally and achieve their effects because they "make sense" within local frames of meaning. For example, Traveling Thunder's prescription of ceremonial practice as the most appropriate mode of intervention for mental health problems requires little from outside professionals and instead privileges the expertise of reservation ritual leaders in meeting the needs of their own communities. Finally, this recognition of effective local resources for addressing emotional distress helps to redefine the role of outside professionals who desire to help. For example, instead of reproducing the expert-client relationship with its inherent power asymmetry, knowledgeable preventionists might enter instead into collaborative and empowering partnerships with tribal communities in which successful prevention projects fundamentally depend on the proportionate contributions of everyone involved. In this reworking of the colonial encounter, such prevention partnerships might actually generate therapeutic benefits in their own right.

IMMIGRANT CHILDREN IN THE UNITED STATES

Over the last several decades, the immigrant population in the United States has increased drastically. Immigrant children and U.S.-born children of immigrants under the age of eighteen are the fastest-growing segment of the population (Capps, Fix, & Murray, 2005; Portes & Rumbaut, 2001). Scholars suggest that migration presents a myriad of challenges to youth development and adaptation (Portes & Rumbaut, 2001; Suarez-Orozco & Suarez-Orozco, 2001; Tartar, 1998; Ulman & Tartar, 2001). Whether they are first, second, or third generation, immigrant youth may face tremendous mental health challenges brought on by the process of acculturation and adaptation. It is important to note that there is great diversity within the immigrant population and immigrant children should not be compartmentalized into one general category due to their diverse ethnic backgrounds, generational classification (e.g. first, second or third generation etc.), immigration status, language proficiency, socioeconomic status, cultural practice, religious background, and other qualities.

BACKGROUND

At present, more than one-tenth (28.4 million) of the U.S. population is foreign-born, and immigrant children make up one out of every five people in America (Portes & Rumbaut, 2001). The first and second generations of immigrants and their children total approximately fifty-five million people (Portes & Rumbaut, 2001). Many of these immigrants come to the United States with children or settle down and have children in the United States. Moreover, it is estimated that by 2010, the foreign-born population may grow to make up more than 42 million people and more than 13 percent of the U.S. population (Capps et al., 2005). Mexico accounts for 9 million (30 percent) of the estimated 28.4 million foreign-born in the United States, Asia accounts for 8 million (26 percent); the remainder of Latin America accounts for 7 million (22 percent); Europe and Canada follow with 6 million (18 percent); and other countries account for about one million (3 percent) (Capps, Passel, Perez-Lopez, and Fix, 2003).

MIGRATION AND ADAPTATION

Scholars suggest that migration presents a myriad of challenges to youth development and adaptation (Portes & Rumbaut, 2001; Suarez-Orozco & Suarez-Orozco, 2001; Tartar, 1998; Ulman & Tartar, 2001). When immigrant children and adolescents leave their country of origin to immigrate to the United States, they often leave behind their nuclear and extended families, familiar language, culture, community, friends, and social systems (James, 1997), all of which play an instrumental role in combating physical and mental health risks while fostering normal development during their adolescence. Immigrant youth may be at risk for undesirable physical and mental health outcomes due to the immigration process, which can result in family instability, diminished social supports, diminished access to health care, and acculturative stress (Aronowitz, 1985; Blacke, Ledsky, Goodenow, O'Donnell, 2001; Harker, 2001; Portes & Rumbaut, 1996; Suarez-Orozco & Suarez-Orozco, 2001), educational and neighborhood segregation, and other social determinants of health. Although research suggests that first generation immigrants tend to be healthier than their American counterparts, it is the second, third, and subsequent generations of immigrants who face numerous acculturative challenges due to assimilation. Studies indicate that the process of acculturation can lead to problems associated with an individual's psychosocial adaptation such as lower levels of self-esteem, depression, happiness, sense of identity, and health (Aronowitz, 1985; Portes & Zhou 1993; Rumbaut, 1996; Sodowsky & Lai, 1997). Furthermore, a large number of immigrant children live in urban communities where the aforementioned challenges are exacerbated due to the likelihood of increased life stressors.

ACCULTURATION

Acculturation theory provides a useful framework when addressing primary prevention of mental health disorders. Acculturation theory refers to changes in an individual's behavior, social activities, thinking patterns, values, and self-identity, as a result of contact with another culture (Gordon, 1964). Acculturation attitudes are deconstructed into four distinct types: *integration, assimilation, separation*, and *marginalization* (Berry, 1986). Integration strategy is when an individual holds on to his or her cultural integrity and maintains his or her ethnic culture but also decides to transition into a host culture and to become an integral part of the larger society (Berry, 1986; Phinney et al., 2006). Assimilation strategy refers to when an individual decides to relinquish practices of his or her ethnic culture but indulge in the mainstream culture by attempting to transition into the mainstream society (Berry, 1986; Phinney et al., 2006). Separation strategy implies that an individual selects to maintain his or her ethnic culture while deciding not to interact with mainstream culture and to have a self-imposed withdrawal from the larger society (Berry, 1986; Phinney et al., 2006). Marginalization strategy refers to an individual's decision not to maintain his or her ethnic culture of origin and not to participate in the mainstream culture (Berry, 1986; Phinney et al., 2006). Generally, integration is perceived to be a less adversarial strategy for immigrant youth to use as it allows them to embrace their ethnic culture and the diverse American cultures. However, due to the recent economic downturn, the events of September 11, 2001, the war on terrorism, and anti-immigrant sentiment, assimilation has quickly gained popularity among mainstream America as the favorable attitude to be adopted by immigrants. An assimilation approach for immigrant children can be detrimental, as they are pushed to adopt mainstream cultures and abandon their ethnic, cultural, and religious values, beliefs, and ways of life, which otherwise protect against the risks associated with being an immigrant and member of an ethnic minority.

RISK AND RESILIENCY

Immigrant youth may be at risk of mental health challenges due to the migration process, cultural differences, discrimination, poverty, and socioeconomic deprivation, such as lack of access to adequate housing, segregated communities, poor access to health care and other preventive services, and segregated education. Some common mental health challenges for immigrant youth are depression, anxiety, stress, low self-esteem, and PTSD, to name a few. When mental health challenges are not addressed, co-occurring behavioral health concerns may develop and can include the following: substance abuse, unsafe sexual behaviors, conduct problems and delinquency, academic failures, and other behavioral challenges. In addition, immigrant youth have been found to be less likely to receive mental health and other health care services due to such factors as lack of access to health care, parental preferences and help-seeking patterns, unrecognized need for services, and other socioecological factors (Kataoka et al., 2003). Difficulties with parental acculturation may also impact immigrant youth. Due to their age at immigration, many parents face challenges such as limited English proficiency and unfamiliarity with mainstream American culture. These challenges often lead to diminished social roles in the family. As a result, children often have to take on adult-oriented roles and may, for example, make appointments for their parents, assist in paying bills, become translators, and raise their siblings—thus launching into adulthood at an early age. Moreover, intergenerational family conflicts leading to familial instability can present acculturative challenges for parents and children. In addition, environmental risks, such as community violence, gang and drug culture, and downtime, can further increase the risks of mental health problems.

Although faced with tremendous challenges, many immigrant youth also come from cultures where protective factors are embedded in family and community systems; these protective factors can prevent and buffer the risk of mental health disorders. Given the humble backgrounds of many immigrant populations, immigrant children can tap into the resiliency produced through their lived experiences. Immigrants overcome adversity and retain a sense of purpose in a future filled with optimism about educational aspirations, achievement motivation, persistence in attaining personal and professional goals, hopefulness about self, family and loved ones, spiritual connectedness, and good health (Benard, 1995). Social and behavioral science need to have a paradigm shift from a risk perspective that focuses on deficits and pathology to a resiliency perspective that is rooted in the strengths of individuals, families, and communities (Benard, 2007; see Chapter Three for full discussion of resilience). Many immigrant children come from cultures where families foster resiliency through social-integration techniques rooted in extended family networks. These extended family networks aim to mentor and monitor children through highly involved and caring relationships. Family networks maintain high expectations for their children and foster self-efficacy through opportunities to participate in activities inside and outside of the home. In addition, for many immigrant children, extended community involvement through recreation centers, places of worship, vocational training, and various other programs foster social integration, thereby building resiliency in combating risk factors (Hull, Kilbourne, Reece, & Husaini, 2008; Nettles & Pleck, 1996).

ADDRESSING PRIMARY PREVENTION

A key in addressing primary prevention of mental health in this population is to shift the paradigm to focus on resiliency and on strength-based approaches rather than on risks and deficits. Many immigrant youth come from cultures where nuclear and extended family play an influential role in the acculturation process. Therefore, family connectedness evidenced by social support and cohesion is critical in combating mental health risks. Another key protective factor in many immigrant communities is their strong sense of spirituality. Therefore, understanding, preventing, and addressing mental health in many cultures is attributed to a strong sense of spirituality and to nontraditional methods of addressing mental health that often involve herbal remedies, supernatural healing methods, modification in diet, and spiritual practices. When we develop community partnerships, this partnership results in a stronger infrastructure, which in turn brings a reduction in mental health problems. Furthermore, resiliency can be reinforced by providing opportunities for immigrant youth to increase their self-esteem and self-efficacy through social skills and social competence development activities (Bell, 2001; Winfield, 1994). A strength of many immigrant groups is their collectivistic culture where family, elders, religion, and community are highly valued; each of these can foster hope, trust, care, and a sense of belonging for immigrant youth.

PROTECTIVE FACTORS

Outside of the home, a key protective factor in addressing mental health challenges is the interaction of immigrant youth with the educational system. Immigrant youth who are able to transition and integrate into the educational system, where they can acquire language proficiency and have minimal academic challenges, will be less likely to endure acculturative stress and the onset of mental health challenges. However, it is essential for schools to provide integrative activities (for example, multicultural events, mentoring programs focused on immigrant youth, and culturally sensitive counseling services) that foster acceptance and respect diversity and are reflective of multi-ethnic, multilingual, multicultural, and multi-spiritual diversity represented in their schools and communities. Moreover, it is pertinent to observe the neighborhood context of the immigrant youth to determine the various assets and risks in the community. Assets such as community centers, youth employment opportunities, places of worship, schools, and various community-based organizations buffer the acculturative challenges faced by immigrant youth.

The role of culture in the prevention and treatment of mental health is to use the existing culturally-based protective factors to ameliorate risk factors (Prado, Szapocznik,

Maldonado-Molina, Schwartz, & Pantin, 2008). In order to understand and address the mental health of immigrant youth it is essential to observe the cultural background of immigrant youth. Many immigrant communities define mental health differently compared to an American context. In order to focus on prevention, the paradigm of preventing and addressing mental health solely from a genetic or medical model needs to shift to a holistic approach. Prevention strategies should aim to modify existing approaches so they are culturally sensitive and treat each immigrant youth on a case-by-case basis rather than prescribe to generic approaches that are rooted in cultural assumptions. Cultural awareness and sensitivity needs to be infused into both macro- and microlevels of prevention so that policies and practice have parallel goals in addressing and preventing mental health.

POLICY RECOMMENDATIONS

Historically, migration to the United States has occurred in a series of distinguishable periods, often referred to as *waves*. The first wave of immigration occurred during the post–Civil War Period; the second wave took place at the end of World War I; the third wave lasted from 1947 to 1960; and the fourth and most recent wave of immigration began after the passage of the 1965 Immigration Act (Public Law 89–236, Smith, 2005). The 1986 Immigration Reform and Control Act attempted to address the issue of illegal immigration by increasing enforcement and creating new pathways to lawful immigration. It was followed by the Illegal Immigration Reform Act and Immigrant Responsibility Act of 1996, which addressed border enforcement and use of social services by immigrants (Congress of the United States Congressional Budget Office, 2006). More recently, the Homeland Security Act of 2002 restructured the Immigration and Naturalization Service by transferring a great majority of its duties to the Department of Homeland Security (Congress of the United States Congressional Budget Office, 2006). The Department has also been scrutinized by critics who suggest it is curtailing the civil liberties of citizens. Although immigration reform has been a hot topic of discussion during the last several years, no major immigration policies have been passed to date.

Current immigration policies largely address issues of "legal" and "illegal" immigration and do not address immigrant transitions and adaptations. The panic-filled rhetoric used to describe immigration reform and the war on "illegal" immigrants has severe short- and long-term mental health consequences for legal immigrants, illegal immigrants, and U.S. citizens. The punitive nature of current immigration policies discourages both documented and undocumented immigrants from accessing protective services and opportunities. True immigration reform should also focus on policies that aim to use familial, cultural, and community assets in transitioning newly arrived immigrants into the United States. These policies should take into account immigrants' socioeconomic contexts and settlement communities by including integration initiatives that aim to educate each immigrant generation regarding the acculturative challenges faced by immigrant youth. Policies should, above all, focus on strengths at the individual, family, and community levels.

In addition, immigration policies and media outlets should focus on disseminating messages of integration rather than assimilation so that public perception and sentiment fosters inclusion of all Americans in reform that targets affordable health care. Private and public sentiment are necessary tools in influencing development of new health policies and in modifying existing health policies that address health disparities among immigrants and other minority groups. Preventing mental health disorders helps immigrant youth and also helps all communities strive to produce healthy and vibrant youth.

URBAN YOUTH

There is growing empirical evidence that low-income urban youth are at heightened risk for stressful life experiences in general and for chronic, uncontrollable stressors in particular (Attar, Guerra, & Tolan, 1994; Bennett & Miller, 2006; Turner & Avison, 2003). Urban environments present with a number of conditions that may interfere with development and increase the risk of mental health problems. For example, low income and social class are well-known determinants of poor health and behavioral concerns. More specifically, poverty brings with it a range of economic stressors that include interpersonal conflict about money, evictions, dilapidated housing, noise, crowding, environmental toxins, inadequate health care, ineffective schools, and disruptions of important services (see Landis et al., 2007 for a review). Beyond the effects of poverty in general, urban poverty in particular is associated with heightened exposure to community violence (Youngstrom, Weist, & Albus, 2003; Morales & Guerra, 2006). Many characteristics of the urban environment, such as community violence, crime, gang activity, drug use, and poverty, are disproportionately experienced by youth residing in these areas, which places them at greater risk for the development of mental health concerns (Bell & Jenkins, 1993; Ritchers & Martinez, 1993). Such trauma exposure has been linked to the development of PTSD, depression, anxiety, conduct difficulties, and adolescent substance use (Horowitz, Weine, & Jekel, 1995). Ethnic minority youth, particularly African American and Hispanic youth, are overrepresented in low socioeconomic status (SES) urban areas (Cooley-Quille, Boyd, Frantz, & Walsh, 2001) and disproportionately affected by community violence and chronic levels of stress (Attar, Guerra, & Tolan, 1994). The economic disparities low-income urban youth face contribute to disparities in the availability of adequate mental health care that may be particularly needed due to repeated exposure to violence. The Surgeon General's report on culture, race, and ethnicity (DHHS, 2001) identified access to care as a major issue involved in mental health service disparities in African American populations. More specifically, the Surgeon General's report identified underrepresented ethnic and cultural groups as less likely to seek treatment for mental health prevention or illness than more privileged groups due to issues of mistrust and stigma.

In general, much attention has been given to the negative outcomes of youths residing in low-income, urban environments. However, many of these youths are able to thrive, engage in successful behaviors, and develop adaptive skills. Urban neighborhoods suffer from stereotyping, which poses a barrier to developing effective health promotion strategies. Stereotypes ignore a neighborhood's diversity and strengths, both of which are important resources for inner-city communities (Leviton, Snell, & McGinnis, 2000). Thus, when discussing the influence of the low-income urban environment, it is important to consider both structural and ecological impact on the well-being of the youth.

THEORETICAL MODELS

The following sections describe the structural and ecological theoretical models.

Community Infrastructure and Structural Model

The inherent structure of urban life confines a vast number of people to a small area, which may unavoidably produce stress, including decreased support for prosocial behavior, disintegration of extended families, and higher tolerance of deviance (Black & Krishnakumar, 1998). Many families living in urban areas are confronted with the challenge of population density and associated problems, including crowding, which may heighten vulnerability to a number of public health concerns. Children and youth residing in urban communities are exposed to illnesses associated with crowding and unsanitary conditions that are coupled with limited access to adequate physical and mental health resources. With limited information on the mechanisms linking urbanization to children's and youth's health and well-being, professionals and policymakers are left with little information to guide interventions to prevent the negative effects of urbanization on youth (Black & Krishnakumar, 1998).

Ecological Models

Although the literature tends to highlight the deleterious effects of urbanization on youth (Fitzpatrick & Boldizar, 1993; Margolin & Gordis, 2000; Rosario, Salzinger, Feldman, & Ng-Mak, 2003), it is important to note protective and resiliency factors. Most notably, it is important to consider the role of familial and social networks that contribute to the psychological development of children and youth residing in low-income, urban environments. Examining the lives of urban youth from an *ecological model* accentuates the strengths and sense of community that may inherently exist within such communities given confined space and limited resources. An ecological model provides a clear understanding of how multiple systems work collaboratively to foster resiliency, adaptive skills, interpersonal relationships, and collective socialization.

Reciprocity and feedback are central concepts of the systems-based ecological model. The interconnections of multiple systems, including caregivers and the social context of youth, are highlighted in this model (Bronfenbrenner, 1981). Because youth do not exist in isolation or as passive agents, a model that accounts for how youth act on their environment is essential. High levels of family and community support have been shown to act as a buffer that predicts positive outcomes and potentially offsets the negative impact of other stressors. Among urban youth, stress resilience is associated with variables such as close family relationships, extended family support, and use of positive discipline strategies (Wyman et al., 1992).

Youths' mental health and well-being are also influenced by their interactions with caregivers in other settings (for example, in schools and churches). Interactions across settings are important because they provide a collective socialization experience that helps children learn to cope with differing sets of activities, roles, expectations, and relationships (Jencks & Mayer, 1990). Research suggests that family support may moderate the effects of life stress on development among children and adolescents (Quamma & Greenberg, 1994). There is also evidence that family support may specifically moderate the effects of youth exposure to violence. Overstreet and Dempsey (1999) found that youth whose mothers were present in the home were at less risk for depression related to exposure to violence than children whose mothers were not present in the home. More broadly, youth may be influenced by systems that impact them indirectly rather than directly. For example, the racial segregation, crime, limited resources, and violence common to many low-income, urban communities may hinder the ability of families to protect themselves (McLoyd, 1998). Finally, larger institutional structures (for example, government and culture) influence the lives of youth with policies that provide or limit resources to low-income, urban communities.

ADDRESSING PRIMARY PREVENTION

Chronic exposure to uncontrollable stressors such as community violence and poverty ultimately takes a toll on those residing in such communities by making individuals vulnerable to additional stressors. Frequent unemployment, financial strain, crime, and overcrowding are only a few of the social mechanisms that may impede the psychological health of residents within low-income communities. The recurring exposures to chronic stressors frequently characterized by such environments contribute to circumstances in which additional stressors are more likely to occur. The continuous exposure may ultimately deplete one's internal resources to cope, thus making one vulnerable to negative behavioral and psychological outcomes. In addition, adding strain to vulnerable systems may limit the protective nature that possibly exists. Thus the deleterious effects of chronic stressors commonly experienced in low-income urban settings are easily identifiable. However, less evident are the social and political bridges that can be built to foster institutional change and to address the societal ills that contribute to mental health disparities evident among underserved and under-resourced communities. Primary prevention can serve as a framework to address the risk and potential hazards for high-stressed urban youth.

Policy as a Mechanism of Prevention for Urban Youth

Urban youth are greatly impacted by the social, economic, and political contexts that threaten their psychological well-being. Racism, mass unemployment, pervasive violence, and police brutality pose serious threats to youth and their families. In addition, urban youth have been disproportionately affected by social and economic conditions that contribute to mental health disparities. For example, the failure of many urban school districts to prepare young people academically, the absence of early childhood education, and the removal of after school opportunities have combined with a growing fear of crime to shape a national consciousness that consistently disregards the injustices negatively affecting urban communities and the youth who live in them (Ginwright, Cammarota, & Noguera, 2005).

In order to fully address the mental health needs of urban youth, policy must be considered as a medium for prevention. Although policymakers express concern about the future of urban youth, few have actually taken steps to address the economic, political, and social conditions that shape their lives. Current policies focus on limiting youth participation in the democratic process, as a result, youth are rendered powerless. The emergence of policies that unfairly target youth as the source of social problems has prompted public policy advocates to rethink their basic assumption about how to support youth development, create educational opportunities, and encourage youth civic participation (Ginwright, Cammarota, & Noguera, 2005). A step toward prevention is to encourage a sense of empowerment and civic engagement to promote psychological well-being among urban youth. One theoretical model that illustrates this approach is *social justice youth development* (SJYD), which is rooted in the following principles: analyzing power within social relationships; making identity central; promoting systemic change; encouraging collective action; embracing youth culture; and developing tools to analyze power (see Ginwright & James, 2002, for a detailed description). This model uses an ecological framework to examine how young people respond within oppressive social systems and identifies a developmental trajectory to foster social justice in youth. By engaging community members in the political, social, economic, and psychological conditions that impact their lives, prevention programs and policies are enhanced. Such participation allows the community's perspectives and experiences to be included in the process of prevention and change.

Fostering Resiliency as Prevention

Urban youth are chronically exposed to stressors that may render them vulnerable to such psychological issues as depression and anxiety. Fostering a sense of resiliency and strength becomes essential to the psychological well-being of these youth. Thus resiliency as prevention serves to fill the gap between policy and tangible change. Existing models of resiliency highlight mechanisms through which protective factors might moderate the relation between negative life events and adjustment. *The compensatory model* suggests that positive factors in an adolescent's life may counteract or neutralize the effects of risk factors (Garmezy, Masten, & Tellegen, 1984). In the *challenge model*, negative life events are linearly related to adaptive behavior only when the number of protective factors is small. When protective factors are high, moderate levels of negative life events may actually enhance adjustment. The *immunity/vulnerability model* asserts that protective factors are more important than the number of negative life events in the prediction of adaptive functioning (Garmezy et al., 1984). Rutter (1987) illustrates a more direct way of understanding the concept of resiliency as it relates to prevention thus:

> Protection does not reside in the psychological chemistry of the moment but in the ways in which people deal with life changes and in what they do about their stressful or disadvantageous circumstances. Particular attention needs to be paid to the mechanisms operating at key turning points in people's lives when a risk trajectory may be redirected onto a more adaptive path [p. 329].

Resiliency must be defined as the relative strength of individual characteristics and external protective processes (supports provided by families, school staff, communities, policies) compared to the influence of risk and vulnerabilities in the external environment (Winfield, 1994). When resiliency is viewed as a developmental process that can be fostered, then strategies for change can be directed toward practices, policies, and attitudes. However, Winfield (1994) reminds us that simply changing practices and policies will not result in a community of resilient youth. The author identifies protective processes that must be reinforced to ensure that youth will remain resilient when faced with risk factors and vulnerabilities. The three characteristics of the process of fostering resilience include (1) a long-term and developmental focus, (2) viewing children with strengths rather than with deficits, and (3) nurturing protective processes so that children can succeed by changing systems, structures, and beliefs within schools and communities.

Fostering resiliency and protective processes in communities that support urban youth requires a major shift in belief systems within larger institutional systems (for example, schools and local and national governments). Policymakers, communities, and parents must examine more broadly how social service agencies and schools, in concert with other youth service agencies, can better operate as protective factors in the lives of youth residing in high-risk, urban conditions. As such, resiliency becomes a pathway to protect, support, and nourish the development of urban youth.

Pathways to primary prevention may include psycho-educational programs delineating mental health and mental illness. Education can be used as a primary prevention tool to decreasing stigma and mistrust while increasing treatment-seeking for underrepresented ethnic and cultural groups. Beyond education, building the reciprocal relationship between communities, schools, and local and national governmental agencies to foster awareness and capitalize on the strengths within these systems may lead to prevention of more severe mental health concerns. Innovative strategies are typically successful for groups like urban youth that are less likely to engage with mental health services. Preventions must include culturally and contextually appropriate approaches to mental health. Such methods as the use of paraprofessionals, as the use of beliefs and values that are identifiable and relatable to urban youth, and as the incorporation of cultural nuances, will prove instrumental in taking steps toward primary prevention.

CONCLUSION

The IOM's *Leading Health Indicators for Healthy People 2010: Second Interim Report* (1998) listed five major goals, including reduction in mortality rates due to illness and disease. Mental health and well-being was nowhere mentioned in those five major goals, and yet, 15 percent of the disability burden of developed countries like the United States is due to mental illness, including uncompleted suicide attempts. This burden is higher than that for all cancers combined (Lopez, Mathers, Ezzati, Jamison, & Murray, 2006). Poor mental health and mental illness are not reserved for the "mad" or the weak. One in ten people in the United States will, in his or her lifetime, experience poor mental health. It is the confluence of equitable access to good and appropriate care, socioeconomic livability, education, social support, and cultural strengths that serve as protective and preventive factors for those who never develop a full-syndrome illness or for those who recover to live productive lives.

The IOM Committee on Prevention of Mental Disorders (1994) delineated primary preventive measures into three categories: *universal interventions* that target the general population; *selective interventions* that target populations determined to be at risk for mental illness; and *indicated interventions* that target individuals displaying signs of an illness. This demarcation efficiently underscores the basic message regarding primary prevention of poor mental health and mental illness. Primary prevention is a relevant concern for the U.S. population as a whole. We highlighted three distinct groups in the United States, each affected by what we viewed to be preventable determinants of mental illness. These examples demonstrate the importance of mental health to individual well-being, to communities, and to society as a whole.

Currently, the nation is plagued with concerns related to financial security and employment. Since the start of the recession in December, 2007, the number of unemployed persons has increased by 7.6 million to 15.1 million and the unemployment rate has doubled to 9.8 percent as of this writing (Bureau of Labor Statistics, 2009). The chronic stressors of unemployment and financial strain expose all to the risk of poor mental health. Therefore, it is imperative to identify preventive measures to sustain positive mental health.

How we understand mental health, whether we recognize its trajectory in relation to some of the social determinants of health, and how we prioritize it in our health policies, funding allocations, and social program designs, will determine whether the disability burden of mental illness increases or declines. Can we begin to conceptualize mental health in terms of illness prevention and health promotion versus disorder treatment? Will we move to a system that permits payment to providers for preventive mental health services?

Martin Luther King Jr., perhaps the United States' most famous social justice activist, stated, "We are caught in an inescapable network of mutuality, tied in a single garment of destiny. Whatever affects one directly, affects all indirectly." This is the truth of mental health and illness. When one is not able to cope with the normal stresses of life, to work productively and fruitfully, and make a contribution to community, many are affected. When those who make policy decisions opt for equitable and inclusive policies, we are all affected. To reframe an individualist notion of mental illness as a public health concern acknowledges the significant impact mental well-being has on overall health. To effectively join mental health to the goals of primary prevention will require social action and policy change.

DISCUSSION QUESTIONS

1. Should primary prevention for mental health be culturally tailored? If yes, why? If no, why not? What would this approach entail for veterans, youth, and immigrants? What challenges would generalist strategies present?
2. How would you adjust current policy regarding veterans and mental health care to make family involvement central to primary prevention?
3. How does an institution (such as the military), or a society (such as that of the United States) go about confronting and eliminating stigma associated with mental distress?
4. What are some helpful solutions to addressing the mental health of immigrant youth in the U.S? Do these solutions vary in regard to the ethnic background of the immigrant youth and the area of settlement?
5. How have September 11, 2001, the subsequent wars in Iraq and Afghanistan, and the Patriot Act of 2001 impacted the mental health and well-being of immigrants in the United States? Is the impact different globally? If so, please describe these differences. If not, why not?
6. Resilience was identified as a mechanism of prevention. Identify protective and risk factors that impact the resiliency of urban youth. Discuss strategies that can enhance resiliency given the stressors urban youth commonly face. What is the role of primary prevention in fostering the resiliency of urban youth?

REFERENCES

American Psychiatric Association. (1994). *Diagnostic and statistical manual of mental disorders: DSM-IV* (4th ed.). Washington, DC: American Psychiatric Association.

Aronowitz, M. (1985). The social and economical adjustment of immigrant children: A review of literature. *International Migration Review, 18*(2), 237–257.

Associated Press. (2009). Military fights stigma of mental care: Officers, vets fear "can do" culture undermines campaign to provide help. Retrieved February 10, 2009, from http://www.msnbc.msn.com/id/30782778

Attar, B. K., Guerra, N. G., & Tolan, P. H. (1994). Neighborhood disadvantage, stressful life events, and adjustment in urban elementary school children. *Journal of Clinical Child Psychology, 23*, 391–400.

Bell, C., & Jenkins, E. (1993). Community violence and children in Chicago's Southside. *Psychiatry, 56*, 46–54.

Bell, C. C. (2001). Cultivating resiliency in youth. *Journal of Adolescent Health, 29*(5), 375–381.

Benard, B. (1995). Fostering resilience in children. Urbana, IL: ERIC Clearinghouse on Elementary and Early Childhood Education. (ED 386 327). Retrieved July 1, 2009, from http://www.athealth.com/consumer/disorders/childresilience.html

Benard, B. (2007). The hope of prevention: Individual, family, and community resilience. In L. Cohen, V. Chavez, & S. Chehimi (Eds.), *Prevention is primary* (pp. 63–89). San Francisco: Jossey-Bass.

Bennett, M. D., & Miller, D. B. (2006). An exploratory study of the Urban Hassles Index: A contextually relevant measure of chronic multidimensional urban stressors. *Research on Social Work Practice, 16*, 305–314.

Berry, J. W. (1986). The acculturation process and refugee behavior. In C. L. Williams & J. Westinmeyer (Eds.), *Refugee mental health in resettlement countries.* (pp. 25–37). Washington, DC: Hemisphere.

Black, M. M., & Krishnakumar, A. (1998). Children in low-income, urban settings: Interventions to promote mental health and well-being. *American Psychologist, 53*(6), 635–646.

Blake, S. M. Ledsky, R., Goodenow, C., & O'Donnell, L. (2001). Receipt of school health education and school health services among adolescent immigrants in Massachusetts. *Journal of School Health, 71*(3), 105–114.

Bronfenbrenner, U. (1981). *The ecology of human development.* Cambridge, MA: Harvard University Press.

Bureau of Labor Statistics. (2009). Employment situation summary. Washington, DC: U.S. Department of Labor.

Burnam, M. A., Meredith, L. S., Tanielian, T., & Jaycox, L. H. (2009). Mental health care for Iraq and Afghanistan War Veterans. *Health Affairs (Project Hope), 28*(3), 771–782.

Capps, R., Fix, M., & Murray, J. (2005). *The new demography of America's schools: Immigration and the No Child Left Behind Act.* Washington, DC: Urban Institute.

Capps, R., Passel, J. S., Perez-Lopez, D., & Fix, M. (2003). *The new neighbors: A user's guide to data on immigrants in U.S. communities.* Washington, DC: Urban Institute.

Commission on Social Determinants of Health. (2008). *Closing the gap in a generation: Health equity through action on the social determinants of health.* Geneva: World Health Organization.

Congress of the United States Congressional Budget Office. (2006). *Immigration policy in the United States.* Retrieved October 12, 2009, from http://www.cbo.gov/ftpdocs/70xx/doc7051/02-28-Immigration.pdf

Cooley-Quille, M., Boyd, R. C., Frantz, E., & Walsh, J. (2001). Emotional and behavioral impact of exposure to community violence in inner-city adolescents. *Journal of Clinical Child Psychology, 30*(2), 199–206.

Cozza, S. J., Chun, R. S., & Polo, J. A. (2005). Military families and children during operation Iraqi freedom. *The Psychiatric Quarterly, 76*(4), 371–378.

Cuijpers, P., Van, S. A., Smit, F., Mihalopoulos, C., & Beekman, A. (2008). Preventing the onset of depressive disorders: A meta-analytic review of psychological interventions. *American Journal of Psychiatry, 165*(10), 1272–1280.

Darwin, J. L., & Reich, K. I. (2006). Reaching out to the families of those who serve: The SOFAR project. *Professional Psychology: Research and Practice, 37*(5), 481–484.

Erbes, C., Westermeyer, J., Engdahl, B., & Johnsen, E. (2007). Post-traumatic stress disorder and service utilization in a sample of service members from Iraq and Afghanistan. *Military Medicine, 172*(4), 359–363.

Feldner, M. T., Monson, C. M., & Friedman, M. J. (2007). A critical analysis of approaches to targeted PTSD prevention: Current status and theoretically-derived future directions. *Behavior Modification, 31*, 80–116.

Felix, R. H., & Kramer, M. (1952). Research in epidemiology of mental illness. *Public Health Reports, 67*, 152–160.

Felner, R. D., & Felner, T. Y. (1989). Primary prevention programs in the educational context: A transactional-ecological framework and analysis. In L. A. Bond & B. E. Compas (Eds.), *Primary prevention and promotion in the schools* (pp. 13–49). Newbury Park, CA: Sage.

Fitzpatrick., A. D., & Bruce, S. E. (1997). Impact of exposure to community violence on violence behavior and emotional distress among urban adolescents. *Journal of Clinical Child Psychology, 26*, 2–14.

Fitzpatrick, K., & Boldizar, J. (1993). The prevalence and consequences of exposure to violence among African American youth. *Journal of the American Academy of Child and Adolescent Psychiatry, 32*(2), 424–430.

FOCUS Project. (2009). FOCUS: Resiliency training for military families. Retrieved October 22, 2009, from http://www.focusproject.org/history.html

Friedman, M. J. (2006). Posttraumatic stress disorder among military returnees from Afghanistan and Iraq. *American Journal of Psychiatry, 163*(4), 586–593.

Garmezy, N., Masten, A., & Tellegen, A. (1984). The study of stress and competence in children: A building block for developmental psychotherapy. *Child Development, 55*, 97–111.

Gibbs, D. A., Martin, S. L., Kupper, L. L., & Johnson, R. E. (2007). Child maltreatment in enlisted soldiers' families during combat-related deployments. *Journal of the American Medical Association, 298*(5), 528–535.

Ginwright, S., Cammarota, J., & Noguera, P. (2005). Youth, social justice, and communities: Toward a theory of urban youth policy. *Social Justice, 32*(3), 24–40.

Ginwright, S., & James, T. (2002). From assets to gents of change: Social justice, organizing, and youth development. *New Directions for Youth Development, 96*, 27–46.

Gone, J. P. (2007). "We never was happy living like a Whiteman": Mental health disparities and the postcolonial predicament in American Indian communities. *American Journal of Community Psychology, 40*(3–4), 290–300.

Gone, J. P. (2008). "So I can be like a Whiteman": The cultural psychology of space and place in American Indian mental health. *Culture & Psychology, 14*(3), 369–399.

Gordon, M. M. (1964). *Assimilation in American Life*. New York: Oxford University Press.

Harker, K. (2001). Immigrant generation, assimilation, and adolescent psychological well-being. *Social Forces, 79*(3), 969–1004.

Hoge, C. W., Auchterlonie, J. L., & Milliken, C. S. (2006). Mental health problems, use of mental health services, and attrition from military service after returning from deployment to Iraq or Afghanistan. *Journal of the American Medical Association, 295*(9), 1023–1032.

Hoge, C. W., Castro, C. A., Messer, S. C., McGurk, D., Cotting, D. I., & Koffman, R. L. (2004). Combat duty in Iraq and Afghanistan, mental health problems, and barriers to care. *New England Journal of Medicine, 351*(1), 13–22.

Hoge, C. W., Terhakopian, A., Castro, C. A., Messer, S. C., & Engel, C. C. (2007). Association of posttraumatic stress disorder with somatic symptoms, health care visits, and absenteeism among Iraq war veterans. *American Journal of Psychiatry, 164*(1), 150–153.

Horowitz, K., Weine, S., & Jekel, J. (1995). PTSD symptoms in urban adolescent girls: Compounded community trauma. *American Academy of Child and Adolescent Psychiatry, 34*, 1353–1361.

Huebner, A. J., Mancini, J. A., Wilcox, R. M., Grass, S. R., & Grass, G. A. (2007). Parental deployment and youth in military families: Exploring uncertainty and ambiguous loss. *Family Relations, 56*(2), 112–122.

Hull, P., Kilbourne, B., Reece, M., & Husaini, B. (2008). Community involvement and adolescent mental health: Moderating effects of race/ethnicity and neighborhood disadvantage. *Journal of Community Psychology. 36*(8), 534–551.

Huus, K. (2007, October 15, 2007). Gut check: Iraq war's impact at home. MSNBC.com. Retrieved March 20, 2009, from http://www.msnbc.msn.com/id/20822561/page/2/print/1/displaymode/1098

Institute of Medicine (IOM). (1994). *Reducing risks for mental disorders: Frontiers for preventive intervention research*. Washington, DC: National Academies Press.

Institute of Medicine (IOM). (1998). *Leading health indicators for healthy people 2010: Second interim report*. Washington, DC: National Academies Press.

Jakupcak, M., Luterek, J., Hunt, S., Conybeare, D., & McFall, M. (2008). Posttraumatic stress and its relationship to physical health functioning in a sample of Iraq and Afghanistan War veterans seeking postdeployment VA health care. *Journal of Nervous and Mental Disease, 196*(5), 425–428.

James, D. C. (1997). Coping with a new society: The unique psychosocial problems of immigrant youth. *Journal of School Health. 67*, 98–102.

Jayakody, K., Danziger, S., & Pollack, H. (2000). Welfare reform, substance use, and mental health. *Journal of Health Politics, Policy, and Law, 25*(4), 623–652.

Jencks, C., & Mayer, S. (1990). The social consequences of growing up in a poor neighborhood. In L. Lynn & M. McGeary (Eds.), *Inner-city poverty in the United States* (pp. 187–222). Washington, DC: National Academy Press.

Jenkins et al. (2008). Debt, income and mental disorder in the general population. *Psychological Medicine, 38*(10), 1485–1493.

Jones, B. J., Gallagher III, B. J., Pisa, A., & McFalls Jr., J. A. (2008). Social class, family history, and type of schizophrenia. *Psychiatry Research, 159*(1–2), 127–132.

Kataoka et al. (2003). A school–based mental health program for traumatized Latino immigrant children. *American Academy of Child & Adolescent Psychiatry, 42*(3), 311–318.

Kendler, K., Prescott, C., Myers, J., & Neale, M. (2003). The structure of genetic and environmental risk factors for common psychiatric and substance use disorders in men and women. *Archives of General Psychiatry, 60*(9), 929–937.

Kessler et al. (2008). Individual and societal effects of mental disorders on earnings in the United States: results from the national comorbidity survey replication. *American Journal of Psychiatry, 165*(6), 703–711.

Keteyian, A. (2007a). Suicide epidemic among veterans. *CBS News Investigates.* Retrieved May 15, 2009, from http://www.cbsnews.com/stories/2007/11/13/cbsnews_investigates/main3496471.shtml

Keteyian, A. (2007b). Veterans' families speak out. CBS News.com. Retrieved October 10, 2009, from http://www.cbsnews.com/video/watch/?id=3504148n%3fsource=search_video

Keyes, C.L.M. (2002). The mental health continuum: From languishing to flourishing in life. *Journal of Health and Behavior Research, 43*, 207–222.

Kolkow, T. T., Spira, J. L., Morse, J. S., & Grieger, T. A. (2007). Post-traumatic stress disorder and depression in health care providers returning from deployment to Iraq and Afghanistan. *Military Medicine, 172*(5), 451–455.

Landis et al. (2007). Urban adolescent stress and hopelessness. *Journal of Adolescence, 30*(6), 1051–1070.

Levine, A. (2009). VA's bold goal: Eradicate homelessness among veterans in 5 years. *CNN U.S.* Retrieved November 3, 2009, from http://www.cnn.com/2009/US/11/03/shinseki.homeless.veterans

Leviton, L. C., Snell, E., & McGinnis, M. (2000). Urban issues in health promotion. *American Journal of Public Health. 90*(6), 863–866.

Lilley, S. (2007). Military went to war; country didn't: Yawning gulf seen between perspectives of military families, general public. Retrieved February 5, 2009, from http://www.msnbc.msn.com/id/20230892

Lincoln, A., Swift, E., & Shorteno-Fraser, M. (2008). Psychological adjustment and treatment of children and families with parents deployed in military combat. *Journal of Clinical Psychology, 64*(8), 984–992.

Link, B. G., Mirotznik, J., & Cullen, F. T. (1991). The effectiveness of stigma coping orientations: Can negative consequences of mental illness labeling be avoided? *Journal of Health and Social Behavior, 32*(3), 302–320.

Lohaus, D. (Director). (2006). *When I came home*. [Documentary film]. United States: New Day Films.

Lopez, A. D., Mathers, C. D., Ezzati, M., Jamison, D. T., & Murray, C.J.L. (2006). Measuring the global burden of disease and risk factors, 1990–2001. In A. D. Lopez, C. D. Mathers, M. Ezzati, D. T. Jamison & C.J.L. Murray (Eds.), *Global burden of disease and risk factors* (pp. 1–13). New York: Oxford University Press and World Bank.

Margolin, G., & Gordis, E. B. (2000). The effects of family and community violence on children. *Annual Review of Psychology, 51*, 445–479.

McLoyd, V. C. (1998). Socioeconomic disadvantage and child development. *American Psychologist. 53*, 185–204.

MCVET. Maryland Center for Veterans Education and Training. (2009). Retrieved October 10, 2009, from http://www.mcvet.org

Military.com. (2009). New GI bill overview [Electronic Version]. Military.com. Retrieved October 20, 2009, from http://www.military.com/money-for-school/gi-bill/new-gi-bill-overview

Milliken, C. S., Auchterlonie, J. L., & Hoge, C. W. (2007). Longitudinal assessment of mental health problems among active and reserve component soldiers returning from the Iraq war. *Journal of the American Medical Association, 298*(18), 2141–2148.

Morales, J. R., & Guerra, N. G. (2006). Effects of multiple context and cumulative stress on urban children's adjustment in elementary school. *Child Development, 77*, 907–923.

National Institute of Mental Health. (2009). Mental health topics: Statistics. Retrieved May 10, 2009, from http://www.nimh.nih.gov/health/topics/statistics/index.shtml

Nettles, S. M., & Pleck, J. H. (1996). Risk, resilience, and development: The multiple ecologies of Black adolescents in the United States. In R. J. Haggerty, N. Garmezy, & M. J. Rutter (Eds.), *Stress, risk, and resilience in children and adolescents: Processes, mechanisms, and interventions* (pp. 147–181). New York: Cambridge University Press.

O'Connell, M. E., Boat, T., & Warner, K. E. (2009). *Preventing mental, emotional, and behavioral disorders among young people: Progress and possibilities*. Washington, DC: National Academies Press.

O'Keefe, E., & Franke-Ruta, G. (2009, November 4). Shinseki cites plight, plan to help homeless veterans. *Washington Post*, p. A23. Retrieved November 4, 2009, from http://www.washingtonpost.com/wp-dyn/content/article/2009/11/03/AR2009110303615.html

Overstreet, S., & Dempsey, M. (1999). Availability of family support as a moderator of exposure to community violence. *Journal of Clinical Child Psychology, 28*, 151–159.

Phinney, J., Berry, J. W., Vedder, P., & Liebkind, K. (2006). The acculturation experience: Attitudes, identities, and behaviors of immigrant youth. In J. W. Berry, J. S. Phinney, D. L. Sam, & P. Vedder (Eds.), *Immigrant youth in cultural transition: Acculturation, identity, and adaptation across national contexts* (pp. 71–116). Mahwah, NJ: Erlbaum.

Pietrzak, R. H., Johnson, D. C., Goldstein, M. B., Malley, J. C., & Southwick, S. M. (2009). Perceived stigma and barriers to mental health care utilization among OEF-OIF veterans. *Psychiatric Services, 60*(8), 1118–1122.

Portes, A., & Rumbaut, R. G. (1996). *Immigrant America: A portrait*. Berkeley: University of California Press.

Portes, A., & Rumbaut, R. G. (2001). *Legacies*. Berkeley: University of California Press.

Portes, A., & Zhou, M. (1993). The new second generation: segmented assimilation and its variants. *Annals of the American Academy of Political and Social Science, 530*, 74–96.

Prado, G., Szapocznik, J., Maldonado-Molina, M. M., Schwartz, S. J., & Pantin, H. (2008). Drug use/abuse prevalence, etiology, prevention, and treatment in Hispanic adolescents: A cultural perspective. *Journal of Drug Issues, 38*(1), 5–36.

Quamma, J. P., & Greenberg, M. T. (1994). Children's experience of life stress: The role of family social support and social problem-solving skills as protective factors. *Journal of Clinical Child Psychology, 23*, 295–305.

Rand Corporation. (2008). One in five Iraq and Afghanistan veterans suffer from PTSD or major depression. [News release.] Retrieved March 8, 2009, from http://rand.org/news/press/2008/04/17/index.html

Ren, X. S., Skinner, K., Lee, A., & Kazis, L. (1999). Social support, social selection and self-assessed health status: results from the veterans health study in the United States. *Social Science and Medicine, 48*(12), 1721–1734.

Renshaw, K. D., Rodrigues, C. S., & Jones, D. H. (2009). Combat exposure, psychological symptoms, and marital satisfaction in National Guard soldiers who served in Operation Iraqi Freedom from 2005 to 2006. *Anxiety, Stress, and Coping, 22*(1), 101–115.

Ritchers, J. E., & Martinez, P. (1993). The NIMH community violence project: I. Children as victims of and witnesses to violence. *Psychiatry, 56*, 7–21.

Ritchie, E. C., Benedek, D., Malone, R., & Carr-Malone, R. (2006). Psychiatry and the military: an update. *Psychiatric Clinics of North America, 29*(3), 695–707.

Rosario, M., Salzinger, S., Feldman, R. S., & Ng-Mak, D. S. (2003). Community violence exposure and delinquent behaviors among youth: The moderating role of coping. *Journal of Community Psychology, 31*(5), 489–512.

Rumbaut, R. G. (1996). The crucible within: Ethnic identity, self-esteem, and segmented assimilation among children of immigrants. In A. Portes (Ed.), *The new second generation* (pp. 119–170). New York: Russell Sage Foundation.

Rutter, M. (1987). Psychological resilience and protective mechanisms. *American Journal of Orthopsychiatry, 57*(3), 316–331.

Sammons, M. T., & Batten, S. V. (2008). Psychological services for returning veterans and their families: Evolving conceptualizations of the sequelae of war-zone experiences. *Journal of Clinical Psychology, 64*(8), 921–927.

Sayers, S. L., Farrow, V. A., Ross, J., & Oslin, D. W. (2009). Family problems among recently returned military veterans referred for a mental health evaluation. *Journal of Clinical Psychiatry, 70*(2), 163–170.

Schoevers et al. (2006). Prevention of late-life depression in primary care: Do we know where to begin? *American Journal of Psychiatry, 163*, 1611–1621.

Seal, K. H., Bertenthal, D., Miner, C. R., Sen, S., & Marmar, C. (2007). Bringing the war back home: mental health disorders among 103,788 US veterans returning from Iraq and Afghanistan seen at Department of Veterans Affairs facilities. *Archives of Internal Medicine, 167*(5), 476–482.

Shanker, T. (2008, April 6). U.S. Army worried by rising stress of return tours to Iraq. *New York Times*. Retrieved February 5, 2009, from http://www.nytimes.com/2008/04/06/washington/06military.html?scp=1&sq=US%20Army%20worried%20by%20rising%20stress%20of%20return%20tours%20to%20iraq&st=cse

Smith, J. I. (2005). Patterns of Muslim immigration. USINFO.STATE.GOV, International Information Programs. Retrieved June 26, 2005, from http://uninfo.state.gov/products/pubs/muslimlife/immirat.htm

Sodowsky, G. R., & Lai, E.W.M. (1997). Asian immigrant variables and structural models of cross-cultural distress. In A. Booth, A. C. Crouter, & N. Landale (Eds.), *Immigration and the family: Research and policy on U.S. immigrants* (pp. 211–234). Mahwah, NJ: Erlbaum.

SOFAR. (2009). Strategic outreach to families of all reservists. Retrieved October 22, 2009, from http://www.sofarusa.org/about_sofar.htm

Stecker, T., Fortney, J. C., Hamilton, F., & Ajzen, I. (2007). An assessment of beliefs about mental health care among veterans who served in Iraq. *Psychiatric Services), 58*(10), 1358–1361.

Suarez-Orozco, C., & Suarez-Orozco, M. (2001). *Children of immigration.* Boston: Harvard University Press.

Tartar, M. (1998). Counseling immigrants: School contexts and emerging strategies. *British Journal of Guidance Counseling, 26*, 337– 352.

Turner, J. R., & Avison, W. R. (2003). Status variations in stress exposure: Implications for the interpretations of research on race, socioeconomic status, and gender. *Journal of Health and Social Behavior, 44*, 488–505.

Ulman, C., & Tartar, M. (2001). Psychological adjustment among Israeli adolescent Immigrants: A report on life satisfaction, self-concept, and self-esteem. *Journal of Youth and Adolescence, 30*, 4449–4463.

U.S. Department of Health and Human Services. (1999). *Mental health: A report of the Surgeon General—executive summary.* Rockville, MD: U.S. Department of Health and Human Services, Substance Abuse and Mental Health Services Administration, Center for Mental Health Services, National Institutes of Health, National Institute of Mental Health.

U.S. Department of Health and Human Services. (2001). *Mental health: Culture, race and ethnicity. A supplement to mental health: A report of the Surgeon General.* Washington, DC: National Institute of Mental Health.

U.S. Public Health Service. (2000). *Report of the surgeon general's conference on children's mental health: A national action agenda.* Washington, DC: Department of Health and Human Services.

Üstün, T. B. (1999). The global burden of mental disorders. *American Journal of Public Health, 89*, 1315–1318.

Vasterling et al. (2008). Posttraumatic stress disorder and health functioning in a non-treatment-seeking sample of Iraq war veterans: A prospective analysis. *Journal of Rehabilitation Research and Development, 45*(3), 347–358.

Wagenfield, M. O. (1972). The primary prevention of mental illness: A sociological perspective. *Journal of Health and Social Behavior, 13*, 195–203.

Winfield, L. F. (1994). *Developing resilience in urban youth. Urban Monograph Series.* Oak Brook, IL: North Central Regional Educational Laboratory.

World Health Organization (WHO). (2007). What is mental health? Retrieved May 20, 2009, from http://www.who.int/features/qa/62/en/index.html

Wyman et al. (1992). Interviews with children who experienced major life stress: Family and child attributes that predict resilient outcomes. *Journal of the American Academy of Child and Adolescent Psychiatry, 31*, 904–910.

Wynn, J. (2007). Issues confronting America's veterans transitioning from the war in Iraq. Paper presented at the Morgan State University 6th Annual Symposium on Eliminating Health Disparities. War Within: The Impact of Trauma and Violence on Black Men's Mental Health, Baltimore, MD.

Youngstrom, E., Weist, M. D., & Albus, K. E. (2003). Exploring violence exposure, stress, protective factors, and behavioral problems among inner-city youth. *American Journal of Community Psychology, 32*(1–2), 115–129.

Zimmerman, M., Bingenheimer, J., & Notaro, P. (2002). Natural mentors and adolescent resiliency: A study with urban youth. *American Journal of Community Psychology, 30*(2), 221–243.

INDEX

Page references followed by *fig* indicate an illustrated figure: followed by *t* indicate a table; followed by *e* indicate an exhibit.

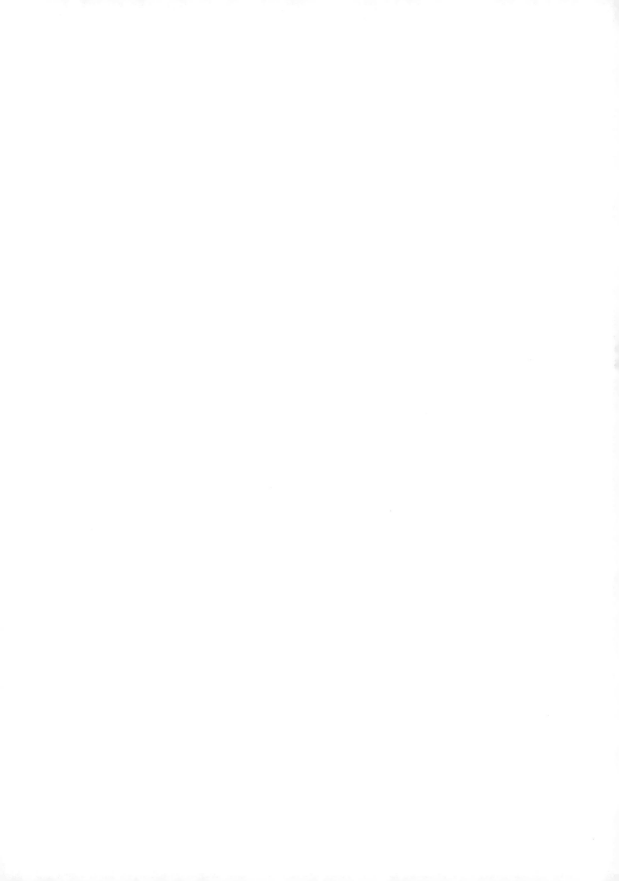